Hallas'
Caring for People with Mental Handicaps

Eighth Edition

Professor W.I. Fraser,
MD, FRCPsychDPM
Professor of Mental Handicap,
Ely Hospital, Cowbridge Road West,
Cardiff

R.C. MacGillivray,
MB(Ed), FRFPS, FRCP(Glas), DPM(Lond), FRCPsych
Second Opinion Doctor,
Mental Welfare Commission for Scotland,
Edinburgh

Ann M. Green,
BA, MA, C PSYCHOL, AFBPsS
Top Grade Clinical Psychologist,
Lothian Health Board,
Gogarburn Hospital,
Edinburgh

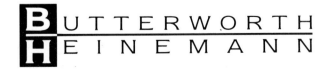

BUTTERWORTH
HEINEMANN

Butterworth-Heinemann Ltd
Linacre House, Jordan Hill, Oxford OX2 8DP

A member of the Reed Elsevier plc group

OXFORD   LONDON   BOSTON
MUNICH   NEW DELHI   SINGAPORE   SYDNEY
TOKYO   TORONTO   WELLINGTON

First published 1958
Second edition 1962
Third edition 1967
Fourth edition 1967
Fourth edition 1970
Spanish translation 1974
Japanese translation 1975
Fifth edition 1974
Spanish translation 1976
Japanese translation 1976
Sixth edition 1978
Reprinted 1980
Seventh edition 1982
Reprinted 1983
Eighth edition 1991
Reprinted 1993
Paperback edition 1995

© Butterworth-Heinemann Ltd 1991

British Library Cataloguing in Publication Data
A catalogue record for this book is available from the
British Library

Library of Congress Cataloguing in Publication Data
A catalogue record for this book is available from the
Library of Congress

ISBN 0 7506 2316 0

Composition by Scribe Design, Gillingham, Kent
Printed and bound in Great Britain by Clays Ltd, St Ives plc

Preface

It is now over 30 years since the first edition of *The Nursing of Mental Defectives* (the original title) was published. Each succeeding edition has been found useful by student nurses, parents and the many others involved in caring for the mentally handicapped in Britain and overseas. The years have brought many changes in patterns of care, in legislation and personnel, and with each change alterations to the text have become necessary.

During recent years there has been a dramatic shift in policy in caring for people with mental handicaps. Hospitals have either been closed, or the number of beds reduced, resulting in more and more patients being cared for in the community. Unfortunately these changes seem to have created a lot of anxiety, particularly amongst the parents of people with mental handicaps. Despite reassurances, anxieties still prevail that those people who await discharge from hospitals to be closed will face deteriorating conditions there or will be sent home to be cared for by their families; if the person is placed in the community, there are worries as to whether he or she will be able to cope and be truly integrated. These concerns are particularly worrying to parents who are becoming elderly.

The care of people with mental handicaps has long since ceased to be the prerogative of doctors and nurses. Now it really is team work with parents, doctors, nurses, psychologists, social workers, teachers, physiotherapists, speech therapists and many more all playing their part with the new emphasis on community care. The title 'patient' has become largely irrelevant and replaced by 'client' or 'resident'. One thing is certain, by whatever the title the handicapped person is known expert care, guidance and planning for the future is needed. This new edition of the book comprehensively reflects the skills required.

For the eighth edition we have a new title, *Hallas' Caring for People with Mental Handicaps*, a new format and new members of the team of contributors. Ronald MacGillivray and Bill Fraser have been with me since the fourth edition, and, as always, I enjoy their partnership and friendship. Joining as editor is Ann Green, Top Grade Clinical Psychologist in Edinburgh.

List of contributors

Karen Allen, *BDS, MSc,*
Dental Officer (Special Needs Dentistry), Westerhailles Dental Clinic, 7 Murrayburn Gate, Westerhailles, Edinburgh

P. Baker, *BSC, MPhil, C Psychol,*
Senior Clinical Psychologist, The Board of Health, Le Vaquiedor, St Martins, Guernsey, Channel Islands

Bronwen Burford, *BA, Dip Ed,*
Research Associate, Gogarburn Hospital, Glasgow Road, Edinburgh EH12 9BJ

S.E. Cheseldine, *BA, PhD, MSc, AFBPsS*
Principal Clinical Psychologist, Royal Scottish National Hospital, Larbert FK5 4EJ

V. Chlebowski, *CQSW,*
Principal Social Worker, Gogarburn Hospital, Glasgow Road, Edinburgh EH12 9BJ

P. Dickens, *BA, MPhil, LHSM, MBIM, C Psychol, AFBPsS,*
Top Grade Clinical Psychologist, Royal Scottish National Hospital, Larbert FK5 4EG

E. Fischbacher, *MBChB, MRCGP,*
Associate Specialist in Mental Handicap, Lothian Health Board, Gogarburn Hospital, Glasgow Road, Edinburgh EH12 9BJ

H.C. Fowlie, *OBE, MBChB, FRCP(Ed), FRC Psych, DPM,*
Formerly H.M. Medical Commissioner, Mental Welfare Commission for Scotland

Professor W.I. Fraser, *MD, FRC Psych, DPM,*
Professor of Mental Handicap, Ely Hospital, Cowbridge Road West, Cardiff

Ann M. Green, *BA, MA, C Psychol, AFBPsS,*
Top Grade Clinical Psychologist, Lothian Health Board, Gogarburn Hospital, Glasgow Road, Edinburgh EH12 9BJ

S.M. Guinea, *MA, C Psychol,*
Senior Clinical Psychologist, Lothian Health Board, Gogarburn Hospital, Glasgow Road, Edinburgh EH12 9BJ

P. Higson, *BA, PhD, Dip Clin Psych,*
Unit General Manager (Mental Health), Clwyd Health Authority, North Wales Hospital, Denby, Clwyd LL16 5SS

M. Holland, Head of Parliamentary Affairs and Secretary to Medical Advisory Panel, Mencap National Centre, 123 Golden Lane, London EC1Y ORT

J. Jancar, *MB, BCh, BAO, FRC Psych, DPM,*
Hon Consultant Psychiatrist, Stoke Park Hospital, Stapleton, Bristol BS16 1QU

P. Kemp, *RNMH, RGN,*
Community Nursing Services Manager, Lothian Health Board, Gogarburn Hospital, Glasgow Road, Edinburgh EH12 9BJ

W.R. Lindsay, *BA, PhD, Dip Clin Psych, C Psychol, FBPsS,*
Top Grade Clinical Psychologist, Tayside Area Clinical Psychology Department, Strathmartine Hospital, Dundee

Ros. Lyall, *MBChB, MPhil, MRC Psych,*
Consultant Psychiatrist, Gogarburn Hospital, Edinburgh

R. McConkey, *BA, PhD, FPsSI,*
Director of Training and Research, Brothers of Charity Services (Borders Region, Scotland), St Aidan's House, Gattonside, Melrose, Roxburghshire TD6 9NN

R.C. MacGillivray, *MB(Ed), FRFPS, FRCP (Glas), DPM (Lond), FRC Psych,*
Second Opinion Doctor, Mental Welfare Commission for Scotland

G. Mackay, *MA, DE Psych, PhD,*
Course Director for Diploma in Recorded, Special Educational Needs, Jordanhill College of Education, Division of Special Educational Needs, South Brae Drive, Glasgow

P. Mathias, *BSc, MA, MSc, PhD,*
Principal of Education and Training, CCETSW, Derbyshire House, St Chad's Street, London WCIH 8AD

Amanda Michie, *MA,*
Research Psychologist, Tayside Area Clinical Psychology Department, Strathmartine Hospital, Dundee

J. Montague, *BMus, Dip Mus Ther,*
Music Therapist, Lennox Castle Hospital, Lennoxtown, Stirlingshire G65 7LB

J.P. Odor, *BSc,*
Senior Research Fellow, CALL Centre, University of Edinburgh, 4 Buccleuch Place, Edinburgh EH8 9LW

L. Renton, *BSc, Dip COT,*
Senior Lecturer, Occupational Therapy Department, Queen Margaret College,
Clerwood Terrace, Edinburgh EH12 8TS

J. Stansfield, *MSc, MCST,*
Senior Lecturer in Pathology, Department of Speech Therapy, Queen Margaret
College, Clerwood Terrace, Edinburgh EH12 8TS

E. Wilkinson, *MCSP,*
Mental Health Unit Superintendent Physiotherapist, Lothian Health Board,
Gogarburn Hospital, Glasgow Road, Edinburgh EH12 9BJ

S. Willoughby-Booth, *MA, RATh,*
Head Art Therapist, Lothian Health Board, Gogarburn Hospital, Glasgow Road,
Edinburgh EH12 9BJ

J.G. Wishart, *MA, PhD,*
Senior Research Fellow, Edinburgh Centre for Research in Child Development,
University of Edinburgh, Department of Psychology, 7 George Square, Edinburgh
EH8 9JZ

P.A. Woods, *BSc, PhD, MSc, Dip Psych, AFBPsS,*
Unit General Manager (Service Development) and Head of Unit, Clinical
Psychology Services, Bryn-Y-Neuadd Hospital, Llanfairfechan, Gwynedd, Wales

Contents

1

Introduction

1.1 Changing perspectives on mental handicap

Bill Fraser and Ann M. Green

Labelling and defining

Definitions and classifications will always be problematic. We learn new terms just as the move starts towards their obsolescence. Mental handicap is in some respects a confusing and unsatisfactory term used to describe a condition of lifelong intellectual impairment and accompanying disabilities in social functioning. It is not simply a clinical diagnosis: it is a social process of changing expectations, labelling, and families coming to some understanding of what handicap means (Booth, 1978).

Labels are ephemeral; not only are the terms 'idiot', 'imbecile' and 'feeble-minded' objectionable, but also 'subnormal' and in English-speaking countries 'defective' and 'retarded' are becoming unacceptable to parents and professionals alike. People whose IQs are under 50 are now referred to as 'people with severe mental handicap' or as having 'severe learning difficulties'. Those with measured intelligence in the 50–70 range are termed 'people with mild mental handicap', or as having 'moderate learning difficulties'. Children who function at a level below IQ 50 are usually still educated within special schools or classes for children with severe learning difficulties. Despite the heated and unproductive controversies about associated stigma, terms and definitions are necessary. Labelling is required if only to provide the statistics on which services are planned and provided. Fryers (1987) has pointed out that the practical objectives of a survey or study usually determine the definition.

The current diagnostic criteria of mental handicap are in the third edition of the Diagnostic and Statistical Manual – DSM III (American Psychiatric Association, 1980):

1. Significant sub-average intellectual functioning – an IQ of 70 or below – on an individually administered IQ test (in the case of infants, a clinical judgement of significant sub-average intellectual functioning).

2. Concurrent deficits or impairments in adaptive behaviour, taking the person's age into consideration.
3. Onset of intellectual impairment before the age of 18 years. (When the impairment occurs after the age of 18 years, this is classified in DSM III as dementia and includes brain damage after head injury, chronic psychosis, presenile dementias).

Prevalence

The prevalence of the generally accepted three grades of mental handicap: (Mild/moderate; Severe; and Profound) are 30/1000, 3/1000 and 0.5/1000. Throughout the developed countries 0.3/1000 will still be in (and currently seem to require) 'health-care' environments (Minns *et al.*, 1989).

The principles and practical problems of fundamental change

Worldwide, the last twenty years have seen services for people with mental handicaps move in a usually faltering piecemeal fashion towards a service that is rationally based. In the UK, since the publication of the White Paper on Better Services for the Mentally Handicapped (DHSS, 1971) and the passing of the 1971 Education Act (Department of Education, 1971), the momentum of transition from a hospital-medical-based service towards a local flexible multi-disciplinary service has increased. Yet the actual change is still far less than the amount written about it; and than the rhetoric and promises of professional service-planners. There still is a debate about the need for some health-care residential provision for a small minority of intellectually impaired people with specific needs: people with profound/multiple handicaps who have concurrent physical illness; those with additional severe physical or sensory disabilities which are deteriorating; and those with very disturbed or challenging behaviours. There is no doubt that an almost total model of community provision for all people with mental handicaps is possible, but whether it is sustainable in terms of society's enthusiasm, resources and skilled manpower requires further examination. So far in the UK the majority of users of the Mental Handicap Service have not experienced any radical difference in the last 15 years; and even if community dwellings were available for all, it is doubtful if the objective of normalization of Nirje (1969), namely ordinary opportunities and experiences and integration into normal patterns of society, is being fulfilled. Wolfensberger (1983) identifies the main problem as people with mental handicaps being devalued by the rest of society because of negative perceptions of their differences. Such attitudes then justify a number of responses including ambivalence about the allocation of resources to their needs. Wolfensberger's solution is radical – 'the use of culturally valued means to enable disadvantaged people to lead culturally valued lives.'

Emerson and Pretty (1987) have identified three important principles in Wolfensberger's interpretation of normalization:

1. A person's experience of behaviour and status is determined by the environment in which they live. The community residences therefore need to reflect the values of the surrounding culture.

2. Full participation in the life of the community is both a right and a need of people at significant risk of devaluation.
3. The essential objectives of community living are to enhance the quality of life experiences of those whose status has been significantly devalued.

O'Brien (1986) identifies five essential accomplishments as being necessary for quality of life: community presence, choice, competence, respect and community participation, to which Kristiansen and Ness (1987) have added expression of individuality and the experience of continuity in one's life. Evans, Beyer and Todd (1988) have incorporated these principles in their evaluation of community living which now is longer by reference to, or by comparison with, handicapped people's former lives (in institutions) but by reference to explicit values (normalization). So at last the issues of integration are being addressed.

Wolfensberger's (1980) concept of normalization – that people with mental handicaps should 'pass' as normal, like anyone of equivalent age and culture – has been a source of widespread misinterpretation and controversy; it has been asserted that it is an attempt to make people normal, to ignore their individual differences, to remove them from contact with their disabled peers and to ignore pathological conditions in disabled people. Although there have been examples of abuse of Wolfensberger's approach, it has been inspirational. It seems that the normalization principle and traditional human service work are still competing concepts (McCord, 1980). The previously unchallenged paradigm of remunerative work has to be replaced by one which asserts that unless physical and social integration are cornerstones of service delivery people will not live valued lives: human service workers must seek out generic service which can replace obsolescent specialized ones.

Naturally, administrative and direct service staff feel that their work and worth is under assault and react accordingly, often by producing an illusion of change; by pouring money into institutions (increasing the hotel-like appearance rather than increasing the home-like facilities); by attacking the basis of normalization as a 'religion'; or by picking out the rare but undoubtedly worrying perversions of normalization and denial of disability from which to attack the application of normalization in general. The problem is not only of changing the view of staff who work with people with mental handicaps but also the mainstream of society. Unfortunately, mass education campaigns in which handicapped people are not visible and not encountered in everyday situations, do not foster an increased acceptance of disability. The process of 'communitization' (Hogan, 1980) of disabled people has hardly begun, yet the public has acquired quickly new outlooks towards disabled people. As McCord says, 'we are faced with the phasing out of a hundred-year-old human service system'. For this to be successful, the new community systems of care must be carefully evaluated in terms of the extent to which they are meeting defined needs. Systems must also be assessed with regard to the cost of their implementation and will require, as Ager (1990) points out, an estimate of their sustainability. 'However important and cost effective a strategy is, if the service can't be sustained its ultimate worth is clearly negligible.' Some services fail to take account of the difficulties in recruiting appropriate staff to sustain the service that has developed. This is particularly worrying in view of the 30% fall in school-leavers projected for the next seven years. Corton, in Derham (1988), has identified, working in an international perspective, three generations of development. The first generation is simply 'rescuing' mental handicap hospitals in desperate need, importing professionals to meet short-term needs. The second generation is small local developments, incremental changes as the UK has experienced in the past 20 years – good ideas being implemented as finance allows. The third generation is concerned with sustainable systems development and the integration of local initiatives into supportive national development. This involves, crucially, 'bottom up' planning from the 'grass roots' with local initiatives fostered rather than 'top down' edicts and strategic planning from central government. In mental handicap services 'top-down' planning is still the usual convention but there have been areas, e.g. North West Regional Health Authority, where the 'bottom-up' approach calls for written plans to be based on individual client needs. The question that Ager reiterates is: how can we be sure that we develop sustainable mental handicap services? He points to three key characteristics of service development: firstly, respect for local strengths and local stakeholders and avoidance of large-scale disruption of local networks; secondly, change built upon existing repertoires of behaviour and the strength of the present systems; and thirdly, incremental change of perhaps small interventions with sustainability as a key factor, and active participation by professional stakeholders. McConkey (1988) has pointed out that in the Third World the professionalization of services acts as a powerful barrier to sustainable delivery of care, and he advises the use of local, partially or unqualified personnel for family support; and the employment of professional expertise as trainers and monitors rather than for direct therapeutic interventions. Thus, the problems outlined in relation to normalization and community care have within them the seeds of their own solution.

Normalization in itself is perhaps most valuable as a philosophy because of its claim for ordinariness and directness in care-giver approaches. Burton Blatt (1987) has written 'my main purpose is to force you to examine not only the dilemmas in their (handicapped people's) new lives but also in your life and to help you understand better that if aspects of their work seem unresolvable it is only because they *are* – if only for the moment – unresolvable.' One such 'unresolvable' question has come from an unlikely source – psychotherapy – the 'acceptance' of normalization cannot be 'taken' simply as an intimate and positive one-to-one relationship between mentally handicapped persons and other people; because of the deep-seated and confusing nature of feelings on which our treatment of people with mental handicap is based. Even a large number of 'heart-changing personal experiences' would not necessarily generalize change in a meritocratic society (Boucherat, 1987). Boucherat suggests that for the ultimate success of normalization, existing materialistic social values would have to be turned upside down. It is important to recognize that people need to accept their limitations and then attain their own ambitions for life in the community.

Recently, moreover, another basic problem which may be similarly difficult to surmount, is how people with mental handicaps now living in the community continue to exist on the fringes of society. Physical integration takes place without social integration (Humphreys *et al.*, 1987). The person with a mental handicap may have few friends, and none of normal intellect. He/she may leave school without the necessary development of social cognition, communication skills and the large number of strategies needed to solve the many problems which face all of us who live in the sometimes 'baffling and problem-strewn battleground that is our social world' (Beveridge and Conti-Ramsden, 1987). People with mental handicaps, even those who are most articulate, appear to live in a world of learned helplessness and even the most genuine care-givers have clear role asymmetry in their behaviours and in their communication with such handicapped people whom they claim to regard as their equals. (One's usual style is to talk to a person with a mental handicap as tutor to pupil.) It may be too much to ask what Boucherat suggests – for a 'change of heart' – but it could begin with changing our communication styles with intellectually disabled people starting in infancy.

Rowitz (1989), editor of the US journal, *Mental Retardation*, has identified several other issues that must be addressed in the 1990s. They will be raised in this volume but not solved. *The Graying of the Population*, including people with mental handicaps. This means there will be less resources proportionately available for the retarded, and the problems of the ageing handicapped population will proportionately increase. *Concern for Adolescents with Mental Handicap* – at present services for this group are not clearly delineated. *Expansion of the Health Care Delivery Service* – the health needs of people with intellectual disabilities have taken a back seat in the push for community care. Health promotion clinics (especially with the threat of AIDS now imminent) and, if a two-tier service develops as the NHS reorganizes, health maintenance and preferred provider companies will flourish. *New Vocational Opportunities* – fewer young people will mean more service-industry vacancies for people with mild mental handicaps. *Expanding Research on Families* – Child psychiatrists and psychologists are now bringing systems theories to bear on the family dynamics of people with handicaps and Expressed Emotion is now a measurable factor in handicapped family relationships. *Biomedical Research* will make significant breakthroughs. There has already been a resurgence of interest in the biological factors associated with mental handicap. Genetic defects will be precisely identified and bioengineering cures will come. Litigation will increase in pursuit of access to ordinary services and also to specialist services. More low-birth-weight children with handicaps will sue their mothers who smoked gestationally.

Plastic surgery will be increasingly requested for Down's syndrome and other conditions where there are stigmata. Such measures should not be considered as 'cosmetic' surgery. The procedures are all standard – exactly what would be done for normal children with fat necks, droopy lower eyelids, flat nasal bridges and hypoplastic ears. The most stigmatizing feature is the open mouth and tongue thrust. Reduction in tongue size improves breathing, reduces respiratory infection and sleep apnoea, which can cause overactivity in toddlers with Down's syndrome. Children who look more normal will have more expected of them. This is a good thing (Howells, 1989).

Fog on the voyage

At the time of writing, it is unclear what the impact of the recommendations of the Government's 1989 White Paper on the future of the NHS will be for people with mental handicaps (the absence of any mention is ominous), but clearly the direction of thinking is towards competition between hospitals and more freedom for the medical practitioners to act as budget holders to buy treatment, tests and non-urgent operations from wherever they shop around: NHS, self-governing or private hospitals. In the case of mental handicap, as for other services, where no alternative exists, the present hospitals, whether self-governing or not, will have to continue to provide services. Audit will be a condition of a hospital being recognized for training. This is fairly straightforward in the case of, for example, surgery but in the case of mental handicap services currently available Performance Indicators only give very crude ideas about how well the mental handicap service is performing, e.g. the rate of discharge from institutions; the quality of service is only judged by the number and type of staff involved; no outcome or quality of life measures are incorporated. Each district will have a duty to buy the best services they can from whatever source. The emphasis on the Government is to continue to have an NHS free at the point of service financed from general taxation and paying increased attention to consumers' wishes. The pitfalls for people with mental handicaps in any reorganization of the Health Service – their vulnerability, the high cost of their care, their inarticulateness, the vast range of their disabilities and the lack of experience of most practitioners in looking after their health care needs – raise questions that cannot be answered in this volume.

The Griffith's Report *Community Care: Caring for People* (1988) has declared that the key responsibility for the 'social', as distinct from the 'health' element in community care for the elderly and people with mental illness and mental handicaps, will go to the local authorities who will be purchasers of care. Health authorities will retain considerable responsibility for those they discharge from long-stay mental illness hospitals. Social security will cease to pay board and lodging costs in council-run homes. The central government grant to services for people with mental handicaps will not be ring-fenced, putting more burden on the community charge.

Social security will pay only the board and lodging costs in private homes, with local authorities paying the 'care' element. That will allow them to spend the money on care for people at home if that is the best choice. Cash will not be forthcoming where councils try to expand their own workforces. Instead they will have to buy in services from the private and voluntary sectors. Councils will thus become in part the paymasters of private home owners but giving the local authority the 'care' element of the cost will help check on whether people with intellectual disabilities are getting – or really need – such care.

Health authorities will continue to be responsible for investigating, diagnosing, treating and rehabilitating, for health education and promotion, for community nursing, and for advising on the Health element in 'care packages'. Authorities can undertake joint action or act as agents for each other. The management of some community facilities and services may be handled on an agency basis.

A crucial person will be the care manager who will co-ordinate needs assessment and multi-disciplinary action planning with individual clients who choose (or shop around) to engage them. They will have a budget to ensure that care packages for clients are sustained.

Thus the future as portrayed by both the White Paper and the Griffiths Report suggests more use of agencies – agencies providing care managers, community carers, agencies providing homes and work or day-care settings; and more packages of care including health care in health management agencies, and 'preferred health provider' services.

History may note that the 1970s gave us a philosophy for human service provision; the 1980s clarified our insight into the importance of sustainability in human service development. The 1990s may offer a framework in which the range, the flexibility and the individuality of services that consumers require can be developed: only when the mist clears can the impact of the current changes be judged.

References

Ager, A. (1990) Planning sustainable services – principles for the effective targetting of resources in developed and developing nations. In *Key Issues in Mental Retardation Research* (ed. W. Fraser) Routledge, London, pp. 385–394

American Psychiatric Association (1980) *Diagnostic and Statistical Manual – DSM III* APA, Washington, D.C.

Beveridge, M. and Conti-Ramsden, G. (1987) Social cognition and problem solving in persons with mental retardation. *Australia and New Zealand Journal of Developmental Disability*, **13**, 99–106

Booth, T.A. (1978) From normal baby to handicapped child. *Sociology*, **12**, 203 221

Boucherat, A. (1987) Normalisation in mental handicap – acceptance without questions? *Bulletin of the Royal College of Psychiatrists*, **11**, 423–426

Burton Blatt, B. (1987) *The Conquest of mental Retardation*, Pro-Ed, Arstin, TX

Department of Education (1971) Education Act, HMSO, London

Department of Health (1989) NHS Act. *Working for patients*, HMSO, London

Department of Health and Social Security (1971) White Paper on Better Services for the Mentally Handicapped. HMSO, London

Derham, M. (1988) The right kind of development. *TEAR Times*, **39**, 4–6

Emerson, E. and Pretty, G.M.H. (1987) Enhancing the social relevance of evaluation practice. *Disability, Handicap and Society*, **2**, 151–162

Evans, G., Beyer, S. and Todd, S. (1988) Looking foward not looking back: the evaluation of community living. *Disability, Handicap and Society*, **3**, 239–252

Fryers, T. (1987) Epidemiological issues in mental retardation. *Journal of Mental Deficiency Research*, **31**, 365–384

Griffiths Report (1988) *Community Care – Agenda for Action*, Department of Health, London

Hogan, M. (1980) Normalization and Commutization. In *Normalization, Social Integration and Community Services* (eds R. Flynn and K. Nitsch)., Baltimore University Press, Baltimore, MD

Howells, G. (1989) Down's syndrome and the General Practitioner. *Journal of the Royal College of General Practitioners* **39**, 470–475

Humphreys, S., Lowe, K. and Blunden, R. (1982) Long term evaluation of services for mentally handicapped people in Cardiff. *Mental Handicap*, **16**, 23–26

Kristiansen, K. and Ness, N.E. (1987) *Hjelpesystenet*; Igar. I dag I morgon. Trondheim

McConkey, R. (1988) Out of Africa: an alternative style of services for people with mental handicaps and their families. *Mental Handicap*, **16**, 23–26

McCord, W.T. (1980) From theory to reality: obstacles to the implementation of the normalisation principle in human services. *Mental Retardation*, **20**, 247–253

Minns, R.A., Brown, K., Wong, K., Fraser, W. (1989) Neurodevelopmental study of profoundly mentally handicapped children in hospital care. *Journal of Mental Deficiency Research*, 439–455

Nirje, B. (1969) The normalisation process and its human management implications. In *Changing Patterns in Residential Services for the Mentally Retarded* (eds R. Kugel and W. Wolfensberger), President's Committee on Mental Retardation, Washington, DC

O'Brien, J. (1986) A guide to personal futures planning. In *The Activities catalogue – A Community Programming Guide for Youth and Adults with Severe Disabilities* (eds G.T. Bellamy and B. Wilcox). Brookes, Baltimore

Rowitz, L. (1989) Editorial: Trends in mental retardation in the 1990s. *Mental Retardation,* **27**, iii

Wolfensberger, W. (1980) The definition of normalisation – update, problems. In *Normalization, Social Integration and Community Services* (eds R. Flynn and K. Nitsch) Baltimore University Press, Baltimore, MD

Wolfensberger, W. (1983) Social role valorisation: A proposed new term for the principle of normalisation. *Mental Retardation*, **21**, 234–239

1.2 Multi-disciplinary care and training

Peter Mathias

Introduction

The purpose of this section is to offer a classification of multi-disciplinary care and to look at its implications for training.

For at least two decades, the principle that care should be provided on a multi-disciplinary basis has been part and parcel of social policy and the way that services are organized.

This applies at several levels from simple devices of attaching social workers to special schools, through the provision of multi-disciplinary community teams to the provision of formal joint consultative and planning committees to enable the health services, local authorities and others to plan together. So, from the simple recognition that people with a mental handicap can benefit from the help and advice of several different disciplines has sprung elaborate machinery to develop the inter-organizational cooperation necessary to allow people from different disciplines to combine their expertise in the service of the client.

This is so, of course, because the disciplines or professions are or have been in a sense, associated with a particular service: teachers and education psychologists by education; doctors, clinical psychologists and para-medical therapists by the health service; and social workers by local authorities and voluntary agencies.

This is beginning to break down as reform of the services and the growth of the private and voluntary sector occurs. The changing face of organizations demands maximum clarity about the benefits and value of multi-disciplinary work and how it can be organized. For example, nurses are no longer necessarily a hospital-bound adjunct of the health service but are finding employment in a variety of situations and settings. In part, this is due to and in part this contributes towards the changing skill and competence base of nursing.

So nothing is static, disciplines change and adapt; and their administrative base can be altered. Simplistic assignment of roles and responsibilities is therefore likely to hold only a relative short-term truth. The processes of multi-disciplinary cooperation, on the other hand, may have a longer term currency. The classification that follows is based largely on process and purpose, but first a word about the disciplines.

Multi-disciplinary care: a classification

The dictionary defines discipline as a department of knowledge, a branch of instruction, or to bring under control. The word applied to the human sciences holds connotations of these three things – a sense of ordered, controlled, disciplined development of knowledge as understanding, in this instance including the effects of intervention with people. Many disciplines have developed a specialism in or paid attention to mental handicap or learning difficulties. Thus teachers with special expertise in learning difficulties, doctors and dentists with applied knowledge, lawyers who specialize and develop particular parts of the legislation, and nurses, social workers and psychologists with special interests.

The person with a handicap, and their family can seek advice from a variety of practitioners according to age and nature of help required.

However, without a focus in a particular aspect of provision, attempts to organize multi-disciplinary care or training can drift towards the abstract. Multi-disciplinarianism for its own sake may lead to preoccupation with the relationship between the disciplines and for example, endless arguments about boundaries and territories, or similarities and differences. The result is often rigid demarcation between the roles and responsibilities of different workers, which is unhelpful, or agreement that everything and everyone is the same and that profession X should merge with profession Y. This has happened in the debate between nursing and social work.

This section examines the place of multi-disciplinary care in the natural and professional helping system available to people with a disability and their families and offers a way of classifying multi-disciplinary care into four levels.

The classification is a variation on one that is commonly used in counselling. In this discipline, the literature suggests that people naturally turn to a hierarchy of support ranging from the informal to the formal. More specifically, Sugarman (1986) identifies a range of support in a hierarchy of formality extending from (1) the natural help system, (2) the mutual help system to (3) the non-professional help system and finally (4) the professional help system. These support systems are in addition to the personal psychological resources of the individual, family or group.

The classification of multi-disciplinary care uses this approach, starting with the client, and extending to more formal inter-disciplinary arrangements such as multi-professional teams.

The natural help system or the kith and kin system is probably the first line of support for most handicapped people and/or parents of children with a disability. A variety of mutual help groups exist for people with a mental handicap or their parents. These may offer support and/or act as pressure groups for the improvement of services. The non-professional help system (Golan, 1981) consists

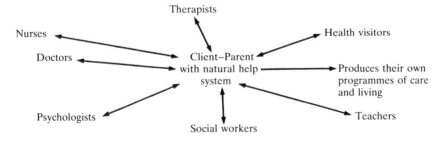

Figure 1.2.1 Multi-disciplinary care level I

of voluntary workers, community care givers and people such as the clergy and the police.

The professional help system is at the extreme of the continuum and consists of those individuals whose training and employment confers on them community or institutional sanction and responsibility for offering help to various client groups.

Pursuing this latter a bit further, Byrne, Cunningham and Sloper (1988) examined the views of parents of children with Down's syndrome about the services they received from different professionals. They found that: '23% of families were in contact with five or more helpful professionals, 56% between 2 and 5, 14% with one and only 6% of families were not in contact with any helpful professionals. Approximately half of the women we interviewed (48%) were completely satisfied with all the services they received. 52% felt that they had at least some needs which were not being met. A sizeable minority (ranging from 7% to 38%) described particular professionals as very unhelpful'.

When the subject of multi-disciplinary care is discussed, the context of the discussion very often centres on the professional and discussion between professionals about how they might work together more effectively in the service of their client. But it is clear from Byrne's study that most parents receive a service from several disciplines or professionals and that they often receive the services separately. In this instance, it is the parent or client who integrates (or sifts) advice and help from different disciplines to produce multi-disciplinary care. They may do this on their own or with the help of the natural support or mutual help systems.

Multi-disciplinary care level I: the client as their own case-manager in the natural or mutual help system

The first level of multi-disciplinary care is therefore, in a sense, naturally occurring. Parents or clients seek out different disciplines or professions for advice, help or support and turn this into a programme of care, perhaps with help from kith and kin or mutual help groups (Figure 1.2.1).

The implications for training or for strengthening this level of multi-disciplinary care are clear: target the clients, help them to become better at seeking out and integrating the help of different professionals. Examples of this sort of activity do exist, mostly organized by mutual help groups, for example, local MENCAP or People First organizations. Alternatively, or in addition, the family or client could be given the resources to buy or purchase the particular combination of multi-disciplinary care or services they consider best suited to their requirements. Experiments of this kind are being made with this and other client groups in the UK and in the USA.

Multi-disciplinary care level II: guides, named people, counsellors

The second level of multi-disciplinary care (Figure 1.2.2) is slightly more formal. It is exemplified by the ideas of a named person or guide who helps the parent or client find their own through the maze of services and disciplines that are available. These are people with some knowledge of the local services, or of particular problems, who are made, or make themselves, available. Sometimes this activity becomes the formal responsibility of a particular professional (a nurse or a social worker), sometimes a professional will extend their role to fulfil this purpose (a teacher, a day-centre worker). In the particular instance of parents with young

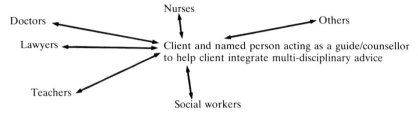

Figure 1.2.2 Multi-disciplinary care level II

children about to enter school, Byrne *et al.* argue the case for a special counsellor, someone to help parents choose. This is an aspect of multi-disciplinary care albeit at one remove from the traditional notions of being the coordinated giving of help and advice.

Strengthening this aspect of care can be achieved through making the named person or guide better equipped or better resourced to achieve their purpose, but again it is essentially the client who coordinates, integrates or makes sense of the advice.

From this point the classification of multi-disciplinary care gives the professional a more central place. There are two further levels.

Multi-disciplinary care level III: key workers, case managers and coordinators in the professional help system (Figure 1.2.3)

A number of professionals find themselves in jobs in which they are called on to coordinate and obtain advice from different sources and translate it into a programme of activity with, or on behalf of, the client. Many management posts carry such responsibility, but it is also a feature of basic activity for some social workers, teachers, nurses and doctors. The disciplines from which advice or help is needed may be called together in a group, may even form a team, but at this level the responsibility for action is usually located very clearly with one person, and a multi-disciplinary approach is necessary in order to discharge their responsibility.

Examples of this are the head teacher who convenes a multi-disciplinary group of speech and physiotherapists and social workers in order to respond to the needs of pupils; the ward sister who has to translate the advice of doctors, psychologists and paramedical specialists into daily programmes of activity for patients; and the day-centre worker or manager who seeks out help from different disciplines to help a client overcome particular difficulties.

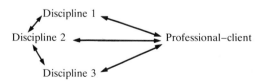

in varying relationship but with professional holding formal responsibility to produce effective multi-disciplinary care

Figure 1.2.3 Multi-disciplinary care level III

Recent ideas about care-management are a formalization of level III activities, in which more formal powers and responsibilities are placed on one person, from whatever discipline, to plan and manage a coordinated service for clients.

Multi-disciplinary care level IV: Teams and committees of the professional help system

Level IV activities refers to those in which the combined powers and expertise of a variety of disciplines are necessary to solve a problem, provide a service, plan a strategy or allocate resources. Such activity is often pursued through a team, group or committee and responsibility is often placed at the level of the group rather than any single person or profession. This is in fact the form of inter-disciplinary work which comes most readily to mind, e.g. the Community Mental Handicap team.

A lot has been written about teams. It is clearly a mistake, however, to equate multi-disciplinary care with teamwork. It is really a specific subset of multi-disciplinary activity which, in common with the other subsets described in previous pages is worthy of study in its own right.

The classification: a summary

Multi-disciplinary care exists in a variety of forms, some of which have not received the attention they should either in the literature or in service provision. This section has so far offered a four-part classification of multi-disciplinary care:

1. Level I of which concerns parents or clients in receipt of separate services from a number of disciplines and who themselves integrate the advice and translate it into a programme of activity informed by various disciplines.
2. Level II is an extension of level I in which parents or clients effect the integration with the help of someone else, a named person, a guide or a counsellor.
3. In level III activities professionals adopt a more central role in managing the inputs from different disciplines and have formal responsibilities to do so – as in case management or the management of a service or unit the staff of which come from different disciplines.
4. Level IV activities describe the work of teams, groups or committees in which the responsibilities are vested at group rather than individual level, although there might be a formal leader.

The product of multi-disciplinary activity is thus varied. It might be the allocation of resources, the planning of a service, individual case management or the formulation of an individual programme plan. The problem is to match form of activity to task and to avoid striving for the complex when the simple will do.

For example, it might be more effective to help parents integrate advice themselves than to set up a multi-disciplinary team to do the same thing; it might be better to simplify the administrative structure and transfer services from one authority to another rather than set up a joint committee; or it may be more effective to vest responsibility in one person rather than several.

Training for multi-disciplinary care: examples from social work, psychology and nursing

Introduction

This section will explore the issues of multi- or inter-disciplinary training with reference to psychology, nursing and social work because significant moves towards shared training in these three disciplines have been made in the last few years.

Shared learning

The relationship between nursing and social work has been more controversial than that between social work and psychology.

In 1982 the General Nursing Council's and the Central Council for Education and Training in Social Work (CCETSW) published *Co-operation in Training, Part I* and published Part II in 1983.

These booklets showed that:

1. In the field of mental handicap some knowledge and skills were common to nurses and social workers.
2. Where the knowledge and skills were different, they were often complementary and nurses and social workers often had to combine their expertise in inter-disciplinary work.

This led to the suggestion that a variety of forms of shared learning were possible for in-service and qualifying training. Many of the recommendations for in-service, in-house cooperation still stand but can now be seen in the context of other trends in training and in particular the growing sophistication of the literature which relates training to organizational change and the development of the services.

The recommendations for qualifying and post-qualifying training have received further attention and some modification. Shared qualifying and post-qualifying training schemes now exist. Recent publications from the nursing boards and CCETSW make further suggestions about how progress might be made (ENB/ CCETSW, 1985, 1988), and the new challenge is to continue the shared learning initiatives within the reform of nurse and social work training manifested in Project 2000 and the new Diploma in Social Work.

All these developments are particularly pertinent to services for people with mental handicap because the services themselves are in a state of reform as practitioners, managers and administrators strive to make them more sensitive to the needs of clients and consumers.

Models of training: interventionist and educational or context embedded – content focused

The 1980s have seen the elaboration of an interventionist approach to training which sets it within an organizational context. This supplements the approach to training which is primarily concerned with individual learning and which some commentators call the educational approach.

Something of these two approaches to training can be seen in the unpublished report made by a group of psychologists and social workers who met together under the auspices of the British Psychological Society (BPS), the British Association of Social Workers (BASW) and the Central Council for Education and Training in Social Work (CCETSW).

The BPS/BASW/CCETSW report argues that there are shared learning needs at post-qualification level for psychologists and social workers, that these are concerned with continuing professional development and that they can best be met in training or professional development programmes, the objectives of which should be derived from an analysis of local trends in the development services. In other words, the group argued that the single most important thing that members of different disciplines have in common is the need to extend, refine, adapt and develop their skills and knowledge in response to service developments. They called this the context-embedded approach.

This is interventionist training by another name but included in any inter-professional development programme might very well be training events designed to help individuals acquire new knowledge and skill using the educational approach or as the BPS/BASW/CCETSW group referred to it – a content-focused approach.

The main differences between the interventionist and educational approach or the context embedded and content focused approaches can be seen in Figures 1.2.4 and 1.2.5, produced by Bramley (1988).

It is argued that the interventionist approach overcomes the shortcomings of the educational one which consist of:

1. Difficulties in transferring, maintaining or applying skills acquired in training sessions in everyday work.
2. The development of, at best, tenuous links between individual learning and organizational effectiveness.
3. The lack of recognition that the setting in which individuals' work affects performance as well as does the possession of skills, abilities and competence.

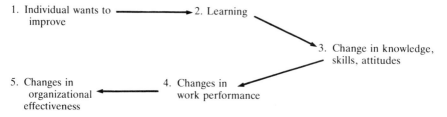

Figure 1.2.4 The educational model

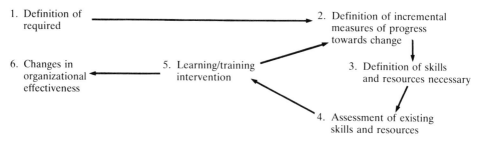

Figure 1.2.5 The interventionist model

Training, organizational change and the development of services

In the interventionist approach learning is seen as instrumental to organizational effectiveness and it is as necessary to think about organizational or group learning and development. The methods of interventionist training include team development, work group training, action learning and on the job facilitation of skill development. It is to these methods that the logic of the BPS/BASW/CCETSW group leads.

A variation on this approach can be seen in a number of training programmes designed to help in changing the services for people with mental handicap in which decision makers:

1. Make clear their values and express them as a consistent set of goals and objectives.
2. Generate and examine the alternatives available for the achievement of the goals.
3. Predict and assess the utility and probability of the consequences that follow from the adoption of each alternative.
4. Compare the consequences in relation to the agreed set of goals and objectives.
5. Select the alternative in which consequences correspond to a greater degree with goals and objectives.
6. Organize training in a cascade throughout the services so that everyone is equipped to play their part.

(Adapted from Legge, 1984.)

Success in this approach depends upon the engagement of all the key decision makers and the development of knowledge about all, or a wide range of, the choices available. Partial engagement or restricted choices can lead to faulty decisions, lack of agreement about ends and means and a refusal by one or more of those disciplines cooperating to change practice.

Hence the BPS/BASW/CCETSW group suggested that regional multi-professional groups be established to plan training but recognized that such groupings would need close links with the service organizations if they were to be effective.

The interventionist or context embedded trend in training leads inevitably to the literature on organizational change which in some ways transcends or subsumes formal inter-disciplinary training.

Nevertheless, it is useful to think of this literature when considering or relating inter-disciplinary training to organizational effectiveness because it adds a further dimension to it.

It can be seen from the preceding pages that multi-disciplinary training is informed by and, in turn, informs more general trends in training as those involved struggle to make training effective for the individual and for the service.

Competence and CATS

There are, however, two further and related trends which are relevant to multi-disciplinary training. They are the growth of the competence movement and the development of credit accumulation and transfer schemes (CATS). Both are significant for the services to people with mental handicap, particularly with respect to shared learning at professional qualifying levels.

A number of occupational groups and professions are beginning to describe the activities of their practitioners in terms of competence, of what it is that practitioners do and the requirements that can be made of them.

This movement reaches its apogee in the work of the National Council for Vocational Qualifications (NCVQ) and the Training, Enterprise and Education Directorate of the Department of Employment (formerly the Training Agency). The remit of the NCVQ has recently been extended to include the professions who, on a voluntary basis, are invited to express their work and the outcomes of any training programmes or awards they might offer in terms of competence. A string of advisory and guidance papers have been issued by the NCVQ and the Training Agency which explain their view of competence and of how awards might be designed. The usefulness of this approach can be illustrated by examining the problems that the Nursing Boards and CCETSW have encountered in answering demands from practitioners and administrators for greater shared or joint training.

The problems were all related to the structure and length of training and the regulations that govern them rather than with the content or outcome of training where it was much easier to see similarities and differences.

Expressing awards and qualifications in terms of competence and concentrating more on the outcome rather than the process of training shifts the debate from a pre-occupation with rules and regulations surrounding learning to consideration of what it is that people are learning to do. The rules and regulations are still there but they are concerned with assessment of students on which it may be easier to reach agreement.

The development of credit accumulation and transfer schemes should also make it easier to provide accredited multi-disciplinary training. There is an acceptance that people acquire competence in a variety of ways and that this should be recognized formally. So, for example, in-house training schemes may count towards degrees, vocational training can be related to general education and people may acquire or accumulate credits towards awards and qualifications through a greater diversity of routes than ever before.

Most of all it should be possible for multi-disciplinary training to focus on content where necessary, rather than form of training.

The future of multi-disciplinary training

What can training do to make multi-disciplinary care more effective? This section has tried to answer the question at several levels.

Training can help the service user become more effective at integrating the separate advice received from different disciplines and professions. It can help a named person, or counsellor become more effective on behalf of the service user. It can help those responsible for managing programmes of multi-disciplinary care become more effective. Finally, it can help teams of people work together to meet service requirements more effectively.

There is one feature of the services that has been barely mentioned. At present, the majority of those offering direct care in the health and social services are without a descriptive, profession or even qualification for what are often complex and demanding jobs.

The establishment of the National Council for Vocational Qualifications will hopefully change this. It is important that whenever possible the same qualifications and awards are available to people on either side of service boundaries so that at the level of direct carers, who will always be in a majority in the workforce, the principle of multi-disciplinary or inter-occupation cooperation is established. Such cooperation will foster or complement multi-disciplinary training at qualification and post-qualification level.

Finally, although most of the examples given in the section have been drawn from nursing, social work, and psychology the same arguments apply to many of the other professions or occupational groups active in the field. Essentially multi-disciplinary training should be based on common understanding of the needs and aspirations of people with mental handicap; and some shared methods and interventions; inter-professional collaboration is most effective at the level of the individual client.

References

Bramley, P. (1988) Evaluating training. *Training Officer*, **24**, July

British Psychological Society/British Association of Social Workers/General Nursing Council/Central Council for Education and Training in Social Work: (BPS/BASW/CCETSW) (1989) *Continuing Professional Development for Psychologists and Social Workers within the Community Services for People with Mental Handicap*. An unpublished report of a working group available from CCETSW, London

Byrne, E.A., Cunningham, C.C. and Sloper, P. (1988) *Families and their Children with Down's Syndrome: One Feature in Common*, Routledge, London

English National Board for Nursing, Health Visiting and Midwifery/Central Council for Education and Training in Social Work:

(1985) *Co-operation in Training*. An unpublished report of a working group.

(1988) *Shared Initiatives in Residential Services – Regulations for Post-Qualifying Programmes of Study*.

General Nursing Council/Central Council for Education and Training in Social Work:

(1982) *Co-operation in Training Part I – Qualifying Training*.

(1983) *Co-operation in Training Part II – Inservice Training*.

Golan, N. (1981) *Passing through Transitions: A Guide for Practitioners*, Free Press, New York

Legge, K. (1984) *Evaluating Planned Organisational Change*, Chapter 2, Academic Press, London

NCVQ (National Council for Vocational Qualifications (1987–89) *Series of Guidance Papers* (available from NCVQ, London

Porter, L., Lawler, E. and Hackman, J. (1975) *Behaviour in Organisations*, McGraw-Hill, Singapore

Sugarman, L. (1986) *Life Span Development. Concepts, Theories and Interventions*, Methuen, London

Training Agency (TA) *Guidance Papers on Competence and National Occupational Standards* (available from the Training Agency, Moorfoot, Sheffield)

2

Assessment

Paul Dickens

Introduction

The whole area of assessment of people with a mental handicap has changed out of all recognition in the past few years. A glimpse at previous editions of this text, as well as other standard books on the subject (e.g. Mittler, 1970), will remind readers that in the early seventies, assessment was limited to the use of intelligence tests and a few pioneering measures of what is termed 'adaptive behaviour'. Compare this with the present situation, with an abundance of sophisticated measures of the latter, as well as exciting developments in computer-generated and scored assessments, self-assessment measures and tests of ability and competence.

There are several reasons for this rapid development. Firstly, there has been legislation in many countries requiring agencies to assess the needs of handicapped people with more detail and accuracy than before. Secondly, there has been an increased emphasis on individual programme plans or similar types of personal service planning. Thirdly, the increasing move of mentally handicapped people from institutional to community living has necessitated the careful assessment of their skills and social capacity. Lastly the increasing use of non-professionals as carers and service providers has meant that the traditional methods of evaluation, which usually required specialist psychological knowledge and intensive training, have been replaced by 'user-friendly' measures designed to be used as quickly as possible with minimal training and maximum practical usefulness.

It has also been recognized that the assessment of people with a mental handicap must focus as much on the environment within which they exist as on their own personal characteristics. Assessment needs to consider the opportunities that the environment offers for growth and development, which may lead into the evaluation of service efficiency, effectiveness and quality. Often this type of assessment is termed an 'ecological inventory' (Browder, 1987) and is used prior to beginning an assessment to find out which skills are important for that person in the environments in which they operate. This involvement of the environment leads us to consider assessment as important on three levels (Dickens, 1984):

1. *Primary* – At a face-to-face level, concentrating on the person.
2. *Secondary* – At an immediate environment level, looking at the social and physical context in which the person operates.
3. *Tertiary* – At a service or agency level, looking at the system within which a person receives services.

This inclusion of environment in assessment enables us to remember not only the fact that a person's skills and attributes are shaped by that environment, but also that a person's behaviour can vary across environments.

The history of the assessment of people with a mental handicap has seen firstly the development of tests that aided detection and diagnosis, such as the Binet and Simon tests of intelligence that were produced in the early part of this century to distinguish between educable and ineducable children. This was followed by the rise of assessment measures that aided prognosis, such as the Vineland Social Maturity Scale (Doll, 1953) which helped predict the outcome of training. This early measure led to the production of more sophisticated measures of social behaviour centred on the idea of 'adaptive behaviour'. This is an age-related set of skills that reflect the way in which any particular individual copes with the natural and social demands of his or her environment, including the skills necessary for personal independence and those needed for following social rules.

The impetus for this development was from the American Association on Mental Retardation, who in 1961 adopted what is known as the dual criteria of mental retardation: a person can be classified as mentally retarded (handicapped) only if they are both intellectually impaired and have deficits in adaptive behaviour. Assessment therefore must take both of these areas into account.

More recently there has been a shift away from tests and measures for classification towards measures that aid the production of individual teaching, programme or service plans. Often these assessments are part of packages that link a dedicated assessment directly to teaching plans or schemes (e.g. the Portage Project, 1975).

When approaching the task of assessing a person with mental handicaps, it is important that the purposes of the assessment are clear. There can be many purposes for assessment, including:

1. Finding out what skill to teach a person, and at what level to start that teaching.
2. Giving information to guide decisions on where a person should live/work/go to school, etc.
3. Providing a baseline for teaching programmes (the so-called 'before and after' measures).
4. Surveying the features of a large number of people with a mental handicap, for the planning of new services.
5. Highlighting a person's strengths and needs, to identify areas for further teaching, or areas where service input is required.
6. Comparing an individual with their peers for the purpose of assessing progress.
7. Providing detailed examination of specific problem areas of skill or behaviour to assist in diagnosis.

There are of course many other uses of assessment for people with a mental handicap. What is important, however, as Dickens and Stallard (1987) have pointed out, is that the professional is clear about which purpose their assessment is serving. If this is not clear then the wrong type of assessment may be used, or results gained that do not provide the information required.

There are a number of types of assessment procedure that are used in the assessment of people with a mental handicap. Many of the procedures described in this chapter are performance tests, that is, tests where the person being evaluated has to perform various tasks in front of the assessor. Most tests of intelligence and other cognitive skills are in this category, and there are also some adaptive behaviour measures that rely on what is also termed 'direct testing'. A second type of assessment tool is the rating scale where a person's performance on a number of measures is rated by an assessor either from real-life knowledge or observation, or by the assessor questioning someone who is familiar with the person being assessed. Many adaptive behaviour measures come into this category of method. Thirdly, there are observational measures that are generally used for the detailed assessment of specific behaviour, and involve the assessor in time-based actual observation of the person. Of course not all assessments described in this chapter fall neatly into one or other of these categories. Indeed many use combinations of all three methods of data collection, whilst others have the option of using different ways, according to circumstances.

Before moving on to look at some of the specific areas of assessment currently important in mental handicap, it is worth considering some factors common to most of the assessment measures and methods that we will be describing.

Firstly, most of them have as their basis the base that what is required is an *objective* assessment of a person. That is the whole purpose of having formal structured tests and measures, and is the guiding principle behind many of the techniques of observational assessment that will be mentioned. This means that the picture we get from our assessment is as unbiased and as accurate as possible. It is very easy to become biased in opinion about someone, in either a positive (the so-called 'halo effect') or a negative way. Most tests and measures try to eliminate bias by being as reliable as possible. This means they will give the same results on a person when used by different testers, or in different environments or on different occasions. Reliability figures are often quoted in test manuals, and should be consulted when selecting a measure, so that one with maximum reliability is used. If the measure does not appear to be reliable, then great care is required in the interpretation of the results. Measures also attempt to eliminate bias by being standardized, usually in the manner of presentation and in the way in which the results relate to other groups of similar people, termed 'norms'.

One very important concept in the area of assessment is that of validity. This is concerned with what an assessment measures, how well it does so, and how the things that are measured relate to real life. It is important that a measure attempting to assess one area of skill, say language, takes into account all the different aspects of that area, and gives them weight according to their importance in a person's functioning. A measure of language that left out the use of nouns, for example, would not be a valid assessment of language, and would also give a biased picture of the person's language skills. The idea of 'social validity' is very important, and concerns the degree to which an assessment reflects the real-life performance of handicapped people or the demands made on them by their environment. If we are interested in finding out how institutionalized people with a mental handicap might function in the community, it is vital that we use an assessment that looks at the important areas in community living and samples the skills that are necessary for that setting. These may be quite different from those required in an institutional setting, so an assessment developed on an institutional population would not be valid.

These and other important basic underlying concepts about assessment are discussed in much more detail in most of the main textbooks on the assessment of people with a mental handicap, such as Mittler (1970), Matson and Breuning (1983), Hogg and Raynes (1987) and Dickens and Stallard (1987).

The remainder of this chapter is taken up with a discussion of the main types of assessment currently available in various important areas of the functioning of people with a mental handicap, including cognitive skills, adaptive and maladaptive behaviour and specific areas of evaluation such as language and memory skills. Where reference is made to a specific test or assessment measure, details of this are included in Appendix 2.

Cognitive measures

As we have already seen, the development of measures of intellectual deficiency was the earliest stage in the history of assessment procedures for people with a mental handicap. These measures are still an important part of practice, as the intellectual handicap aspect of this group of clients cannot be minimized. Intelligence tests as such are still used in everyday practice, not so much for their role in diagnosis, given what has been said about the dual-criteria approach to this above, but more in the study of specific areas of performance, with a view to providing remedial programmes. There are a number of general intelligence tests in use, including the Stanford–Binet Intelligence Scale and the Wechsler Scales. Both of these are really for use with a non-intellectually impaired client group, and so suffer from a bias towards educational achievement and the use of language. They are not standardized on a mentally handicapped population and have a high-ability baseline so that their use with people of lower levels of intellectual skill is limited to providing basic intelligence quotients (IQs). To overcome these problems more recent tests have been developed. In Great Britain the British Ability Scales has a number of subtests that are a good source of information on cognitive abilities, whilst the Woodcock-Johnson Psycho-Educational Battery is used widely in the USA. It covers memory, reasoning and language skills.

All the above tests require the person being tested to have a degree of language capability, which is often not the case with people with a mental handicap. There are, therefore, a number of tests that use non-verbal means for acquiring data. The main one of these is the Coloured Progressive Matrices, a picture reasoning test, which is standardized on British mentally handicapped people. The British Picture Vocabulary Scale is often used a test of intelligence, although it is really a measure of word knowledge. It also requires no language to be used, and is very useful as a quick (though not too accurate) measure of functioning. The Columbia Mental Maturity Scale is a test of intelligence that relies on non-verbal input, and has the added advantage of not needing any motor movements from the person being assessed, making it invaluable when assessing multiply handicapped people.

Likewise the Leiter International Performance Scale is a purely non-verbal measure of intelligence, which can be presented without speech and requires no speech from the person being assessed. It is used mainly with deaf clients for this reason. The problem with many of these specialized tests is that to be non-verbal they sample only a restricted set of cognitive skills, when compared with the big test batteries such as the British Ability Scales. As with all intelligence measures, their use with people with a mental handicap is fraught with difficulties of interpretation and validity. Many of them sample educational skills, and mentally handicapped people do not receive the same type of educational provision or input as the general population. Many of them rely heavily on language and verbal concepts, and mentally handicapped people are not usually as verbally fluent as the general population. Lastly they put an emphasis on logical deductive reasoning, and most people with a mental handicap are lacking in precisely these skills.

There are two ways of getting round these difficulties and providing accurate and worthwhile information on people with a mental handicap. The first is to focus exclusively on specific cognitive skills such as memory. The Wechsler Memory Scale is often used with this group of people although it is not really intended for them and suffers from the usual verbal bias. The Rivermead Scale is a more recent test of memory functioning and can be used successfully with quite handicapped people. Similarly the area of language skills can be considered as a subset of general cognitive functioning. Here there are a number of standard tests that form a regular part of psychologists' and speech therapists' working practice, including the Reynell Developmental Language Scales (Revised) and a new assessment specifically standardized on a handicapped population, the Communication and Speech Profile (CASP).

The second approach is to focus on what might be termed 'functional intelligence', that is those intellectual skills that are necessary for handicapped people to function in everyday life (that is, they are valid) and yet take into account the difficulties in assessment that most conventional tests pose. A good example of one of these types of measure is the Paton's Assessment Schedule, Form C, which assesses literacy, numeracy, orientation in time and place and other vital skills for survival particularly in a community setting. Most clinical psychologists have some similar clinical measures of functional intelligence in their kit.

Whichever of these ways is chosen, the emphasis is firmly on using intelligence tests and measures of cognitive functioning as parts of a comprehensive assessment package, rather than as an end in themselves. The days of routine intelligence assessment are gone.

Measures of adaptive and maladaptive behaviour

The assessment of adaptive behaviour is probably the most important and flourishing area of assessment in the field of mental handicap. We have already seen that the adoption in the late 1960s of the dual criteria system of diagnosis led to the production of relevant measures, and these have become more numerous as their usefulness has been shown, particularly in the move from institutional-based services to community based alternatives.

The generally accepted definition of adaptive behaviour is: 'the degree to which an individual meets standards of personal independence and social responsibility expected of their age and cultural group' (AAMD, 1961).

This is discussed further in later chapters, but it generally is considered to be a collection of skills, reflecting the ability of a person with a mental handicap to adapt to the natural and social demands of their environment. It is often subdivided into two areas: adaptive behaviour, which is the area of personal skills of independence; and maladaptive behaviour, which is concerned with the standards of social behaviour and conformity with social norms. This subdivision is reflected in the construction of many of the standard measures of adaptive behaviour.

The two pioneering efforts at measuring this concept came from Doll (1953) and Gunzburg (1968). The former devised the Vineland Social Maturity Scale which measured eight areas that Doll thought vital to the success of training and habilitation with handicapped people. Building on this work, Gunzburg devised the Progress Assessment Charts (PAC) which were a practical tool for staff to use in the assessment and teaching of handicapped people, particularly in institutional and day-centre settings. They are still popular today in six alternative forms, and all are divided into four areas of skill, self-help, communication, socialization and occupation. Data are gathered by a combination of interviews and direct-testing. A pictorial representation in the form of a circle is the output, which enables an easily understood profile of abilities and guides the formation of teaching plans. This type of representation of results has been used in other measures, particularly the STAR Profile (Social Training Achievement Record), although this is divided into 16 areas of skill.

One of the main scales in use to measure adaptive and maladaptive behaviour, particularly in the USA, is the AAMD Adaptive Behavior Scale. This scale was originally developed to cover the adaptive behaviour side of the dual definition criteria, and drew on the early measures such as the Vineland and PAC as the source of much of its content. The ABS is in two parts, adaptive behaviour and maladaptive behaviour, each of which is subdivided into domains representing major skill blocks (e.g. 'Independent Functioning' and 'Antisocial Behaviour'). In the adaptive section, the domains are further divided into subdomains (e.g. 'Toilet Use') and these are then further divided into items (e.g. 'Self-Care at Toilet'). The maladaptive domains are just divided into items. Information is gathered by interview, and each item is really a rating scale of that particular piece of behaviour. There is a lot of published literature on the ABS, and it is widely used because it is reliable in diagnostic use. It is limited as a source of information for programme planning, however, and there are significant problems concerning the maladaptive section that makes its use unreliable.

Of the similar scales to the ABS (that is those more concerned with diagnosis than programme planning), the most up to date and comprehensive are the Vineland Adaptive Behaviour Scales and the Scales of Independent Behaviour. The first of these is an update of the Vineland Social Maturity Scale, but with a radically different content and scoring method. It exists in two forms, a survey form for quick diagnostic use and an extended form, which gives more information for programme planning. The second is split into the same two sections as the ABS, but it has a more reliable section on maladaptive behaviour. It can also be used in a short form for surveys, or for the assessment of early development in children. Both of these scales represent the most up-to-date application of population sampling and test construction. They are also both paired to related tests of intelligence, so that results are compatible in terms of the dual criteria of mental handicap. They also feature computer scoring, interpretation and report produc-tion, one of the exciting developments in assessment at present, and can also be used to give input to individual programme plans.

The latter point is of vital importance, as the concept of adaptive behaviour is of great use when planning and producing teaching programmes for people with a mental handicap in service setting of many kinds, whether on an individual or a group basis. There has, therefore, been a rapid recent development of 'dedicated' assessment tools linked directly to a set of pre-prepared teaching guidelines or plans that take the assessment information as a baseline for intervention. In Great Britain there are a number of these in current use, some of which owe their inspiration to the package developed in the USA in the late 1970s known as the Portage Guide to Early Education. This was a combined assessment and teaching kit devised for use by teachers working advising parents on teaching tasks for pre-school children with mental handicaps. The assessment was colour and number coded, and each item on the chart cross-referred to a similar item on a set of similarly indexed teaching cards. The assessment therefore leads directly to the specification of a relevant teaching goal for the child.

Most of the assessment packages that use this sort of approach do not specify the teaching task in their accompanying material as specifically as the Portage does. The Beereweeke Skill Teaching System, for example, contains a detailed observational and direct-testing checklist that can then be used as the basic information for deriving individual specific teaching goals, reflecting the areas on the chart that were not well performed by the client. The other notable systems include the Step system and the set of measures devised in Hampshire, England that include the Hampshire Assessment for Living with Others (HALO) and the Hampshire Assessment, New Curriculum (HANC). The last two are part of an assessment and programme planning system featuring inter-linking assessment measures designed for various settings including residential, day care and home environments. Their aim is to provide information for the implementation of individual programme plans. One interesting feature of the Hampshire assessments is the involvement of clients in the assessment process by asking them to judge how important a particular skill is for them, whilst care workers are asked to judge how easy it would be for the person to learn a skill. This enables the setting of training priorities by the person responsible for the individual plan.

This type of assessment lends itself to an observational and direct-testing type of data collection. Mention should also be made of an assessment instrument that is purely observational in its method of assessing adaptive behaviour, the Balthazar Scales of Adaptive Behaviour. This is in two parts: the BSAB-1 which looks at self-help skills; and the BSAB-2 which looks at adaptive and maladaptive personal and social behaviour. It is particularly useful in institutional settings where observation is easier to accomplish, and with more severely and profoundly handicapped people. The Behaviour Assessment Battery is another measure that relies totally on direct testing for information on handicapped people. This test battery consists of a number of areas, each of which is subdivided into specific skills. Assessment and teaching are combined in an experimental approach to the discovery of a profoundly handicapped persons' skills and potential. This test is very useful with people who are functioning at very low levels of adaptive behaviour because it covers very basic areas of skill.

There are also a number of scales that focus exclusively on maladaptive behaviour rather like the BSAB-2. These include the Aberrant Behaviour Checklist and the British Behaviour Disturbance Scale. Both measure the extent to which an individual carries out specified maladaptive behaviours, with what severity and frequency, and are of help in providing baseline information prior to treatment programmes, as well as being general measures of behaviour problems. It is more usual, however, to use specific observation techniques when evaluating problem or challenging behaviour. Typically a general measure of maladaptive behaviour might be used to pinpoint the areas causing most concern. These areas would then be explored in detail, probably using natural observation. This might involve various methods of recording, including time-sampling, where a person is observed at a regular interval and occurrence of the problem during that interval noted, or event-sampling, where the behaviour in question is recorded at each occurrence, and the circumstance under which it occurs identified. The chapter in this book that covers challenging and difficult behaviour will consider how this assessment information is used to devise treatment programmes.

Although there are a number of measures of maladaptive behaviour available, there are few that examine the presence and nature of psychiatric symptoms in people with a mental handicap. Senatore, Matson and Kazdin (1985) have devised an experimental scale that assesses psychiatric symptoms called The Psychopathology Inventory for Mentally Retarded Adults (PIMRA). This has two forms, one of which can be given as an interview with the person, the other being a checklist for care staff to complete. The items include ratings of various types of psychiatric symptoms, including psychotic disorders, anxiety-based conditions and generaly personality disorders. It is an experimental tool that should be used with care, given the difficulties attached to describing and defining mental illness in people with a mental handicap. There are also a number of reports in the literature of attempts to devise scales of specific psychiatric conditions, such as depression and anxiety (e.g. Kazdin, Matson and Senatore, 1983), but there remains a dearth of available standard tests for this purpose.

Assessing the person and their environment

Mention was made earlier in this chapter of the recent development of assessment systems that not only evaluate the individual person with a mental handicap, but also the environment in which they function. This is based on the realization of the effects of environmental variables on the behaviour and development of people with mental handicap that has arisen from the background of a behavioural approach to human problems (e.g. Dickens, 1980). In terms of assessment this has often focused on a parallel assessment of the characteristics of living and working environments. The Scale for Assessing Coping Skills (Copewell) Scales) has in it sections that ask the assessor to rate the availability of opportunities to practise skills in their environment. The Chart of Initiative and Independence is based on the assumption that it is not enough just to possess skills, but that the handicapped person must be able to show initiative in using these skills in the correct circumstances, and that the environment within which they exist contains adequate opportunities for them to do so.

Another way in which the role of environment is recognized in assessment is the very recent development of systems that produce what are called 'individual service plans'. In other words this is an individual-based approach that firstly defines what a person's needs are then examines the extent to which their present situation meets these needs, and lastly prescribes services that are necessary for the unmet needs to be satisfied. The best example of such a system is called 'Getting to Know You', and was developed in the USA by Brost and Johnson (1982). This is a completely different type of assessment tool than the others mentioned in this chapter, as it stresses the importance of subjective evaluations of an individual as well as objective ones. The system provides a framework and method for constructing a picture of the life and circumstances of a person with mental handicap to enable a service plan for them to be written.

Lastly there are many scales used to evaluate environments themselves, and the service systems within which handicapped people exist. Program Analysis of Service Systems (PASS) is such a device that examines how close a service is to meeting the ideals and principles of the philosophy of normalization. Using PASS a team of raters visits a service and using many techniques including interviews and observation, rates the degree to which the service meets these ideals, and the needs of its clients, on a number of dimensions. The specific subsection that measures adherence to normalization has been developed into a scale in itself, called PASSING (Program Analysis of Service Systems Implementation of Normalization Goals). Other more experimental and research orientated methods for evaluating services and environments include those produced by King, Raynes and Tizard (1971) for their studies of institutional and non-institutional care.

Conclusion

Assessment in the field of mental handicap is a vital topic in both senses of the word. It is vital in the sense that it is an area that is of great importance in any setting where care is provided, in that it serves many functions, some of which have been mentioned above. It is also vital in the sense that it is a live issue, where new developments are providing ever more sophisticated ways of gaining information about people. At the same time the new techniques are being developed within a framework that puts great importance on dignity, confidentiality and the full participation of handicapped people in mapping out their own futures. The emphasis is also shifting to the evaluation of people as part of systems, and the examination of strengths and weaknesses in those systems as being of influence in the development of handicapped people. Part of these environments is the type of care and training provided, and the development of the combined assessment and treatment package is an attempt to ensure that the assessment of a person with a mental handicap leads directly to a beneficial outcome for them.

References

AAMD (American Association on Mental Retardation) (1961) *Manual on Terminology and Classification in Mental Retardation*, 2nd edn. AAMR, Washington

Brost, T. and Johnson, V. (1982) *Getting to Know You*, Wisconsin Coalition for Advocacy, Madison

Browder, D.M. (1987) *Assessment of Individuals with Severe Handicaps*, Paul Brookes Publishing Co, Baltimore

Dickens, P. (1980) A radical behaviourist looks at mental handicap. *Apex*, **8**, 60–61

Dickens, P. (1984) The evaluation of services for mentally handicapped people using PASS. *Journal of Mental Handicap*, **12**, 102–103

Dickens, P. and Stallard, A. (1987) *Assessing Mentally Handicapped People: A Guide for Care Staff*, NFER-Nelson, Windsor

Doll, E.A. (1953) *The Measurement of Social Competence*, American Guidance Service, Circle Pines

Gunzburg, H.C. (1968) *Social Competence and Mental Handicap*, Bailliere Tindall and Cassell, London

Hogg, J. and Raynes, N.V. (1987) *Assessment in Mental Handicap*, Croom Helm, London

Kazdin, A.E., Matson, J.L. and Senatore, V. (1983) The assessment of depression in mentally retarded adults. *American Journal of Psychiatry*, **140**, 1040–1043

King, R.D., Raynes, N.V. and Tizard, J. (1971) *Patterns of Residential Care: Sociological Studies in Institutions for Handicapped Children*, Routledge, London

Matson, J.L. and Breuning, S.E. (1983) *Assessing the Mentally Retarded*, Grune Stratton, London

Mittler, P. (ed.) (1970) *The Psychological Assessment of Mental and Physical Handicaps*, Methuen, London

Senatore, V., Matson, J.L. and Kazdin, A.E. (1985) An inventory to assess the psychopathology of mentally retarded adults. *American Journal of Mental Deficiency*, **89**, 459–466

3

Education and training

3.1 Early intervention

Jennifer Wishart

Being told that your child is mentally handicapped must rate as one of the worst moments in a family's life. In some cases, such as Down's syndrome, the diagnosis can be confidently made at birth. In other cases, the presence of handicap may go unrecognized for some time, unsuspected until it becomes increasingly evident that the child is consistently failing to reach significant milestones in development on time. While some professionals might maintain that an earlier diagnosis makes it easier for parents to come to terms with their child's handicap, in either case parental hopes are inevitably dashed and their plans for the child's – and indeed the family's – future will need re-assessment.

Very few children with handicap are now raised in hospital settings; the vast majority live at home with their parents or with foster parents. The rise in overall levels of ability seen after this change in practice in the sixties led to considerable optimism that even greater improvement might be possible. Given that the move from an institutional to a home setting had in itself been found to be beneficial, it seemed highly plausible that developmental prospects might be further improved by even more careful tailoring of the mentally handicapped child's learning environment to his or her particular needs and skills. Results from psychological and genetic research clearly showed development to be the result of a complex interaction between the environment in which an individual grows up and his or her genetic inheritance. Although any genetic disorder or neurological damage underlying the handicap could not be corrected, it seemed reasonable to argue that it could to some degree be compensated for by supplementing the child's learning experiences and providing added environmental support for attempts at learning. Much of the research on normal developmental processes suggested that if any environmental enrichment programme was to be implemented, then it should start at the earliest possible moment: if the early years were of disproportionate significance in normal learning, it seemed even more likely that these years would be of critical importance to the success or failure of learning in children with mental handicap.

Early intervention programmes were first introduced in the late sixties and their use and popularity has burgeoned in the seventies and eighties. Instead of the previous feelings of isolation and of lack of support services, some parents of young handicapped children now in fact find themselves bewildered by the array of professionals who turn up on their doorstep offering help. A huge variety of early stimulation programmes are now commercially available and these are widely used in many countries. Although parental satisfaction is high, professional opinion is very much divided as to whether early intervention actually *works*, that is, whether it in any way alleviates the mental handicap at which it is directed. Before evaluating the success or non-success of early intervention, however, it might be helpful to describe the content and approach of typical programmes.

Early intervention programmes

Most intervention programmes are based on encouraging and promoting the earlier development of those abilities and skills that normally emerge in the first few years of life, skills which are often considered to be the foundation blocks for all subsequent learning and which are reliably slow to appear in children with mental handicap. Teaching methods generally draw heavily on normal developmental theory and practice, often breaking down the target skill into smaller, more easily achieved steps and then encouraging the child through the use of a variety of activities to combine these sub-stages into the higher level skill. Two typical examples of early intervention programmes will be described here: the Portage Guide to Early Education and the University of Washington's Model Preschool Centre.

The Portage Guide to Early Education

This is a home-based early intervention programme aimed at pre-school children whose development can be expected to be significantly delayed (this includes all categories of at-risk children, not only children with mental handicap). It was validated as a model programme in 1975 by the United States Joint Dissemination and Review Panel and after initial pilot studies, Portage services were also made widely available in the eighties to parents in the UK. The Portage programme is also widely used in other parts of the world (Shearer and Shearer, 1972; Portage, 1985).

In the Portage programme, teaching is mainly carried out by the parent, under the supervision of a 'Home Visitor' (usually a health visitor, speech therapist, psychologist, community nurse or teacher) who visits the child's home at regular intervals, ideally weekly. Home visits start at the earliest possible age. Having ascertained the child's developmental level, the home visitor helps the parents to select from a developmental checklist a small number of new skills to be targeted over the next week; the targeted skills will be close to but just above the child's current developmental status. A number of activity cards suggest ways in which the development of these skills can be promoted during normal, day-to-day activities such as play, feeding or bathtime. Parents are given advice on teaching behaviours and the child's progress is recorded on the developmental checklist. Six areas of development are focused on: response to stimulation, motor skills, cognitive ability, self-help skills, socialization, and language. Development in all areas is closely monitored and goals are set on the basis of each child's own particular progress in each area. The small size of the steps involved and the range of areas covered increase the likelihood that it will be possible to register success on some new developmental step at each visit.

The University of Washington's Model Pre-School Centre

This was first established in the early seventies and has been widely copied as a model for early intervention, both in the USA and around the world (Hayden and Dmitriev, 1975). Its aim was to accelerate and maintain the motor and cognitive skills of young handicapped children, with a view to keeping their developmental progress as close to the developmental norms for non-handicapped children as possible.

The Washington pre-school programme is centre-based with children entering the programme at 18 months and progressing according to age and ability through five levels of classes: Infant Learning, Early Pre-school, Intermediate Pre-school, Advanced Pre-school and Kindergarden. In this intensive early education programme, parents are closely involved with the teachers and with classroom activities and are also encouraged to participate in parent–parent groups. Teaching focuses on five main areas: motor skills, communications skills, social skills, cognitive skills and self-help skills, with training goals drawn from schedules of normal development such as the Gesell Scales and the Denver Developmental Screening Test. Goals are set on the basis of the child's progress and teaching methods are devised on the basis of input both from the parents and from the various multidisciplinary professionals involved with the child at the Centre.

Evaluation of the effectiveness of early intervention programmes

Many of the early intervention programmes now available are being used with a wide variety of children considered to be at risk for developmental delay. In many cases, impressive results have been gained, both in terms of immediate returns and longer-term benefits. In most intervention studies where success has been unequivocal, however, the children involved have not been biologically at risk; they have been identified as at risk because of an inadequate home environment, one unlikely to provide the necessary stimulation to allow satisfactory developmental progress to be made (e.g. children being brought up by parents of very low intelligence, who are drug or alcohol dependent, or who are living in conditions of extreme poverty). In these cases, the intervention programme aims at preventing retardation. This is very different from intervention studies aimed at children with mental handicap. Children in this latter type of programme are not 'at risk' for mental handicap – mental handicap is already present, the only unknown being that of degree. Results from intervention studies with such children are much more mixed. Whereas those who design and implement the programmes claim impressive gains, independent reviewers are more critical of the level of success achieved (Gibson and Harris, 1988).

Improvements in cognitive ability in children in intervention programmes

Some early intervention studies have claimed gains in IQ of up to 30 points. Others have claimed that children who would previously have been expected to fall into the profoundly handicapped category have, with intervention, been able to score instead in the moderate to mild range. In these studies, success has typically been evaluated by the team carrying out the intervention programme. Independent reviewers are quick to point out that in many such programmes, training has concentrated on exactly the sorts of skills that make up tests of early intelligence. It is not surprising, they argue, that such training leads to improvements in IQ/DQ (Developmental Quotient) scores. Although basic self-help skills and fine coordination skills do seem to be responsive to training, critics point out that only small effects have been found on levels of cognitive skills, on language acquisition and on gross motor skills. Little evidence of the generalization of skills and successes to other areas has been found and any advantage gained in early years seems to decline over time until the child is once again performing at the level that would be expected given his or her degree of handicap.

Evaluating effectiveness is not easy. Whose evaluation of programme success are we to accept – that of those running programmes or that of reviewers? What are the criteria for success or failure? Although vast amounts of developmental data have been collected from intervention programmes, the quality of that data has often made it virtually impossible to assess the success of a programme or to compare one programme with another. Children have often entered intervention programmes at different ages, intensity of intervention has differed across children, the division of responsibility for teaching between parent and professional has varied within and between programmes, and the content and methods of individual programmes have often been under revision during the period of intervention.

Evaluation has been further complicated by the fact that very few intervention studies to date have met even the most basic requirements in terms of scientific design. To assess scientifically whether any intervention strategy has been successful, it is essential to compare the developmental progress of the group of children who are taking part in the intervention programme with the progress of a group of children who are not taking part in the programme; this latter group, the control group, has to be matched with the intervention group on any and all relevant factors that might influence developmental outcome.

Few studies have even attempted this, although it must be acknowledged that this is not an easy requirement to meet. Mentally handicapped children are not a homogeneous group of children. In many cases, the aetiology of the handicap is unknown and the nature and extent of the handicap cannot be confidently assessed. As a result, only the most obvious factors, such as current level of functioning, age and family background can be matched with any degree of accuracy. Even then, there can be problems. Although every effort can be made to match important family variables such as parental education and socio-economic background, it is impossible to control for the factor of self-selection: parents who wish to take part in intervention programmes are likely to have different attitudes to their child and to support services from parents who do not wish to participate. When comparing outcome measures obtained from children from these two types of families, any differences found may result from the different home environments being provided rather than from intervention itself.

Very few intervention studies have in fact attempted to make direct use of a matched group of 'untreated', mentally handicapped children. Performance profiles from the children in the intervention study have more usually been compared with normative performance profiles from the literature on development in children with mental handicap. There are two huge problems with this method. The first is that these types of sources usually provide only minimal information about the medical and social histories of the children who provided the developmental data; many of these normative studies, for example, drew their data from hospital populations only, a grouping that is perhaps likely to contain a disproportionate number of the more severely handicapped. More important, however, is that almost all of the databases being used in this way are considerably out of date, having been drawn from studies of the handicapped population carried out in the fifties and sixties.

The past two decades have seen considerable improvements in medical care and general support services for the mentally handicapped and there have been significant changes both in public attitudes to children with handicap and in parental expectations of the level of ability that might be attainable by their handicapped child: irrespective of involvement or non-involvement in formal, structured intervention programmes, the learning environment of the young, handicapped child is considerably more favourable than in earlier decades. It is simply not valid to compare the developmental profiles of children in intervention studies in the eighties with those of handicapped children in the sixties.

Unfortunately, however, we now find ourselves in the scientifically untenable position that it is highly unlikely that any future evaluation studies of early intervention will be able to make use of a 'true' control group of children, a group drawn from exactly the same population as the intervention children but who have not been given any form of intervention. This difficulty stems partly from ethical considerations – the unacceptability of withholding early educational help from any group of children if we believe it to be beneficial. Since it has not been conclusively proved that early intervention *is* beneficial, this is an argument that can – in theory – be overcome. In practice, however, this would not be so easy. Although there is considerable division in scientific ranks over the value of early intervention programmes, the consumers – the parents – are in no doubt and would not countenance their withdrawal. Early intervention programmes – whatever their true worth – are here to stay.

One way round this problem might be to vary the intensity of the intervention, an ethical compromise which draws attention to another problem in evaluating the success of many early intervention programmes. Even within the same intervention programme, the frequency and intensity of intervention has often varied across families, either because of unavoidable circumstances (periods of illness, failure of transport) or because of differences in degree of involvement requested by the target families. Only one study, it would appear, has taken advantage of this naturally occurring variation and incorporated it into its design, using it to evaluate the relative effectiveness of different levels of intervention (Sloper, Glenn and Cunningham, 1986). In this well-controlled study, it *was* found that infants who were trained more intensively on a particular set of tasks succeeded earlier than infants given less training; their gains, however, were relatively slight, short term and proved to be highly specific. This study in fact is fairly representative in outcome of an overall trend in the intervention literature: in general, where more rigorous scientific controls have been applied, evidence of any long-term cognitive benefits has been less convincing than that claimed on the basis of more weakly designed studies in which evaluation has been less stringently carried out. While all of us would wish early intervention to work, the case is far from proven.

Non-cognitive benefits of participation in early intervention programmes

All of the above notwithstanding, it is not being suggested that early intervention is of no value whatsoever to the handicapped child and his or her family. While cognitive gains are of dubious longevity and appear reliably in only certain, fairly circumscribed areas of development, there can be little doubt that the sort of positive feedback on developmental progress that underlies early intervention programmes has to be beneficial – to both child and parent. For the child, the potentially adverse effects of constant experience of failure are to some extent lessened as he or she is coaxed and supported throughout the development of important early skills. For the parent, the commitment of one-to-one professional time must nurture and reinforce the belief that their child's development is worth the effort, that progress *will* be made. By increasing the parents' sensitivity to their own child's particular learning style and by heightening their perception of each step in development being made, parental motivation is kept high and their teaching skills are likely to be considerably enhanced. For many parents, the first months after diagnosis are months of great anguish and often of isolation. Even for experienced parents, there is considerable doubt that they will be able to provide for the needs of their new, handicapped child. Their expectations of what is achievable are often unnecessarily low. The reassurance of an experienced professional that they are indeed doing everything necessary and doing it correctly can relieve at least some of the pressures they must be experiencing at this time.

One of the major benefits of participating in early intervention is undoubtedly that parents are at some point likely either to meet or to be put in touch with other parents who have a child who, although not necessarily of the same age, may have similar problems to those of their own child. Many parents find this form of contact the most beneficial of all. No amount of professional experience can equate with the direct experience of being the parent of a child with a mental handicap and no matter how approachable and sympathetic the professional, another parent is far more likely to be able to help the family to come to terms with their child's handicap.

Early intervention – future directions

Although the balance of evidence suggests that the major aim of ameliorating cognitive deficits is not being met by present methods of early intervention, terminal pessimism is not yet warranted. Research is increasingly providing evidence supporting the view that developmental processes in the handicapped child differ in qualitative as well as quantitative ways from normal developmental processes – that is, that early development in children with mental handicap is not simply a slowed-down version of normal development. Many of today's intervention programmes have simply assumed that theory and practice drawn from research on non-handicapped children can be superimposed onto theory and practice for a handicapped population, with only the rate of learning and the endpoint of development distinguishing the two groups.

If this turns out to be a false assumption, the lack of impact of present methods of early intervention on developmental processes in the handicapped is not surprising. As, however, more detailed research provides us with a better understanding of developmental processes operating in handicap, it will hopefully become easier to identify more accurately the precise processes that are impeding learning, enabling us to develop teaching strategies that can to some degree compensate for these deficiencies. If development in handicapped children *is* indeed different, effective teaching methods are likely to differ fundamentally from those developed to help non-handicapped children to learn.

Conclusions

The fact that an increasing number of young children with mental handicap are being integrated into mainstream schools should not be misinterpreted as evidence of the success of early intervention programmes. Integration has come about through the exercise of parental pressure and through welcome changes in public and political attitudes to the handicapped and a revision of views on their place in society. While little harm can come from being optimistic about the chances of improving developmental outcome in young children with mental handicap, this optimism should be tempered by reality. It must be recognized that in the majority of mentally handicapping conditions, there will inevitably be an upper limit on the facilitative effects that any programme can have. This is especially true where cognitive deficits are genetic in origin or result from neurological damage, whether at birth or in later years.

It *is* possible, however, to supplement the mentally handicapped child's experience in ways that will encourage and promote the maximum gains from whatever level of cognitive functioning is available to that child and which will encourage the child to make full use of his abilities, no matter how limited these might be. In this respect, it should be emphasized that intervention, irrespective of its timing, should not focus too narrowly on promoting the development of cognitive skills – there are many, many other skills which are at least as important if one wishes the person with mental handicap to lead a happy and fulfilling life and to be able to take part in the life – and work – of the community.

To those parents who have not participated in early intervention programmes, whatever the reason, it should be emphasized that their child's developmental prospects have not been irretrievably compromised by this choice. Parents' rights to decide on the best ways of coping with their child's handicap should be respected and no parent should be made to feel guilty that they are depriving their child of the 'proven' benefits of early intervention. While intervention has helped the vast majority of parents through the earliest and possibly most difficult years, some families value privacy more highly; some also find that focusing so intensively on their child's handicap undervalues other attributes of their personality and intrudes unacceptably into normal day-to-day family life. What is important is that any decision, whether to participate or not to participate in early intervention, should be properly informed. It is essential to encourage parents to help their child to develop to his or her full potential, but care must be taken not to instil false hopes that intervention can somehow reverse the effects of the handicap.

References

Gibson, D. and Harris, A. (1988) Aggregated early intervention effects for Down syndrome persons: patterning and longevity of benefits. *Journal of Mental Deficiency Research*, **32**, 1–17

Hayden, A.H. and Dmitriev, V. (1975) The multidisciplinary preschool program for Down's syndrome children at the University of Washington Model preschool center. In *Exceptional Infant: Vol 3. Assessment and Intervention* (eds B.Z. Friedlander, G.M. Sterritt and G.E. Kirk), Brunel/Mazel, New York

Shearer, M.S and Shearer, D.E. (1972) The Portage Project: A model for early childhood education. *Exceptional Children*, **36**, 210–217

Sloper, P., Glenn, S.M. and Cunningham, C.C. (1986) The effect of intensity of training on sensorimotor development in infants with Down's syndrome. *Journal of Mental Deficiency Research*, **30**, 149–162

3.2 The school years

Gilbert Mackay

Introduction

All developed societies have education systems for helping children and young adults to learn. People with difficulties offer a challenge to these systems, and few offer a greater challenge than those who have difficulty learning. As a result, the educational systems of many countries have been expanded in an attempt to make provision for pupils and students with learning difficulties.

The most influential event in the recent history of special education in Great Britain was the publication of the Warnock Committee's report, *Special Educational Needs*, in 1978 (Committee of Enquiry, 1978). This marked the critical change in the official philosophy of the state system of special schools from having an emphasis on pupils' disabilities to an emphasis on their special educational *needs*. This section takes examples from the educational systems of Great Britain, in particular that of Scotland, to describe the provision of schooling for children who have marked learning difficulties, and to consider some of the changes that have taken place in this provision in recent years.

In particular, the section will consider the major groups of pupils with learning difficulties and the provision that is made for them. It will then outline the system that is used in Scotland to record that pupils have special educational needs. Finally, some brief comments will be made on current developments in educational provision.

The pupils

Background

The Education (Scotland) Act 1981 removed the need for official labels for pupils' disabilities. Yet, for the purposes of this section, it is still quite useful to recall the three levels of pupils with marked learning disabilities for whom a place has been made in the Scottish educational system.

In 1906, an act of parliament gave local authorities the power to provide special schooling for pupils who were 'not merely dull and backward', but who were 'not imbecile'. Today, the group of pupils covered by the 1906 Act would be described as pupils with 'moderate learning difficulties'. Those classified in 1906 by the dreadful label 'imbecile' were eventually provided with 'training', as opposed to 'education', during the years 1947–74. They too receive 'education' now, and are described as pupils with 'severe learning difficulties'. Pupils whose difficulties were so great that no provision for them was made in 1906 or 1947 are now often described as having 'profound', or 'severe and complex', learning difficulties. Their right to education was assured by the Education (Mentally Handicapped Children) (Scotland) Act 1974, implemented in 1975.

In some areas it is possible to find local authority day-schools specializing in educational provision for each of the three groups of pupils. In others, there are greater or lesser degrees of integration of pupils with learning difficulties, especially those with moderate learning difficulties, within mainstream education. There are also many examples of pupils with severe and profound difficulties being taught in the same schools. For the purposes of this chapter, however, the three groups will be considered separately, with an outline of the educational provision that is presently made for each in Scotland.

Pupils with moderate learning difficulties

This group is very difficult to define by any easy measurement. Traditionally, they were considered to be in the IQ range 50–70, the mainstream population being in the range 70–140 and beyond. However, this numerical definition is not satisfactory. For instance, it assumes that pupils with IQs of more than 70 may not have moderate learning difficulties, that pupils of 50–70 will have difficulty with school subjects, and that IQ tests contain useful and reliable material for classifying children's levels of difficulty with learning.

None of these assumptions can be accepted confidently. In the past, many children who were failing at school were transferred to special education on account of behaviour which disrupted teachers and pupils in mainstream classes, and on account of difficulties with learning which were as likely to have resulted from social disadvantage or a poor curriculum as from innate personal disabilities (Galloway and Goodwin, 1987). Yet in the same group of pupils with moderate difficulties, there are also pupils whose difficulties are caused by some clinical syndrome, genetic abnormality or central nervous dysfunction.

Despite the problems of describing the population accurately, and despite some moves to integrate them within mainstream education, these pupils remain the largest single group receiving special education in Great Britain. In many respects, a special school for pupils with moderate difficulties seems similar to a mainstream school. Like mainstream primary pupils, for example, pupils with moderate learning difficulties follow a curriculum which includes the main subject areas of communication, environmental studies, expressive arts and problem solving. However, the pupils will need more time to make progress than their age peers in mainstream education, and some will always have difficulty with literacy and mathematics. Some secondary schools for pupils with moderate learning difficulties provide courses that lead to presentation in open examinations, such as Standard Grade, which are taken by pupils in mainstream schools. Others teach short, 'modular' courses which lead to credits from the council which oversees the work of further education colleges.

Not all pupils are able to undertake coursework which leads to examinations or examinable project work, but all can receive an education that enables them to cope more confidently and successfully with the demands of living as independent adults in the community. For this reason, many schools have established 'leavers' units' for their oldest pupils. These units are referred to again in Section 3.3.

Pupils with severe learning difficulties

Traditionally, pupils with severe learning difficulties have IQs in the range 30–50, though the same reservations about the use of IQs as a useful measure of functioning apply to this group as applied to those with moderate learning difficulties. However, the learning difficulties of this group are certainly much more evident. In most cases, the pupil's difficulty with learning can be associated with some congenital condition, or with damage to the central nervous system.

In passing, it should be said that the existence of a syndrome or CNS damage is not, of itself, a reliable indicator of the level of a person's ability or disability in learning. The example of Down's syndrome illustrates this point well. Most children with Down's syndrome have severe difficulty learning, but some have moderate difficulty only, and a few have attainments within the range of pupils in mainstream schools (Cunningham, 1982).

Pupils with severe learning difficulties have problems understanding the complexities of language, and understanding concepts and problems that pupils in mainstream schools are expected to take in their stride. Many will also be less adept in the expressive arts and in skilful movement, though parents and teachers should recognize that performance in activities like these may be weak because we may expect too little of the pupils, or give them few opportunities of challenges in which they may experience success as well as failure.

The educational provision in schools for pupils with severe difficulties will often appear markedly different from that in mainstream schools or in schools for pupils with moderate difficulties. Yet, underlying their curriculum may still be detected some of the aims of a typical curriculum for pupils in mainstream schools. Thus pupils with severe learning difficulties should be expected to develop knowledge, skills, the ability to relate to other people successfully, and a fulfilling expression and growth of their own personality.

Some pupils with severe learning difficulties do learn to read, write and use basic mathematics. However, many do not, and the staff of their schools would not see the acquisition of literacy and numeracy as matters of high priority for the majority of pupils. For them, the aims of education stated in the Warnock Report seem more important: to increase knowledge, and to encourage development of independence and self-sufficiency. For this reason, the curriculum for pupils with severe learning difficulties often places an emphasis on the development of communication, social and self-help skills, practical problem-solving and leisure pursuits.

Young pupils will often take part in communicative and perceptual training activities that are similar to the activities of the pre-reading and pre-mathematics syllabus of mainstream primary schools. But as they get older, the community outside the walls of the school will be used much more as a learning resource as it is the location in which knowledge, skills and attitudes learned in school will eventually be put into practice. In the later stages, pupils in some schools are now being given experience of the world of work and commerce through 'mini-enterprise' schemes in which they may produce and market items such as garden furniture and moulded plastic goods.

Pupils with 'profound', or 'complex', learning difficulties

Pupils in this category were considered to have IQs below 30. This numerical classification is satisfactory as a means of noting that they have the most severe learning difficulties of all, but it does little else: the range of pupils covered by the category, and the regional variations in the way that the label is interpreted, make the identification of this group as difficult as that of any other. If there is a common factor among them, it is that there is not usually much difficulty in identifying a clinical problem that is the cause of their difficulties.

Generally speaking, a child will be considered to have profound difficulties if his or her disabilities fall into one, or both, of two categories. The first category is severe developmental delay: the pupil's ability to solve problems and communicate is years lower than his or her age. One helpful way of setting the difficulties in context is to think of a child who has reached school-entry age still functioning at the level of child in the first year of life. Children with profound difficulties are likely to understand and produce little or no speech, and problems with mobility, vision and hearing are also common (Browning, 1983). The children with the greatest degrees of developmental delay often seem to spend much of their lives asleep.

The second group of pupils who are often described as having profound difficulties are those who have a marked developmental delay and also have behaviour that is under poor control. This type of difficulty is most noticeable in the case of children who act violently and unpredictably, often causing injury to other people and to themselves. However, there is another extreme of behavioural difficulty, namely an 'isolation syndrome', or difficulty in forming relationships, which compounds the problems of severe developmental delays by making the pupil less responsive to the approaches of other people, and to stimuli from his or her surroundings. Sometimes, the developmental level of this group of pupils may be well above the one-year level, but their behavioural difficulties are so severe that the overall effect is as disabling as a greater degree of developmental lag.

The last complication of the use of 'profound' or 'complex' category is that it is interpreted differently in different areas. Thus children who attend schools or classes for pupils with profound difficulties in one part of the country might be considered to have severe difficulties only, if they lived in another. This helps to show the problems that are inherent in any set of classifying labels. More positively, the apparent confusion may be evidence of a breaking down of barriers between categories and part of a movement to create educational settings in which a variety of needs may be met, or in which specialist provision may be located. An example of such specialist provision is that there is an increasing group of schools that provide experiences based on the Hungarian system of 'conductive teaching' (MacKay, 1990), to improve children's functioning in the routines of daily living.

The curriculum for pupils with profound difficulties is determined by the nature and degree of severity of these difficulties. Those with the most severe developmental delays may hardly be aware of their surroundings. Therefore, to increase their awareness, they will have many activities in the form of stimulation of their senses of vision, hearing, movement, taste and smell. Children whose difficulties are less profound will take part in activities that are similar to those for pupils with severe learning difficulties, namely activities aimed at helping them to communicate, to form relationships with other people, to make decisions, to improve their levels of self-help in areas such as feeding, toileting, dressing and grooming, and to find leisure activities.

Recording needs

The degree of severity of a child's difficulty with learning is usually determined formally by a process known as 'recording' in Scotland, and as 'statementing' in England and Wales. This process involves the assessment of the child by a professional team of at least a psychologist and a medical officer. The team will include a teacher if the child is already at school, and may include other professionals, such as social workers, speech therapists or physiotherapists, if they are already working with the child. It is common for the team to meet to discuss their findings and their opinions about the most appropriate educational provision for the child. Sometimes parents take part in these meetings. Even if they do not, parents are expected to express their views about their child's needs on one of the parts of the Record (or Statement) of Needs which is produced by the process of assessment.

When this process is complete, an education officer draws up a final Record of Needs which will take account of the views of the multi-professional team, but which need not adhere to the team's opinions. For example, the team may have recommended the provision of some educational or other service which the education officer, ultimately, does not agree to include in the formal Record. Parents are provided with a copy of their child's Record, and they have certain rights of appeal concerning its content. However, these rights do not extend to appealing for provision which is not cited on the Record. More important, perhaps, parents have no right of appeal if provision which is recommended on the Record is not actually provided by their local education department or other agency.

In addition to an assessment of the child's needs and the statement of how to respond to them, the Record includes the identity of the Named Person, an unpaid adviser to parents. It is clear in the Warnock Report that this role was envisaged as a type of citizen-advocacy, though in law, the duties of the Named Person are quite obscure. Perhaps this was inevitable as, ultimately, the Named Person is a nominee of the education department and not someone chosen by the parents. At the moment, the history of the emergence of the Named Person is a sorry saga, with a future that may now be problematical in view of a clause in the Disabled Persons (Services, Consultation and Representation) Act 1986 which entitles parents not to have a Named Person if that is their wish.

Like the concept of the Named Person, many other aspects of British special education have roots in the USA. However, one important difference between the British and United States systems is that an annual review, re-programming and setting of objectives, is compulsory under the law of the United States (Public Law 94–142) for every pupil who would fall within the 'recorded' or 'statemented' categories. There is no legal compulsion for this annual review in the United Kingdom, though many schools do carry this out voluntarily, and perhaps more effectively than they might in a compulsory system. However, parents do have the right to request an annual review of their child's Record of Needs if, for example, they are not satisfied with its contents or if they feel that it does not reflect progress that their child has made.

The only compulsory review of a Record of Needs is the 'future needs assessment' which is carried out during a pupil's last 2 years at school. The procedure is similar to that used at Recording, but its purpose is to take stock of what pupils have achieved during the school years, so that the time remaining at school may be used as satisfactorily as possible to prepare them for life after school.

It should also help to ensure continuity between the work of the school and the services of adult agencies, such as adult training centres and further education colleges which are considered in greater detail in Section 3.3.

Finally, it should be noted that, although unusual, it is not necessary for a pupil to have a Record of Needs in order to be admitted to a special school or class. Similarly, it is possible to find many pupils with Records of Needs in the classes of mainstream schools. In this respect, recording is quite different from the previous practice of 'ascertainment' which, in effect, was a means of transferring pupils from mainstream to special education.

Developments in special education

In the 1960s and 1970s, perhaps the main influences on developments in the teaching of pupils with severe and profound learning difficulties were the objectives approach and behaviour modification. At the end of the 1980s, however, it became clear that the education of all children in Great Britain, including those with learning difficulties, was being shaped powerfully by approaches that have their roots in the new technologies. One of these approaches, namely, the mini-enterprise, has been mentioned already in this chapter. It can be a useful method of coordinating a number of educational experiences for older pupils through the business technology of creating and marketing products and services.

However, the technology that has affected the education of a wider group of pupils is the micro-computer. There is a multitude of programs for assisting pupils with learning difficulties in areas such as mathematics, problem-solving, perception and communication. Of course, many pupils with learning difficulties cannot use a standard keyboard, especially if their difficulties are profound. However, they still can have access to the computer through the use of special switches. For instance, children who can reach out to touch the computer's screen can make the visual display change, and even those with great physical difficulties may still be able to interact with the computer if they have sufficient mobility to activate a mercury gravity-switch attached to one of their arms or legs, or a pressure pad laid within their range of movement.

Developments in the philosophy of services for people who are disabled are also exercising an important influence on special education. In particular, reference should be made to the philosophy of normalization (Wolfensberger, 1972), which aims to improve the quality of services by ensuring respect for clients' dignity, by taking account of their ages, and by helping them to become integrated within the normal routines of the community. Often, integration seems to be the most difficult of these three principles to meet in the area of education. However, there are examples of movement towards integrated educational provision. Some pupils attend mainstream schools part-time for school-certificate work, or for the use of resource areas such as those in technical, physical and home economics education. Also, some mainstream pupils visit special schools regularly for the experience of knowing people with disabilities, and for the practical tasks of constructing special apparatus or of learning how to care for those who need a lot of personal attention.

It is sometimes said that we should be less concerned about whether education is 'integrated', 'segregated' or 'special', and more concerned about whether or not it is 'appropriate'. There is fundamental truth in this statement, but it may be used too easily to shore up the existing special and mainstream systems. Those who believe that pupils with recorded special needs have a right to be integrated in mainstream education are likely to be disappointed by recent research which shows that advances of this type are still quite patchy in Scotland (Thomson, 1990). Probably there would be little problem about integration if we did not have an established special education system in Great Britain, for then it might be straightforward to make provision for all pupils, including those with the most severe disabilities, in the mainstream schools. But we do have a system. This system grew up as a response to the needs of pupils, and many of its schools continue to meet pupils' needs well. Paradoxically, the system is being questioned as our understanding of the concept 'needs' develops.

References

Browning, M. (1983) *Identifying and Meeting the Needs of Profoundly Mentally Handicapped Children* (Project Report), Jordanhill College, Glasgow

Committee of Enquiry (1978) *Special Educational Needs (the Warnock Report)*, HMSO, London

Cottam, P. and Sutton, A. (1986) *Conductive Education*, Croom Helm, London

Cunningham, C.C. (1982) *Down's Syndrome*, Souvenir, London

Dyer, S. and Thomson, G.O.B. (1988) *Legislating for Partnership with Parents– an Effective Strategy?* (Interim Report 3, Children with Special Needs: Policy and Provision), Department of Education, University of Edinburgh

Galloway, D. and Goodwin, C. (1987) *The Education of Disturbing Children*, Longman, London

MacKay, G.F. (1990) *Moving on Conductive Teaching*, Jordan Hill College, Glasgow

Thomson, G.O.B. (1990) The placement of pupils recorded as having special educational needs: an analysis of Scottish data, 1986–88. *Oxford Review of Education*, **16(1)**, 159–177

Wolfensberger, W. (1972) *Normalisation*, National Institute on Mental Retardation, Toronto

3.3 Adult education

Gilbert Mackay

Introduction

This section reviews three types of educational provision which are open to Scottish young people with learning difficulties when they reach school-leaving age. These types of provision are: (1) continued attendance at school, (2) attendance at a college of further education and (3) attendance at an adult training centre. The discussion aims to draw attention to some general issues about adult education which are applicable beyond the narrow limits of the country in which the provision is set.

No reference will be made to educational provision which is made by nurses, occupational therapists and teachers in hospitals for adults with severe and profound learning difficulties. Hospital provision is sometimes quite similar to provision made in adult training centres. In others, its aim is to enable people to leave hospital permanently and live in the community, and thus it resembles the provision that is made in the community and housing projects which are mentioned at the end of the chapter.

Education beyond 16 years at school

The school-leaving age for all pupils was raised from 15 to 16 years in 1972. Before that, however, pupils who had moderate learning difficulties and attended special schools already had to remain at school until they were 16. Not many seemed to see the extra year as a privilege, judging by the stream of 15-year-old pupils who used to apply for 'de-ascertainment' from special education, so that they might transfer to their local secondary school, and leave it at the same time as everyone else. An additional benefit of de-ascertainment was that the school named on a pupil's leaving record would be a mainstream school rather than a special school, a matter that might have restricted job opportunities in the eyes of unenlightened employers.

Nowadays, attitudes towards continued attendance at school have changed. Young people with learning difficulties will often remain at school until they are 18, and some may still be found in school at the age of 20 and beyond. Undoubtedly, continued attendance at school will often be the result of lack of suitable adult provision. However, continued attendance has also been seen by many schools as an opportunity for building new courses for the needs of young adults.

Two schools, one in Central Region and one in Strathclyde, have been opened for young people of 14 years and above who have severe learning difficulties. Many other schools have created 'leavers' units' for those who are 16 and above. Such units are sometimes sited in different parts of the school from those used by younger pupils, and a different ambience is created by the provision of furnishings and decoration which are more informal than those of ordinary classrooms. However, such changes can be cosmetic only, unless the experiences offered to the pupils are worthwhile. For this reason, leavers' units are aimed clearly at increasing the self-reliance of pupils in the world outside school.

For some pupils, especially those with moderate learning difficulties, opportunities are created for taking nationally accredited courses. Some of these courses are in areas of personal independence, such as cookery and home-management, while others are related to skills that are useful in employment. Even if no formal courses are studied, the practical orientation of education in leavers' units is usually very clear, and indeed much use is made of out-of-school experiences as a source of learning. For example, one leavers' unit disperses its students, individually, for part of each week to approximately 20 shops, factories and other work-places, so that they may have experience of the routines of employment, and may acquire skills and interests which may increase their chances of finding work in the open market.

Mention should also be made of TVEI, the Training, Vocational and Educational Initiative, which aims to increase pupils' and students' knowledge of new technologies, and the part that these play in learning, work and life in the community. The ideas of TVEI have begun to influence the types of experience offered in leavers' units in a variety of ways. These include the use of computers, introduction to manufacturing technology, and the setting up of 'mini-enterprises' in which pupils have experience of creating and marketing products. In the case of the last example, schools recognize the dangers of sacrificing the educational aspects of the experience for the sake of meeting production targets. At the same time they are aware of the possibilities the mini-enterprise offers for enhancing the self-esteem of young people, by showing them that they need not see themselves as a dependent group, because they can produce goods and services that other people wish to have.

Finally, the leavers' units may also help to build the maturity of their pupils by providing social experiences which give them confidence to be away from home and thus see themselves less as children and more as adults. Some schools provide opportunities like this early in pupils' careers by taking them to residential schools in term time. With older pupils, however, there are now many examples of school groups having holidays abroad.

Further education

The education committees of local authorities in Scotland, like those in the rest of Great Britain, make provision for adult learners through a system of further education (FE) colleges. These colleges provide qualifications in commercial, industrial and technical subjects, and many also cover subjects that are taught in schools. However, a number of colleges have departments, or courses, for students with special educational needs. Who, then, attend these colleges, and what are they taught?

The students

The students who attend FE special needs departments will usually have attended a special school in their earlier years. The recommendations that they should attend further education college will often be made at the assessment of 'future needs' which takes place in their last 2 years of school education. In fact, it would be expected that informal links between the school and the further education college would have encouraged the college to make contacts with its future students while they were still at school. In addition, through schemes such as TVEI, mentioned earlier, it would be common for many older pupils to have links with their local FE colleges before they left school.

The students themselves represent most of the wide range of people with learning difficulties. Some have moderate learning difficulties, and therefore may enter further education with abilities that are very similar to those of some entrants from mainstream schools. For them, there may be the chance of integration into classes outside the special needs departments. Other students will have severe learning difficulties. Provision for them in colleges of further education has been established more recently than it is for those with moderate learning difficulties, and may still not be available, even in colleges that have special needs departments.

People with profound learning difficulties do not attend FE colleges. However, some will receive attention from FE lecturers if they attend adult training centres in which an 'outreach' lecturer from an FE college is based. Recently, there has also been a proposal that an FE model of training, with teaching aimed towards clear learning outcomes, is the way in which people with profound disabilities may benefit most from their attendance at adult training centres (Seed, 1988).

The courses

Generally, the course that a student attends in an FE college will be determined by the degree of his or her learning difficulty. Some people with moderate learning difficulties will attend mainstream college classes because skills that they have acquired on their way through school enable them to be integrated satisfactorily with students from mainstream schools. However, the principal provision for pupils with moderate learning difficulties, and even more so for pupils with severe difficulties, is that of special courses (SCOTVEC, 1988).

The types of special course available differ throughout Scotland. Generally, a course will last from 1 to 3 years. Generally, also, the aims of these courses are the same as the Warnock Committee's aims for school pupils: increasing knowledge, experience and understanding, and participation in the life of one's community. The colleges attempt to achieve these aims through courses that promote:

1. *Skills of self-reliance* – To enable students to attend to their bodily needs, personal appearance, health, their ability to travel, their ability to care for other people, and so on.
2. *Social skills* – To enable students to have satisfactory and appropriate relationships with other people in a variety of everyday settings such as shops, public offices, recreational facilities and casual encounters with strangers, and in making and maintaining friendships.
3. *Basic education* – Thus continuing work that was begun in school in literacy, numeracy, environmental studies and so on, or indeed to give students the chance of a fresh start in these areas.

4. *Work practices* – Including physical skills such as the ability to handle materials, use implements, utensils and other tools, and the development of awareness of the importance of punctuality and regularity.
5. *Leisure skills* – So that students may be able to make full use of the resources in their own communities, and may also become aware of a wider range of interests, and thus have the chance of discovering pursuits which will continue to interest them after they have left the course.

The activities that have been described above seem, superficially, to concentrate on helping students to acquire knowledge and skills. However, all of them intend students to undergo a development of attitude that will make them see personal independence as something that is desirable. This may be a difficult attitude to foster if a young person has been conditioned from childhood to see himself or herself as dependent on parents and other adults in authority.

Some courses are heavily timetabled so that students have a clear sequence of classes to follow in the course of the week. This experience may, to a visitor, seem very like a school. Others have classes in the special needs departments, but also spend part of their week with lecturers from mainstream courses in other departments of the college. One of the problems that should be recognized with this latter type of course is that it assumes that lecturers in the mainstream departments have an understanding of the difficulties which students have learning, and a commitment to adapting their course-work accordingly. This problem is just one aspect of the more general issue of supporting learning in FE colleges. For example, Dumbleton (1989) suggests that all FE lecturers have a need to have a much greater understanding of the difficulties that any of their students, and not just those with marked learning difficulties, may present. He recommends that there is a case for the colleges adopting the same approach that operates in the schools (SED, 1978), namely, that there should be a college-wide policy to support the learning of all students who may be having difficulty. This policy could be made to work by in-service training to raise the awareness of all lecturers to the issues, and by using special needs lecturers in roles of consultation, team-teaching and so on, to support their colleagues in making courses as accessible as possible to all students.

It is worth remembering that a number of students encounter experiences like those of FE colleges by moving to 'leavers' units' in their schools between the ages of 16 and 19. This raises important issues. If the provision is similar, should not the FE colleges be providing something different if pupils from leavers' units transfer there? Or, if pupils in general are entitled to leave school at 16, would it not be more age-appropriate if pupils of special schools were given the same right? This issue is not easy to resolve, for there is no FE provision in some areas, especially the rural ones. In addition, the school staff of some leavers' units would argue that the intimacy of their units enables them to provide a more supervised and intense level of training than is possible in the impersonal surroundings of a large college.

Adult training centres (ATCs)

It is important to begin this section by saying that ATCs are not 'educational establishments', strictly speaking, for they come under the control of local authority social work departments. However, they have a place in this section because the service they provide is often clearly educational. In particular, there are three aspects of ATC provision which seem worth considering here.

First, some FE lecturers spend part, or all, of their time working in ATCs. Second, the nature of the provision that is made in ATCs, and other comparable services, can often be understood in educational terms. Third, developments which have been proposed recently for the service of ATCs seem to be particularly appropriate to the educational needs of adult learners.

It should also be said here that ATCs are intended primarily for people with severe and profound learning difficulties. People with moderate difficulties have attended ATCs, certainly, but this is likely to have resulted from the absence of more suitable provision for them.

Educational staff in ATCs

Throughout Scotland, a number of lecturers from special needs departments in FE colleges spend most, or all, of their week working in ATCs. Some years ago, it was common to find that these 'outreach' lecturers spent much of their time teaching elementary reading and number to their students in the centres. For lack of appropriate materials, and perhaps for lack of imagination too, the books and other materials they used were sometimes the same as those in infant classrooms for 5–7 year olds.

The teaching of elementary school subjects still has a place for adults who are motivated and sufficiently able to acquire these skills. There can be no objection to helping them to become literate, or even just to be able to read and write a selection of useful words. Moreover, it is fair to assume that an FE lecturer who has been trained to teach elementary subjects will be able to do this more efficiently than someone who has not been trained. However, there cannot now be many lecturers who see the teaching of literacy and arithmetic as their principal task. Instead, their skills are more likely to be used in teaching the wide range of social and self-help skills mentioned in the next section, and in helping their social work colleagues to design courses for clients.

Course content

The main aim of adult training centres is to enable their clients to become as self-reliant as possible. To achieve this, the staff of the centres follow programmes of activities which are similar to those in leavers' units in schools. Thus instruction is provided in the areas of home-care, preparation of food, grooming, travel, shopping, finding agreeable leisure pursuits, and so on.

Staff in centres have been helped to find direction in their work by using checklists which rate the attainments of their clients in areas such as self-help, communication and so on. One of the earliest of these scales, which is still in use, is the PAC scheme (Progress Assessment Charts) (Gunzburg, 1969), but there are several others. For example, there is the Copewell Battery, based on a manual of fostering independence in adults with learning difficulties (Whelan and Speake, 1979), and *Pathways to Independence* which uses a series of developmental ladders to rate people's attainments across a range of skills which are related to independence (Jeffree and Cheseldine, 1982).

A number of centres are facing up to the challenge of providing sex education, either directly, or as part of a programme in developing and maintaining relationships. Consideration of this topic is bound to create controversy in any culture with a variety of religious traditions, and in which the rights of people with handicaps are seen in terms of stereotypes which often seem to be based on eugenics or simple prejudice.

Less controversially, a growing number of centres are building up resources in electronic technology. They have been assisted in this by the development of a '16+' section within SEND (the Special Educational Needs Database), a national (British) resource located in Glasgow, and accessed through the Campus 2000 network (formerly, Prestel). There are also examples of ATC clients undertaking light manufacturing, catering and other work, either at their centre, or elsewhere in the community.

Future directions?

In a recent review of ATCs in Scotland, Seed (1988) has proposed that current provision should be delivered in terms of three 'models'. These are:

1. The 'work resource centre', in which the ethos is that of a workplace or training workshop, but which also takes clients' home circumstances and needs into account.
2. The 'further education resource centre' model, which has close links with FE colleges, and which is seen primarily as a resource for teaching clients skills and developing their personal and social competence.
3. The 'community resource' model, which uses the community as a source of opportunities for enabling clients to reach out beyond their families, and participate in the routines of daily living as citizens in their local area.

Seed considers that there should be a place for all three types of centre in large conurbations. However, even in areas where this is not possible, he recommends that social work departments should be aware of the three types of emphasis, and make a place for all of them in the services provided by a single centre. The reason for the differentiation of types of provision is that every adult with learning difficulties does not have the same set of post-16 needs, and the needs of any adult may change with the passage of time. For example, Seed sees the FE model of provision having a particularly useful role for school leavers (Seed, 1988, p. 281), but that part-time attendance on a community resource, or work resource, programme might be more appropriate for older adults.

Part-time attendance is a feature of provision in some ATCS already. It is one significant step away from the tradition that ATCs were places that adults with learning difficulties attended for life. For most of us, training is something with definite starting points and end-points, and situations in which the content of training is then tried out. Attendance at an establishment from the ages of 16 to 65 may be appropriate for people who need constant care. Those who do not require care should not have restricted opportunities for participating as full members of their communities.

One exciting outcome of breaking down stereotyped views of people with learning difficulties is that ventures such as the Pathway employment scheme are showing how open employment is possible if individuals are supported, and if the help of management and co-workers is enlisted carefully.

Coda

It is not just the statutory educational and social work services that make provision that is deliberately, or incidentally, educatioinal. For example, voluntary organizations, such as the Scottish Society for the Mentally Handicapped, have created day provision and residential provision. There are also special programmes which use the experience of being a member of a community group, or living in a housing project, as a means of learning self-help activities such as shopping, preparing food, home maintenance and independent travel. The staff of these programmes are also concerned with enhancing social and personal skills in areas such as sexual development, personal responsibilities and things as mundane as living peaceably with other people. Both social work departments and various non-statutory organizations, such as Key Housing, Barnardo's and the churches, provide facilities of this type.

Perhaps it is not too mischievous to end the section with a note of concern that it is possible to have too much education!

Imagine a person with a severe learning difficulty who spends the working day between attendance at both an ATC and some classes at an FE college, then returns home, through an independent travel programme, to a special housing project in which the business of training in self-help and social skills is carried on until it is time to go to bed. If one of the aims of education is preparation for life, when does life begin?

References

Dumbleton, P. (1989) How FE can meet today's challenge, *Times Educational Supplement Scotland*. 17 February 1989, p. 2.

Gunzburg, H. (1969) *The P-A-C Manual*, National Association for Mental Health, London

Jeffree, D.M. and Cheseldine, S. (1982) *Pathways to Independence*, University of London Press, London

SCOTVEC (Scottish Vocational Education Council) (1988) *The National Certificate: Students with Special Needs – a Guide for Teachers and Lecturers*. SCOTVEC, Glasgow

SED (Scottish Education Department) (1978) *The Education of Pupils with Learning Difficulties in Primary and Secondary Schools in Scotland*, HMSO, Edinburgh

Seed, P. (1988) *Day Care at the Cross-Roads*, Costello, Tunbridge Wells

Whelan, E. and Speake, B. (1979) *Learning to Cope*, Souvenir Press, London

4

Teaching new skills

William R. Lindsay and Amanda M. Michie

Many of the methods used to train self-help skills, social skills, leisure skills and work skills are common to all areas. Therefore, before detailing specific applications of work in these areas, this chapter will outline the general methods of training. The methods include didactic teaching, roleplay methods, modelling, sequencing skills, cognitive methods, practice and various behavioural techniques.

Didactic teaching

A skills training programme will often include sections where the therapist teaches the clients about social skills, community skills, work skills, etc. Included in this teaching will be the important components of the abilities or tasks in question and the ways in which they are integrated to enable a more complex performance. The reason for this is that while many community skills and social skills are used by us all in all sorts of everyday situations, it is highly unusual to analyse one's skills in a reflexive way. Most of us are unaware of how we use and organize our abilities, e.g. at work. Therefore when training such skills to people with deficits it is a useful technique to first explain what the skills are. Work skills, leisure skills and other community living skills would be split up according to the sequences of behaviour which constitute competent execution of the ability (see later).

In many ways teaching about the skills is information that is important for the background of a training course in skills training. It is certainly essential for the therapist to have a firm knowledge (for example) of the various social abilities and the way in which they are coordinated to produce complex social interactions. However, the information contained in the teaching sections of the programme are obviously fairly complex and at first, a knowledge of (for example) gaze direction can actually interfere with the natural and automatic nature of social interaction. This complexity of information creates a problem when dealing with people with a mental handicap. Many individuals who have a mental handicap have difficulty in grasping more complex conceptual ideas and need more time to fully comprehend material. With normal adolescents or out-patients this teaching would take three or four sessions. Even with people who have a mild mental handicap it would take a great deal of time to convey the full meaning of all aspects of social skill.

In addition to this many of our clients have difficulties with concentration and attention span so understanding this material becomes even more problematic.

Teaching about the nature of social skill with mentally handicapped people may be annoying and boring to them. Much more than 5 or 10 minutes on the nature of skilled interaction has produced a fidgeting and inattentive group. Therefore, with all but the most able clients it is better to drop formal didactic teaching from the programme. With some thought, material can be incorporated into roleplays, modelling and other aspects of group work. With people with a mental handicap it is easier to understand question asking in the context of a conversation or asking someone out, than it is to understand it in a more abstract way during a teaching session. It is easier to grasp tone and loudness of voice when saying 'no' to strangers, than it is in a teaching session. Therefore while it is essential for the therapist to have a working knowledge of the information which one would teach during a training programme, to include this material in a formal way with a group of mentally handicapped people, may in fact interfere with training.

Roleplay

Roleplay is an essential method when teaching community living skills or social skills to people with a mental handicap. The methods of roleplay have been used for many years in psychotherapy going under various titles from psychodrama (Moreno, 1946) to behaviour rehearsal (Friedman, 1972). The essential aspect of the method is that it allows the group or individual to practise the various skills concerned before going into the real setting. Therefore, the therapist should arrange for as many characteristics from the real setting to be available during the roleplay. In this way clients can learn how to respond to the important aspects of the situatioan before they are actually faced with it. They can learn how to interact at a disco or in a café without having to risk the embarrassment of practising in that setting. Roleplays can be one small aspect of a behavioural or skills sequence or it can include the whole sequence.

The main feature of roleplaying is that it includes the important stimuli from the real setting, but remains under therapist control. Both of these aspects are essential for a roleplay to be effective. If the roleplayed setting does not include the main features of the real setting then it will not be therapeutic. One example of this comes from a study in which pedestrian skills were taught to four subjects with a severe mental handicap (Michie *et al*, 1990). In some of the initial attempts to teach pedestrian skills, these authors tried to organize roleplay settings within the hospital grounds. However, although there were some fairly realistic stimuli – roads, pedestrian crossings, a small amount of real traffic, etc. – it was found that the essential aspect of crossing a road was absent. Crossing roads is a dangerous activity and clients must learn to cope with the danger. You can be seriously injured or killed when crossing a road and this is one of the most important aspects of pedestrian situations. If this aspect is absent then it was found by the authors that the roleplay setting was unrealistic. Therefore, in order to include the important stimuli from the real setting it was necessary to go on to actual roads, quiet roads and busy roads, to ensure that the essential aspect from the real setting were included in the roleplaying setting.

One might then argue that this was not a roleplay setting, it was in fact the real setting. However, this is not the case because of the second requirement mentioned above. The roleplay setting is under therapist control. To continue with this example: when individuals are crossing roads in real life they do not have a guardian on hand to stop them if they are going into a dangerous situation. For the study conducted by Michie, Lindsay, Baty and Smith (1990) the therapist was present to teach skills and to ensure safety during all the training sessions which were held on actual roads. Therefore, they were in fact roleplays, they were not 'real life' road-crossing situations.

If a particular piece of roleplayed behaviour does not go very well it can be done again and again until both therapist and client are happy that the whole sequence is satisfactory. Alternatively, a small piece of the sequence which the client finds particularly difficult can be extracted and practised on its own until the client is happy to try it again in the context of the whole interaction. A further advantage of roleplaying is that failure is relatively less important than it would be in the real situation. Where the client is having difficulty with a certain skill it can be roleplayed in several different ways until the client is more successful. Anxiety provoking aspects of an interpersonal situation can be introduced slowly, as the therapist judges. Roleplaying is such an important method that a short illustrative case example is presented below.

The present authors have conducted a long series of clinical trials on community living skills and social skills, most of the therapy sessions were videotaped. Therefore a record exists of every roleplay attempt with individuals during a treatment session. The following example is of a group which was learning the appropriate skills for interrupting a conversation. In this case a nervous man (Tom) was interrupting a conversation between two women so that he could ask one of the women out. The important first step was how to interrupt the conversation without being rude and how to speak at the appropriate time. This part of the group began with others who were more skilled, showing the rest of the group how they would go about the interruption. Over the course of an hour Tom made six roleplayed attempts at interrupting the conversation. Each time he was rated by an independent assessor on a scale of 0–6. For example, a score of 1 on an item indicates that Tom was very poor at that skill, while a score of 5 would indicate that he had good skills.

Between each roleplay the group discussed how Tom had done. On a couple of occasions another group member modelled the skill again. Once he had successfully interrupted the group, Tom found it impossible to join the conversation. Instead he would rub his hands together nervously and look away from the group. Therefore we paid particular attention to the moments after he had broken

Table 4.1 Roleplay of interrupting conversation

Skills rated						Roleplays
	1	2	3	4	5	6
General presentation	1	1	2	1	3	3
Appropriate gesturing	1	1	1	1	1	1
Confidence of interruption	1	1	2	1	3	4
Effectiveness of interruption	1	1	2	2	3	4
Acceptance of others in group	1	1	2	2	4	4
Ability of joining in conversation	1	0	1	1	3	4
Gaze direction	1	0	1	0	3	3
Voice clarity	–	1	2	2	3	4
Pace of speech	–	2	3	3	3	3
Overall skill	1	1	2	2	3	4

into the group and had a chance to join the conversation. Table 4.1 shows Tom's development through the roleplays. From a very poor baseline the skills increased until by the sixth roleplay he was managing to interrupt and talk to the girls quite successfully. One area that did not reach the level of his other skills was appropriate use of gestures (rubbing his hands together). We were able to stop inappropriate gesturing but were not able to replace it with more appropriate use of gesturing. It can be seen that in this way roleplaying is a flexible technique which will develop a person's skills as the session progresses.

Modelling

The essential aspect of modelling is that a series of complex skills can be demonstrated without going into confusing and tedious explanations of how the skill is sequenced together. Therefore it is particularly useful with people with a mental handicap who may have difficulty following explanations about social interaction as was indicated in the section on didactic teaching. It is a technique that can be used in a variety of different ways during a treatment session. With groups of clients with a mental handicap, perhaps the best way to organize modelling is for one member of the group, who is more competent at a particular skill, to show the rest how he would approach a situation. Alternatively, if no member of the group is at all skilful then a resident from the hostel, ward or resource/training centre who is a friend could model the sequence of skill.

The therapist can also model aspects of behaviour and this is especially useful where it is appropriate to show the group how not to do something. It can be difficult, even threatening, for group members to model inappropriate behaviour and it is often safer for the therapist to do it. For example, if the group is dealing with the importance of gaze direction then the therapist can demonstrate talking to someone while looking at the floor. Alternatively he or she can engage in continuous, close eye contact, while talking. When demonstrating problems in voice volume the therapist can whisper or shout while conversing. Such exaggerations of interpersonal problems can underline the importance of appropriate skills and, if used correctly, can introduce a great deal of humour into the group.

One method of modelling which has been used extensively with other populations is the use of pre-recorded videotapes demonstrating various aspects of interpersonal skill. The authors have found that with people with a mental handicap this is probably less effective, since it is not immediately relevant to the situation that is being rehearsed at the time.

Roleplaying and modelling go together in most group sessions. Normally a group member or therapist would model some part of a social exchange and the group would be able to discuss it. The group members could then roleplay this skill and decide to what extent they are achieving the skill of the model.

Cognitive techniques

This will be dealt with in more detail in Chapter 13. However, it is worthwhile noting in this chapter that there has recently been an upsurge of interest in treatments for psychological problems which are caused by or exacerbated by negative cognitions and thinking.

Perhaps because of the intellectual handicaps of the clients involved there has been a relative neglect of mentally handicapped populations in this literature. This is true despite the fact that those working with people with a mental handicap recognize that very often problems will arise because of these very difficulties in confidence and self-perception rather than lack of ability in the situation. So a man who is able to ask for a drink in a pub may never do so because he is afraid what others might think or is anxious that he will fail and look ridiculous in a public place. A woman who is being forced to go out with someone who has asked her is reluctant to tell him 'no' because she is worried that he might become angry and she is afraid of his disapproval. In this way thoughts about the demands of the various situations and about oneself can undermine the ability of the person with a mental handicap to interact effectively in the community or work setting. These arguments will be outlined in more detail in Chapter 13.

Sequencing

In all community living situations the first thing that has to be done is to break the skill or ability into its component parts. This is extremely important and enables training to be done in smaller, more understandable sections. In this way complex skills can be broken into simple trainable units. The following example highlights the method in relation to an essential community living skill.

Using the bus – This might first be split into fairly large sequences:

1. Leaving the house and walking to the bus stop.
2. Waiting for the bus.
3. Recognizing and stopping the bus.
4. Getting on the bus.
5. Paying.
6. Finding a seat.
7. Recognizing where to get off.
8. Standing up and pressing the bell.
9. Waiting for the doors to open.
10. Getting off.

This sequence might be too detailed for some clients and might not be detailed enough for others. For example, 'getting on the bus' may have to be further broken down into:

1. Waiting until the bus stops.
2. Waiting for the doors to open.
3. Understanding that the doors will not close on you until you are on the bus.
4. Climbing the stairs.
5. Walking to the pay point.

In this way it may be necessary for some clients to use a more detailed series of skills for individual sections of the whole ability.

It is also used in assessment of skills in that we can assess the ability of the individual at each stage in the sequence of the skill. This is doubly important since it may be that the person is only having difficulty in one small section of the skill and therefore there is no need to train the whole sequence. In the previous example, if someone is only having difficulty in paying once on the bus, then the treatment programme should focus on only this section, rather than training the whole ability.

Practice

Practice is included here as a separate method for training because it refers to the repetition of certain aspects in the sequence in a far more intensive way than routine roleplay. Here the therapist would take one particular skill and extract it from the whole sequence of skills. We can then develop exercises for improving the ability almost in isolation of the whole sequence to be taught. One example from Baty, Michie and Lindsay (1989) is an eye contact game included in a training programme to develop skills for using a cafeteria. Here it was found that eye contact was a particularly difficult skill to maintain when the clients were giving the assistant their order.

A game was therefore developed which involved the use of eye contact. The group leader would hold the picture of an item up at her face and the client would have to look at her face and say what the item was. The person who got the item right while looking into the therapist's face got the picture. The person who had the greatest number of items at the end won the game. This simple game proved to be enjoyable for the clients in the group and increased eye contact considerably. Similarly, Michie et al. (1990), on teaching pedestrian skills, developed practice exercises for specific items in the sequence such as walking and looking simultaneously, because certain individuals found it difficult to cross roads and look for traffic at the same time. In this practice sequence the client has to walk and look from side to side at the same time. Other aspects that have required practice are walking on a moving bus. This has been particularly necessary when some group members have become anxious when the bus starts to move and they have not yet found their seat. We would simply require the client to walk up and down the bus while it is moving so that they get used to the various physical sensations of walking on a moving vehicle. Therefore, intense practice of certain aspects of the sequence can be used to help clients gain mastery of that particular element of behaviour.

Behavioural techniques

Although several of the training methods already mentioned would be considered behavioural techniques, there are further techniques that are not used with all clients but are appropriate on certain occasions.

Prompting

Prompting is an extremely useful technique especially at the early stages of training. In a two-person social interaction one client may find it difficult to look at the other person while talking. In this case it is perfectly reasonable to stand beside the person and give them a soft verbal prompt 'look at his face' while he is talking. In this way clients have an immediate instruction to develop a particular social skill in coordination with the other skills which they are using. In extreme cases it has been necessary to lift the client's face so that they are looking into the face of the other person in order to prompt gaze direction. One of the most common prompts is telling the person what to say in a given situation. Therefore if someone is taking something back to a shop because it is faulty, it is perfectly acceptable to prompt the client in what to say during the training sessions. Therefore, if a client is unable to think what to say themselves, the therapist might suggest, 'why don't you say "these biscuits are soft" or "these biscuits are mouldy"?'

Physical prompts can also be used in the early stages of training. For example, in training pedestrian skills clients may be completely unsure about whether it is reasonable to cross a road. In this case physical prompts might be used to start the client off crossing the road. Physical prompts might also be used to guide a client in work skills when they are reluctant to begin because of lack of confidence in their own ability.

Where physical prompts are being used it is important to establish that the subject does not mind being touched. Several individuals object to being touched at first and it is necessary for the therapist to lead slowly into physical prompting so that the client does not become too upset or too anxious.

Fading

An essential consideration when employing prompting is to build in to the training session the fading of prompts. Clearly it is most unhelpful if the client becomes dependent on the therapist's prompts. It is not possible for a therapist to follow a client round town prompting work or leisure abilities. Therefore, as soon as prompts are employed the therapist should have a plan to begin fading the prompts. Prompts should be faded as soon as possible.

As has been mentioned, some subjects object to physical prompting, and if it is felt that such a technique is necessary the prompts may have to be faded into training as well as being faded out of training.

Shaping

Shaping is commonly used in training in that subjects rarely achieve an adequate level of ability on their first attempt. Therefore any approximations towards a reasonable level of skill will be encouraged by the therapist. In this way the therapist is shaping the subject's response through no ability, to poor abilities, to moderate or adequate abilities and even on to good skills. It is important to accept any initial attempt towards gaining the skill and encourage clients' subsequent attempts at improvement.

Shaping is also used as a direct training technique. Here the therapist will establish one response and gradually shape the response increasingly towards the desired response. One example seen later is by Simpson and Meaney (1979) in training the ability to ski. They started with short skis and when trainees became more comfortable with these, they then shaped them by inches towards normal length skis.

Chaining

Chaining is a method that is limited to the sequences of skills. Once the sequence has been established it is useful to train the ability at one or other end of the chain. Then the next step in the sequence will be trained and linked in to the previous one, and so on until the whole complex ability has been learned. When training begins with the first aspect in the sequence this is called 'forward chaining', when it begins with the last it is 'backward chaining'. It is felt that backward chaining is more generally useful since the final aspect is always present and successful completion can always be reinforced.

Reinforcement

In some of the projects that have developed on social skills or leisure skills, one of the methods has been tangible reinforcement. In these studies clients have been reinforced with token, sweets or other reinforcers for the successful accomplishment of certain aspects of social or community living skill. On the other hand, often trainers have used no tangible reinforcement contingent on the successful completion of any particular section or sequence of skills. In these cases many of the skills that are taught, and which shall be reviewed in this chapter are intrinsically reinforcing. Therefore, clients look forward to the training sessions. Perhaps the main point to be made here is that while groups designed to train skills can be a powerful technique in adapting to community life, they are also good fun.

In addition to intrinsic reinforcement in the groups, social reinforcement is a major component of the methods. When clients make attempts to develop new skills or begin to gain confidence in their abilities, then the therapists are genuinely delighted and encouraged to show their delight to the clients. Where possible, social reinforcement should be used to develop and maintain clients' abilities in various skill areas. It is very difficult to teach therapists in the formal use of social reinforcement but individuals should be encouraged to use their natural humour and sensitivity to help clients gain confidence and skill in each situation.

Problems in skills training

Generalization and maintenance

The problems of generalization and maintenance have dogged skills training since its inception. Skills learned in one situation are not readily used in another situation. So someone who is taught to interact in one setting may not use these skills in another area of their life. Also, once the training programme stops there is a tendency for the newly learned skills to fall into disuse and be poorly maintained. While the issues have been well documented over the years the problems remain with us. Therefore when developing any programme of skills training it is essential to plan how the abilities will generalize to the target situations in the client's life and how they will be maintained by the client after the training programme has finished.

One of the simplest methods to ensure generalization to target situations is to do the training in the target situation. In this way the stimuli and events in the environment will gain control over the person's responses. The individual will learn how to cope with the target surroundings, and, in the end, the only difference between the training situation and the target situation is that the teacher/therapist is absent in the latter. For example, if the individual is learning how to cope with a supermarket it will be best to do the training in the local supermarket so that the requirements of this situation will maintain the person's skills. The main drawback of this approach is that it is not always possible to train a group of people in their local situation because of the demands this may make in time and travel.

A less time-consuming approach is to use similar stimuli in the training and target (generalization) situations. The person will learn to respond to the salient stimuli in the situation irrespective of where they are. Baty, Michie and Lindsay (1989) taught cafeteria skills in a therapy room on a ward which then generalized to the real setting. Here, the salient stimuli from the real setting were incorporated into training.

Another strategy to promote generalization is training across several exemplars. A number of authors have written that by teaching in several related situations rather than a single situation, generalization is enhanced. In one example by Michie *et al.* (1990) pedestrian training was done on several quiet and busy roads and skills generalized to new roads. Stokes, Baer and Jackson (1974) used two therapists to train greeting responses which then generalized to all adults in the unit.

A further approach is to train self-control techniques so that the individual is able to use self-statements, self-monitoring, etc., in various situations. Storey and Gaylord-Ross (1987) have used self-monitoring techniques to maintain behaviour after the experimental manipulations have ceased. Meichenbaum (1977) encourages the use of self-instructional training to help generalize learned coping strategies beyond the immediate teaching situation.

The authors cited above have set out in more detail these strategies for promoting generalization and maintenance of newly learned skills.

Social validation

An important concern for those of us who do skills training is the extent to which skills being taught fall within the range of ability shown by people who do not have a mental handicap. This is particularly true for social interaction but is also relevant to other aspects of training leisure and work skills. Bellack (1979) wrote that 'the identification of appropriate target behaviours is probably the most critical task facing workers in the area of social skills' and Trower (1980) stressed the need for 'a body of scientifically validated knowledge of normal social behaviour to provide training targets and assessment criteria'. Lindsay (1982) compared conversation skills of a group of manual workers and three groups of psychiatric patients before and after social skills training. He found that although patients' social behaviour generally moved towards the level of ability displayed by the manual workers, there remained significant differences after treatment with the patients' falling outside normal ranges. In one case the training programme made the patients' ability even more discrepant from the norms than before. Therefore valuable insights into the effect of treatment can be made from a social validation comparison. Van Hauten (1979) gives an example of a programme that was designed to bring about a simple increase in a classroom ability (question asking). This resulted in the child asking far too many questions and so the child's ability remained well outside normal limits.

As people with a mental handicap are encouraged to live normal lives in the community so the need for normative goals for training and rehabilitation becomes paramount. Kazdin and Matson (1981) wrote that there are several main aspects to social validation. One is that the focus of intervention or skills to be taught should generally be considered important for helping the subject cope with everyday life. Therefore they will have to be valid in terms of the living skills needed by normal people who do not have a handicap. Another is that the outcome of treatment should be similarly judged as to how it helps the client to cope with everyday living and the extent to which it approximates the functioning of non-handicapped peers. There are two basic ways of conducting a social validation exercise – subjective evaluation and social comparison.

Subjective evaluation involves using specially qualified judges to rate aspects of competent and incompetent performance as a means of providing appropriate target behaviours and assessing change. Therefore, policemen have been used to identify important skills and to judge the appropriateness of youth/police interactions (Werner et al., 1975), and socially competent individuals have been used to select socially important behaviours and to assess social performance (Wildman, Wildman and Kelly, 1986).

In the method of social comparison, subjects' performance is compared with the behaviour of peers who are considered competent in the skills being treated. Observation of competent individuals can provide specific behavioural targets for training and can also establish a normative range of behaviour to assess the effectiveness of treatments. The methods have been used to compare childrens' problem behaviours after treatment with their non-deviant peers (Patterson, 1974) to compare the problematic eating behaviour of adults with a mental handicap with employees eating habits (Azrin and Armstrong, 1973) and to assess the social behaviour of clients with co-workers in an industrial setting (Chadsey-Rusch et al., 1989).

Social validation is an essential consideration in any skills training programme and studies below will give examples of socially validated outcomes after training.

Training social skills

Several case studies have now shown the feasibility of training social skills in people with a mental handicap. Using a multiple baseline strategy Bornstein et al. (1980) trained several social skills using the methods of modelling, roleplay, instructions, feedback and social reinforcement. They also found that the gains in skills maintained to a 1-month follow-up assessment. Other aspects such as assertion and cooperation skills have been successfully trained by several researchers. Bradlyn et al. (1983) trained five adolescents with a mental handicap in conversation skills using instruction, modelling, roleplay and social reinforcement. They trained the skills of using conversational questions, making self-disclosing statements and making reinforcing and interested comments to others. Improvements in ability were seen in unstructured and extended conversations between subjects and also towards unfamiliar non-handicapped partners. The improvements maintained to a 5-month follow-up assessment. Downing (1987) trained conversational skills with three adolescents with moderate to severe mental handicap. She found substantial increases in initiation of conversation and ability to cue others to continue the conversation. However, these improvements did not generalize to new non-mentally handicapped adults. This type of study indicates that despite the methods recommended to promote generalization of skills to new situations, the problems remain with us.

Group comparison studies suggest that gains produced by social skills training are consistent and effective when compared with alternative group therapies and no treatment controls (Bates, 1980; Foxx, McMorrow and Schloss, 1983; Matson and Senatore, 1981).

More recent studies have addressed the question of generalization, maintenance and social validation of improvements made after social skills training.

Wildman, Wildman and Kelly (1986) used social skills training with seven adults with a mild or a moderate mental handicap who were living in community settings. They concentrated on the conversation skills of asking questions, giving compliments and disclosing information about themselves and made assessments of subjects talking to familiar and unfamiliar non-retarded peers. They found substantial improvements in all subjects after training and these improvements maintained to 1-month, 3-months and 6-month follow-up. Community volunteers also rated the assessment tapes to ascertain the extent to which changes were socially valid. They judged that subjects had made positive adaptive changes in their social interaction.

Storey and Gaylord-Ross (1987) reported three studies with groups of adolescents with mixed mental handicaps in a work training setting. They used a social skills training package to increase positive verbal statements while playing a game during breaktime. They then withdrew several aspects of the treatment package and found that contingent social reinforcement and self-monitoring were sufficient to maintain improvements at a substantial level for up to 8 weeks. They also found that the post-treatment levels of social interaction shown by the subjects were no different from levels shown by groups of non-handicapped peers. Thus validating treatment improvements using the method of social comparison. There was, however, little generalization of improved social abilities to other leisure activities. Matson and Senatore (1981) also found that improvements in social skills maintained a 3 month follow-up assessment following a social skills training programme.

It seems that the methods of modelling, roleplay, instruction, teaching and social reinforcement can be used to train social skills in the short term and in the long term. Some studies have linked changes in social behaviour to naturally occurring events in the environment while others have trained within a social context or embedded social skills in a larger sequence of community integration skills. By using these approaches, various authors have found social skills to maintain for 3, 6, 12 and even 24 months. Improvements in skill have generalized to new individuals and have been shown to be socially appropriate and valid.

Leisure activities

Much of the work to teach people with a mental handicap leisure skills has been done on domestic activities such as playing with toys and other home-based pursuits.

Wehman, Karan and Rettie (1976) compared skills training methods with a condition in which toys were simply available. They found large increases in the use of the toys and a lower incidence of stereotyped mannerisms when the methods of skills training were used to train play. Other researchers have found similar results when investigating methods of increasing play with toys in people with a mental handicap in that active training procedures produce improvements when compared with simple availability of toys procedures. Conditions that include all active procedures tend to be most successful (Wehman, 1978).

While there have been many studies in increasing play skills there are fewer studies on more complex community based recreational pursuits. As an example of leisure facilities which are used frequently in the community several authors have investigated the use of cafés and cafeterias for people with a mental handicap. Van den Pol et al. (1981) taught restaurant skills in a fast food establishment using 'classroom based' instruction. They used roleplay, modelling and coaching methods to teach the skills involved in eating out. After training, subjects' performance in the restaurant improved markedly. Baty, Michie and Lindsay (1989) used a similar procedure to train three women with a severe mental handicap to use cafeterias. The skills of using a café were first broken down into smaller sequences. The subjects were assessed and taught on how to collect a tray; move along the serving counter looking at items on display; make their choice; give the order to the assistant; pay for the items; move from the serving point to the table carrying the tray; make a request to join someone at a table if the cafeteria was busy; take the items off the tray; return the tray and sit down.

All assessments were done in the real setting, while training was carried out in the establishment where the subjects lived and the methods of roleplay, modelling, prompting, shaping and verbal feedback were used. They also used specific practice sessions aimed at the behavioural deficits of poor gaze direction and the ability to carry a full tray. For all subjects their ability to use a cafeteria improved after training. The most salient skills of using a cafeteria were trained and generalization was assessed in a particularly busy city centre cafeteria in which subjects had to be fairly able and adaptable with their new skills. This setting also had a completely different system of use to the one that was used for baseline and post-training assessments. Nevertheless, most of the subjects' abilities generalized to the new setting, indicating that skills gained during training were being used in a durable and flexible fashion. Therefore, there seems a growing body of evidence that the leisure skills of using a cafeteria or fast-food restaurant can be trained effectively in people with a mental handicap.

In one interesting study, Simpson and Meaney (1979) taught skiing skills to 20 adolescents with a moderate or mild mental handicap. They used the graduated length method of snow ski instructioan over 5 weeks. This involved teaching the subjects to use very small skis and slowly increasing the length until they were able to ski on normal size skis. Therefore, one of the essential aspects of instruction is to establish an appropriate response on a small ski and shape the subject's ability closer and closer to the desired response through increasing the length of the skis. They reported considerable improvements in self-concept of subjects and anecdotal improvements in skiing ability of all subjects.

Other authors have investigated the use of physical training and leisure on people with a mental handicap. In general, people who live in institutions (as do many individuals with a mental handicap) are in poorer physical condition than people in the normal population and as such it may be all the more important to make use of local facilities for physical recreation.

Tomporowski and Ellis (1985) assess the effects of a 7-month health-related fitness programme which included jogging, callisthenic and mat exercises, circuit training using motorized treadmills, rowing machines, stationary bicycles and weight-training equipment. This was a large-scale study employing 86 subjects with moderate to profound mental handicap. The programme significantly improved physical fitness and cardiovascular efficiency of subjects but there were no improvements in cognitive or adaptive ability.

It seems that people with a mental handicap show significant improvements in physical fitness, endurance, strength and cardiovascular efficiency after a prolonged period of fitness training. It remains to be seen whether clients will maintain their use of physical recreation facilities when the programme is withdrawn.

However, these studies have not addressed some of the essential issues in using recreational facilities. While they have shown that people with a mental handicap will respond to exercises and will generalize and maintain skills, some of the most important skills in the use of physical recreation and indeed any recreational facility have not been investigated. Organizing your time to allow for recreational pursuits; arriving at a facility at an appropriate time (e.g. if you have booked a session or avoiding times when the facility may be closed); planning to book or organize a recreation session; getting there either on foot or using public transport; paying at the kiosk or desk; perhaps taking responsibility for a locker, etc., are all essential skills necessary prior to the use of the recreational facility itself. It would seem essential to teach all these other skills while investigating the effects of any training programme.

Maintenance of leisure skills

The issue of maintenance of skills has been addressed on several occasions during this chapter and the maintenance of leisure skills is of no less importance than in the other areas already mentioned. Several authors have shown that by approaching the area in ways already outlined, e.g. training across several exemplars, training to a target situation, reducing the difference between the training situation and the generalization situations where skills may ultimately be used, training essential aspects of the situation, skills can be maintained in new settings after treatment.

Lindsay *et al.* (1991) have shown the continued use of library facilities at assessments 3 months and 1 year after the cessation of a short training programme. A group of adults with a mild and moderate mental handicap was given 3 hours training in a local library on how to use the library, the systems of checking books in and out, who to ask for help, how to look for a book section in which you are interested, how to browse through the section to find a book you like and other relevant skills for using the library. Before training began only two of the group of 18 subjects was able to use the library, and after training everyone could use the library. A control group showed no such increase in skill. The authors made two points in relation to this particular leisure activity.

Because the books have to be taken back every 3 weeks to avoid a fine, the library system has an excellent inbuilt maintenance procedure. Every 2 or 3 weeks subjects had to return to the library to renew or return their books. While they were there they always got another book out, thus continuing to foster the maintenance of skills.

A second point was that although very few of the subjects could read well, they undoubtedly enjoyed going to the library, picking a book, taking it home and looking through it at home. It seemed to have a very positive effect on self-image that subjects were able to engage in a responsible community leisure activity.

Conclusion

It is now recognized that full use of free time and leisure activities are essential for the successful integration into the community of people with a mental handicap. In order that individuals are able to do this several issues have to be addressed. The leisure facilities have to be available to the person with a mental handicap. In general this is no longer a problem and clients usually have ready access to any of the leisure facilities available to the general public. Once available, they have to be able to use the facilities and we have seen that through the methods of teaching, roleplay, modelling, prompting, fading and verbal feedback/reinforcement, several leisure skills have been taught to people with a mental handicap. There remains, however, a shortage of studies in which clients are encouraged to use general community facilities, such as libraries or sports centres, rather than to improve personal play or interaction skills. It is also important that once established, these skills are maintained following the cessation of the training programme.

For many people without mental handicap in the community, use of leisure is a planned regular activity, e.g. weekly dancing sessions, keep-fit classes, playing weekly football matches, going to regular sports events, regular visits to the library, etc. Therefore use of leisure time becomes almost a habit and in this way leisure is planned into the routine of the week. It appears that no work has been done on how the person with a mental handicap might plan their time so that leisure pursuits can be fitted around other activities in the week.

General conclusions

This chapter has reviewed the method of skills training in relation to leisure, social skills and general community living skills. Over a wide range of abilities and settings it is clear that by using modelling, roleplay and other methods, clients can be taught to increase their skill and function in these various settings.

The problem of generalization and maintenance of skill remains an issue to be dealt with and we have reviewed several methods designed to help clients continue to use abilities in a range of previously untried settings. It is also important to consider the social validity of abilities which have been trained to ensure that they are useful in the target settings.

Social interaction is a basic skill which cuts across all situations. Good interpersonal skills are necessary in various community living settings such as shops, cafés, etc. They are also necessary in settings designed for leisure and in other areas. Therefore good social skills are a primary goal for various interpersonal settings and a secondary goal for work, recreation etc. Because of this it would seem essential that clients have access to social skills training programmes to ensure that they can rely on a sound set of basic social abilities in various living settings.

As individuals move into the community there is an increasing need for programmes helping them to use community facilities. Therefore, it is increasingly important for services to organize a wide range of skills training programmes. The methods of training are effective across various settings and there are excellent guidelines on the issues of generalization, maintenance and social validation.

References

Azrin, N.H. and Armstrong, P.M. (1973) The mini meal – a method for teaching eating skills to the profoundly retarded. *Mental Retardation*, **11**, 9–13

Azrin, N.H., Flores, T. and Caplen, S.J. (1975) Job finding club: a group assisted programme for obtaining employment. *Behaviour Research and Therapy*, **13**, 17–27

Bates, P. (1980) The effectiveness of interpersonal skills training on the social skill acquisition of moderately and mildly retarded adults. *Journal of Applied Behaviour Analysis*, **13**, 237–238

Baty, F.J., Michie, A.M. and Lindsay, W.R. (1989). Teaching mentally handicapped adults how to use a cafeteria. *Journal of Mental Deficiency Research*, **33**, 137–148

Beck, A.T., Laude, R. and Bohnert, M. (1974) Ideational components of anxiety neurosis. *Archives of General Psychiatry*, **31**, 319–325

Bellack, A.S. (1979) Behavioural assessment of social skills. In *Research and Practice in Social Skills Training* (eds A.S. Bellack and M. Hersen), Plenum Press, New York

Bornstein T., Back, P., McFall, M., Friman, P. and Lyons, P. (1980) Application of a social skills training programme in the modification of interpersonal deficits among retarded adults: A clinical replication. *Journal of Applied Behavioural Analysis*, **13**, 171–176

Bradlyn, A., Himadi, W., Crimmins, D., Christoff, K., Graves, K. and Kelly, J. (1983) Conversation skills training for retarded adolescents. *Behaviour Therapy*, **14**, 314–324

Chadsey-Rusch, J., Gonzalaz, P., Tines, J. and Johnson, J. (1989) Social ecology of the work-place: contextual variables affecting social interactions of employees with or without mental retardation. *American Journal of Mental Retardation*, **94**, 141–151

Crouch, K.P., Rusch, F.R. and Carlan, G.P. (1984) Competitive employment: utilising this correspondence training paradigm to enhance productivity. *Education and Training of the Mentally Retarded*, **19**, 268–275

Downing, J. (1987) Conversational Skills Training: Teaching adolescents with mental retardation to be verbally assertive. *Mental Retardation*, **25**, 147–155

Foxx, R., McMorrow, M. and Schloss, C. (1983) Stacking the deck: teaching social skills to retarded adults with a modified table game. *Journal of Applied Behaviour Analysis*, **16**, 157–170

Friedman, P.H. (1972) The effects of modelling, roleplaying and participation on behaviour change. *Progress in Personality Research*, **5**, 42–80

Greenspan, S. and Schoultz, B. (1981) Why mentally retarded adults lose their jobs: social competence as a factor in work adjustment. *Applied Research in Mental Retardation*, **2**, 23–38

Kazdin, A.E. and Matson, J.L. (1981) Social validation in mental retardation. *Applied Research in Mental Retardation*, **2**, 39–53.

Lindsay, W.R. (1982) Some normative goals for conversation training. *Behavioural Psychotherapy*, **10**, 253–272

Lindsay, W.R. Michie, A.M. Stewart, J. and Smith, A.H.W. (1991) Learning how to use a library: Training generalisation and maintenance of abilities. (In press)

Matson, J. and Senatore, V. (1981) A comparison of traditional psychotherapy and social skills training for improving interpersonal functioning of mentally retarded adults. *Behaviour Therapy*, **12**, 369–382

Meichenbaum, D. (1977) *Cognitive Behavioural Modification: an Integrative Approach*. Plenum Press, New York

Michie, A.M., Lindsay, W.R., Baty, F.J. and Smith, A.H.W. (1990) Teaching pedestrian skills to adults with a severe mental handicap. *Mental Handicap*, **18**, 74–77

Moreno, J. (1946) *Psychodrama*, Vol. I. Beacon House, New York

Patterson, G.R. (1974) Interventions for boys with conduct problems: multiple settings, treatments and criteria. *Journal of Consulting and Clinical Psychology*, **42**, 471–481

Simpson, H.M. and Meaney, C. (1979) Effects of learning to ski on the self-concept of mentally retarded children. *American Journal of Mental Deficiency*, **84**, 25–29

Stokes, T., Baer, D. and Jackson, R. (1974) Programming the generalisation of a greeting response in 4 retarded children. *Journal of Applied Behaviour Analysis*, **7**, 599–610

Storey, K. and Gaylord-Ross, R. (1987) Increasing positive social interactions by handicapped individuals during a recreational activity using a multi-component treatment package. *Research and Developmental Disabilities*, **8**, 627–649

Tomporowski, P. and Ellis, N. (1985) The effects of exercise on the health, intelligence and adaptive behaviour of institutionalised severely and profoundly mentally retarded adults: a systematic replication. *Applied Research in Mental Retardation*, **6**, 465–474

Trower, P. (1980) Situational analysis of the components and processes of behaviour of socially skilled and unskilled patients. *Journal of Consulting and Clinical Psychology*, **48**, 327–339

Van den Pol, R., Iwata, B., Ivancic, M., Page, T., Neef, N. and Whitley, F. (1981) Teaching the handicapped to eat in public places: acquisition, generalisation and maintenance of restaurant skills. *Journal of Applied Behaviour Analysis*, **14**, 61–69

Van Hauten, R. (1979) Social validation: the evolution of standards of competency for target behaviour. *Journal of Applied Behaviour Analysis*, **12**, 581–591

Wehman, P. (1978) Leisure skill programming for severely and profoundly handicapped persons: state of the art. *British Journal of Social and Clinical Psychology*, **17**, 343–353

Wehman, P., Karan, O. and Rettie, C. (1976) Developing independent play in three severely retarded women. *Psychological Reports*, **39**, 995–998

Werner, J.S., Minkin, M., Minkin, B., Fixsen, D., Phillips, E. and Wolf, M. (1975) Intervention package: an analysis to prepare juvenile delinquents for encounters with police officers. *Criminal Justice and Behaviour*, **2**, 55–83

Wildman, B.G., Wildman, H.E. and Kelly, W.J. (1986) Group conversational skills training and social validation with mentally retarded adults. *Applied Research in Mental Retardation*, **7**, 433–458

5

Individual programme planning

Sandra Guinea

Introduction

Traditionally, many people with a mental handicap, particularly those living in institutions, were regarded as passive recipients of care, and looked upon in terms of what they were unable to do, or labelled according to their perceived problems.

However, a positive shift in emphasis has developed from principles of normalization and the promotion of care in the community. Individual Programme Planning has developed from the movement to recognize that each person with a mental handicap is unique, and should receive assistance and support according to his or her individual needs, regardless of the type or severity of handicap.

It is recognized that people with a mental handicap will develop at differing rates, and that the direction of individual development can be influenced by systematic training. Planning for such training should always be individualized, based on the specific strengths and needs of the person. Therefore, it should not be a case of fitting the person to the programme, but rather designing the programme with, and on behalf of, the person.

People with a mental handicap may require assistance in making informed choices and decisions in their lives, and may need specialist help from a variety of service providers in order to effect some positive change and increase their quality of life.

No doubt everyone working in this field has attended meetings and case conferences (usually in the absence of the person in question) to learn of duplication of work and shortfall in service delivery, so that particular goals are left unaddressed. Because of this deficit in communication, it is desirable to develop a coordinated approach to planning whereby key people can meet regularly for shared discussion and decision making. The Individual Programme Planning system can act as a regulated forum to promote such aims.

Key elements of the IPP process

An Individual Programme Plan (IPP) is a written plan of action containing practical and realistic goals and the strategies for achieving these relating to different areas of an individual's life. IPP meetings are held regularly where key people discuss and agree the means to build on or improve the strengths of the individual and to meet identified needs. Recording of such information is an integral part of the IPP system, and a written plan is drafted at the meeting which identifies the goals to

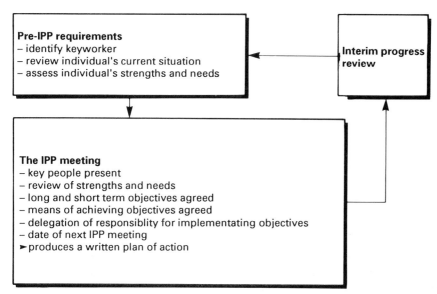

Figure 5.1 The IPP process

be achieved before the next meeting, the methods of achieving them, and the key people responsible for helping the individual reach these goals. The IPP format is therefore valuable in making decisions about priority needs, and for the planning and development of future resources.

The IPP process can be represented as a feedback loop (Figure 5.1).

Prior to the IPP meeting

Identifying the keyworker

The coordinated approach to Individual Programme Planning can be facilitated by identifying a keyworker who will take responsibility for collating information prior to the meeting, and for ensuring that decisions reached at the meeting are acted upon. The keyworker will be someone who knows the individual well and, depending on particular circumstances, this role is likely to be assigned to a member of direct care staff, the keyworker at an Adult Training Centre, or a community service provider such as a nurse or a social worker.

Assessment

The first step in planning an individual programme is to review the current status and level of performance of the person concerned. This can be undertaken in a variety of ways. For example, Green-McGowan and Kovacs (1984) argue that the traditional approach to individual service planning has usually resulted in a painfully short list of strengths and a much longer list of needs or problems that may result in the person being perceived as the problem. They call for a shift in emphasis to look at those characteristics of people with a mental handicap that indicate how they are presently controlling their physical and social environment. By examining how their needs are met from others and situations in the environment during their 24-hour day, discussion and planning can take place regarding how particular strengths can be used to direct the person towards a lifestyle closer to that experienced by non-handicapped peers.

Crosby (1976) outlined essentials of active programming in which the goal is to increase the adaptive behaviour of the individual, and therefore evaluation of the individual's current status should focus on assessment of adaptive behaviour. In addition to the use of psychometric measures such as the American Association on Mental Deficiency Adaptive Behaviour Scale (Nihira et al., 1975), the assessment should also determine what the individual actually does on a day-to-day basis, so that it can indicate the next steps in development towards which programming efforts can be directed. Similar considerations apply to assessments conducted by medical personnel and other therapists, in that each evaluation should specify the person's current developmental status in terms that are pertinent to the areas of concern. These assessments should also identify the next developmental steps to be attained, and propose ways of accomplishing these.

The IPP system in use in Andover, Hampshire, involves the completion of a Needs List in preparation for the IPP meeting (Figure 5.2).

The individual's keyworker uses the Needs List to collate the views of other significant people regarding priority needs. The comprehensive format of the Needs List covers areas such as major day and residential services required; training priorities in activities of daily living, e.g. independent self-care, interpersonal relationships and leisure pursuits; and increased opportunities or broader experiences in any of these areas, which will lead to positive change. The keyworker should also involve the individual with a mental handicap, or an advocate, to make a personal contribution.

Specific assessments or clinical evaluations from professionals involved may also be requested if practitioner opinion is valuable in aiding the goal planning process.

The IPP meeting

Participants

The IPP meeting should be attended by key people in the individual's life, who are in regular contact, and know the person well. Composition of the planning team will be determined by the particular needs of the individual, and will usually include the individual, a family member or advocate, representatives from residential and day service facilities where appropriate, the designated keyworker, and any other significant people who are relevant to meeting the individual's needs.

An important role in the IPP process is that held by the chairperson, whose job is to facilitate the goal planning process, and 'shape up' aims where necessary to produce behavioural objectives leading to clarity of approach and evaluation.

Frequency of IPP meetings will depend on the situation and priorities of the particular individual, but would normally be held at 6–12 month intervals, with interim updates as required.

**Individual Programme Planning
NEEDS LIST**

Individual's name: ....   Keyworker: ....
IPP meeting to be held on:............................ (date) .... (time)
at: .... (place)

Programme Planning Team

The Programme Planning Team should be made up from the following list of people:

Individual	Social worker
Family member/advocate	General practitioner
Residential care person-in-charge	Psychiatrist/other medical
ATC manager/employer	specialist
Special Care Unit manager	Speech therapist
Head teacher/class teacher	Physiotherapist
Psychologist	Occupational therapist
Community nurse	Other

The keyworker should establish which of the people listed have been in contact with the individual since the last IPP meeting. Each of these people should be asked what they would like to put on the Needs List as priority areas for work, and be invited to the meeting.

SECTION 1

Predicted requirements and Current Need For Major Services

Long term accommodation

Short term care

Day care/training

Education

Work

Finance

SECTION 2

**Teaching or Learning Priorities
skills to be acquired in the next few months**

Self care

Domestic

Daily living/work/community living

Communication

Improved behaviour

Close personal relationships

Use of leisure

Physical development

SECTION 3

Improved Life Style and Opportunities

Heath/Hygiene

Physical appearance/coordination

Additions or changes to patterns of activities:

Household activities

Day care/work

Social contact/relationships

Leisure pursuits

Figure 5.2 A Needs List

Selecting objectives

Following a review of the current circumstances regarding the individual concerned, the meeting will then discuss the objectives or goals to be set. Each goal is a statement of intent about what the individual or relevant service will achieve within a specified time period, and is written in performance terms.

For example, a concern shared by those present may be that while the individual is involved in a variety of activities during the day, the evenings and weekends are largely unstructured and empty. The person concerned may complain of boredom, or spend time in fairly passive pursuits which do not lend themselves to meeting other people. A priority goal therefore may be to engage in leisure activities, and while this is a worthwhile aim, it remains non-specific and the individual is likely to require assistance in doing this. The goal would be better re-stated in terms of 'engage a volunteer befriender to take John out twice a week' or 'John will visit the local Sports Centre'. Thus, clear parameters are defined.

As the process of Individual Programme Planning can be viewed as an ongoing system of planning, implementation and evaluation, realistic goals should be set that can be accomplished within the agreed time.

Depending on the methods of assessment used, short- and long-term goals will become apparent from discussion of the individual's strengths and needs, taking account of his or her own personal wishes, by working through a 'Needs List' type format, and by sharing views on shortfall in service delivery.

It may aid the planning process to prioritize goals by examining emerging or prerequisite skills that the individual presently has. For example, a long-term, or terminal goal may be that the person will carry out personal hygiene skills independently. This may seem somewhat unrealistic in a short space of time, so planning can be aided by breaking down the terminal goal into smaller, consistent steps which can be set as individual objectives.

Perhaps through a training programme of task analysis and forward chaining, the individual ('Mary') can now wash her hair with minimal physical assistance. The next step may be set as 'Mary will wash her hair independently three times a week'. The relationship between this and the long-term goal can be clearly seen, and if successfully achieved, will become a prerequisite skill for future objectives such as hair-drying.

The planning process can be further assisted by selecting goals within the overall framework of the five accomplishments from the principle of normalization, thus ensuring that goals have purpose and meaning on a long-term basis. For example, objectives could be considered in the following areas:

1. *Community presence* – The experience of sharing the ordinary places that define community life. Objectives may include selecting settings and activities in the community that will offer a positive experience to the individual concerned.
2. *Choice* – The promotion and protection of individual autonomy and interests both in decisions concerning daily living, and other significant areas such as work settings and living arrangements. Objectives may include enabling the individual to make informed choices and pursue their own interests, and not those that service providers deem most appropriate.
3. *Increasing competence* – The experience of growing ability to perform a variety of skills and activities. Objectives in this area may include promoting and teaching new skills to augment the individual's existing skill repertoire.

4. *Respect* – The experience of holding a valued place among a network of significant people, and a valued role in community life. Objectives may want to address activities which will enable existing negative stereotypes to be challenged, and promote a positive reputation.
5. *Community participation* – The experience of being part of a growing sphere of personal relationships. Objectives may include enabling the individual to meet others in the community and design services so that people have the opportunity to be active participants with non-handicapped groups in a variety of community settings.

In this way, the IPP system is not viewed as a means of legitimizing inadequacies in service provision, and should include objectives that aim at increasing the person's independence, and lessen unnecessary dependence on 'special' services. While resources may not be presently available, interim goals can be set in their absence to move towards a desired resource, and identified shortfall in service delivery can be brought to the attention of service planners.

Meeting objectives

Once objectives have been agreed and prioritized depending on the needs of the individual, the methods of achieving these goals, and the person(s) responsible for implementing the process should be identified.

Specifying the conditions necessary for achieving goals can be enabled by asking the question 'what would it take. . .?' The use of this form separates the identification of goals from an evaluation of the cost of making them.

For example, in considering 'what would it take for the person to travel on his own by public transport to the ATC'?, this may include specifying and setting up a training programme based on detailed task analysis, staff time to assist with training, money for bus fares, or applying for a travel pass. The 'what would it take'? format can therefore identify how goals will be met, under what conditions, and by whom. This leads to identification of a range of items such as specialist services, equipment, finance, timetables, community resources, and what the individual concerned and the key people involved have to do in order to achieve the agreed goals. Specific training programmes can then be designed which include a clear description of the target steps involved and the methods used to meet them to promote consistency of caregiver approach over time.

Evaluating outcome

After decisions on how goals will be met, appropriate and objective criteria for evaluating success should be included in the planning process. A review of present circumstances, including strengths and needs, is an important starting point, as this can serve as a baseline against which future progress and change is compared.

Stating goals in behavioural terms will allow for objective measurement and avoid ambiguity. However, it is not a simple question of a 'pass–fail' situation. Rather, programme planners should consider evaluation in terms of what the desired outcome would be of making the proposed changes, and what the consequences would be for the individual if the present situation remained the same. In this way, forward planning is built in to the IPP meeting, rather than concluding with little more than a static description of the individual's current circumstances.

If success criteria have not been met, the reasons should be recorded and discussed at interim reviews or the next IPP meeting, in order that remedial action can be taken. This may entail reviewing the steps involved in training procedures, or examining deficiencies in service provision.

Recording methods

Because the IPP meeting results in a written plan of action, a method of recording information accurately should be devised. The format chosen should not be another form filling exercise to add to perhaps already voluminous case notes with no further action taken. While it should contain an accurate summary of the meeting's discussion, it is more than a set of minutes. It will include such items as the agreed objectives, the name of the person responsible for implementing those objectives, and the target date for their achievement.

A completed IPP may look like Table 5.1.

As part of an ongoing record to aid future planning, the form may include space to record outcome at some later date. This last section can act as a springboard to begin discussion at the next IPP meeting. For people involved in the care and training of individuals with a mental handicap, rate of progress may appear slow.

Name:	Alison Beveridge		
Date of IPP Meeting:	23 May 1989		
Summary of Current Action:	_____		
Objectives	*Person(s) responsible*	*Target date*	*Outcome*
1. Alison will use the hostel washing machine independently	Key Worker Hostel Staff	Nov 1989	
2. Alison will have her anticonvulsant medication reviewed	Keyworker GP	June 1989	
3. Application will be made for Alison to attend a part time Adult Education course at the local F.E. College	Social Worker	July 1989	
4. Alison will be taken along to the local Photography Club	Keyworker	July 1989	
Signed:	**(Alison Beveridge) (Chairperson)**		

Having accurate records will allow planners to review progress over time, and maintain the direction of a variety of inputs to ensure that they do not lose sight of longer term objectives.

Recording methods chosen will be forms that best reflect the requirements and style of those involved in IPPs. One example is the format outlined in the handbook of IPP guidelines produced by the British Institute of Mental Handicap.

This is a Personal Priority list (Figure 5.3), which is used in conjunction with the Needs List described earlier, and is completed by the Chairperson during the meeting.

Another format based on the AAMD Adaptive Behaviour Scale is used in a residential facility in Ontario (Schachter *et al.*, 1978). Here, individual programme planning is used to designate the broad strategy to be employed in working with residents with a mental handicap, as well as to establish a developmental progression for dealing with a succession of training needs to maximize an individual's capabilities. Programme planners complete a Master IPP, which is a developmentally oriented form listing areas in which an individual may require intervention. The Master IPP form includes six dimensions of behaviour arrived at from factor analysis of the Adaptive Behaviour Scale. These are Personal Self-Sufficiency, Community Self-Sufficiency, Personal Social Responsibility, Physical Development, Personal Maladaptation, and Social Maladaptation. These last two dimensions are placed at the end of the form to promote emphasis on considering

Individual's name: .... Date of meeting:				
People present:				
Areas	**Discussion**	**Objectives**	**Person responsible**	**Outcome** **nine months later**

Figure 5.3 IPP personal priority list

the training of adaptive skills, rather than adopting a problem-oriented approach. Each of these dimensions is further divided on the form into their component domains or sub-domains as presented in the Adaptive Behaviour Scale. For example, under the heading of Community Self-Sufficiency are sub-headings of travel, money handling and budgeting, and shopping skills. Terminal objectives are entered in an adjacent column (e.g. teach resident to make minor purchases with supervision by . . . (Date)).

Looking ahead

Having recorded the plan of action, the chairperson should set the date for the next IPP meeting, and any interim progress reviews if required. Administrative details such as where the plan of action is kept should be decided, and copies given to those involved with implementing objectives. At some point prior to the next IPP meeting, key people should be contacted to prepare their updated review of progress to start the planning process again.

Beyond the IPP

Shared action planning

The Open University, in collaboration with Mencap, has produced a course, 'Mental Handicap: Patterns for Living', which is part of their programme of Continuing Education (The Open University, 1986). The package is designed for people involved with individuals with a mental handicap, such as parents and carers from professional and voluntary organizations. The main aim of the course is to support those involved in preparing and implementing positive change in the lives of people with a mental handicap. Part of the course content is devoted to the concept of Shared Action Planning.

This has a dual focus on the two key elements of relationships and communication. The process is described as one that begins with key relationships in the lives of people with a mental handicap, and extends outwards from this central starting point. The focus on communication arises from the premise that difficulties in this area may account for lack of understanding and sensitivity in relation to the particular needs of the individual. As the title suggests, Shared Action Planning involves joint decision making and collaboration with the individual concerned to produce a coordinated approach to planning.

In similar vein to the IPP system, the mechanisms include a continuous assessment process to negotiate the direction of desired change, and the steps involved to achieve agreed goals. Progress evaluation is also built in. The course authors point out that while Shared Action Planning incorporates many of the aspects of Individual Programme Planning, it involves a shift in approach by involving the perspective of the individual from the outset.

Also recognized is the need to be aware of possible areas of conflict that may arise from different ideas about goals, so that these issues can be resolved. This format also acknowledges the dangers outlined by Green-McGowan and Kovacs (1984) of arriving at a static list of needs, by detailing what requires to happen to achieve the goals, and taking an outward looking approach from the individual's stand point in making decisions about change.

A set of five forms are used to record the planning process. These include summary details of present circumstances, written objectives, constraints and opportunities in meeting objectives, detailed planning steps, and progress records. These outline a comprehensive structure to lead participants through the process of Shared Action Planning. The aim of the approach is to promote greater control by individuals over different aspects of their lives.

Personal futures planning

Another approach which extends the IPP model is that of Personal Futures Planning (O'Brien, 1987). This is a system that plans a desirable future for a person with mental handicap, and describes the conditions that will facilitate a move towards that future. The process can be set in operation prior to planned major life events, such as starting or leaving school, moving home, or starting work. It can also be used to manage unplanned, or crisis events following placement breakdown or the death of a parent. Similar to Individual Programme Planning, it can be used as a method of progress review to identify positive change in areas of the person's life.

The Personal Futures Planning model places emphasis on the quality of the individual's life experiences, which form the basis for discussion at the planning meeting. The aim is to improve these life experiences by involving key people whose cooperation is important to the development of the individual concerned.

Defining what is meant by 'quality of life' may imply value judgements by service providers based on what they consider to be enriching or meaningful experiences. Raynes (1986) defines quality of life as a reflection of the extent to which we perceive our needs being met. This perception is influenced by our particular personality characteristics, the values of our society, and the opportunities afforded by our living and working environments. The individual with a mental handicap may become lost in this process, as opportunity may not have been available to make informed choice about a variety of experiences. Personal Futures Planning provides a framework for describing quality of life experiences by taking the five accomplishments from the principles of normalization as the terms of reference. Activities and experiences which are valued will enable the individual to have increased community presence and participation. Valued activities will also lead to a variety of choice and increased competence, and will provide access to valued roles, while challenging negative stereotypes. Personal Futures Planning aims to provide these experiences by examining change in the individual, change in service delivery, and change in opportunities offered by the community.

The format used to implement these changes is similar to that used by Individual Programme Planning. The lifestyle planning process is agreed during a planning meeting, when the individual's current situation is reviewed, a desirable future is described, and activities selected which will enable the individual to move towards that future. A follow-up meeting is held 2 weeks after to review the individual's situation within the framework of the directions set at the planning meeting.

The aim of the review of present circumstances is to describe the quality of the person's current relationships within community settings. Using the five accomplishments, the quality of the person's present experiences are described. For example, community presence is assessed by identifying settings and resources that the person uses regularly; the significant people that the individual spends time with are identified, and the amount and degree of choice available is examined by describing daily or weekly decisions made by and on behalf of the individual. When the overall picture has been described, the 'what would it take. . .?' format is used to suggest ways in which the individual's quality of life can be enriched.

This current review is taken to the planning meeting, where participants discuss ideas regarding desired change for the future. Opportunities, constraints and critical barriers to improved quality life experiences are discussed, and strategies are agreed to overcome constraints and meet the objectives set for expanding the individual's experiences.

At the initial review meeting 2 weeks later, the frequency, variation and balance of activities which the individual is involved in are evaluated to ensure that they are in line with the changes agreed during the planning process. Again, the 'what would it take. . .?' format is utilized to identify any modification in activities that would lead to better quality of life in terms of increased or improved status, choice, competence, community involvement and integration. One month after the lifestyle planning meeting, the convenor contacts key people involved to review progress to date, and take remedial action if required.

Conclusion

Many people with a mental handicap require help and guidance in the daily activities that we take for granted. Because of the nature of their handicap, they may need others to advocate on their behalf to ensure that opportunities are created to develop normal relationships and lifestyles. Support services of varying kinds are likely to assume an important role in the lives of these individuals, and a coordinated approach is necessary to implement planned change.

Individual Programme Planning facilitates the movement from a passive model of care, to one that is action oriented, with the individual concerned as the focus of planning. The IPP process allows the individual and key people in his or her life to agree on cooperative action towards future change, and provides a structured framework for shared communication and decision making.

Once established, the IPP process should be ongoing, allowing for regular evaluation of progress, and the setting of new objectives according to the particular needs and wishes of the individual.

Service provision can thus be tailored to the requirements of the person concerned, and this will assume increasing importance with the continuing move from hospitals to alternative community placement. For people with a mental handicap who, for whatever reasons, may not exert much control over their lives, Individual Programme Planning can provide an important starting point.

References

Beswick, J., Zadik, T. and Felce, D. (eds) (1986) *Evaluating Quality of Care* (Proceedings of a conference held at Holme Pierrepont, Nottingham), British Institute of Mental Handicap, Kidderminster

Crosby, K. (1976) Essentials of active programming. *Mental Retardation*, **14**, 3–9

Fleming, I. (1988) Making individual plans for change. *Mental Handicap*, **16**, 77–79

Green–McGowan, K. and Kovacs, M. (1984) Twenty four hour planning for persons with complex needs. *Canadian Journal on Mental Retardation*, **34**, 3–11

Houts, P. and Scott, R. (1975) *Goal Planning with Developmentally Disabled Persons: Procedures for Developing an Individualised Client Plan*. Milton S. Hershey Medical Center, Pennsylvania

Jenkins, J., Felce, D., Toogood, S., Mansell, J. and de Kock, U. (1988) *Individual Programme Planning: A Mechanism for Developing Plans to Meet the Specific Needs of Individuals with Mental Handicaps*, British Institute of Mental Handicap, Kidderminster

Nihira, K., Foster, R., Shellhaas, M. and Leland, H. (1975) *Adaptive Behaviour Scale*, American Association of Mental Deficiency, Washington

O'Brien, J. (1987) *A Guide to Personal Futures Planning*, Responsive Systems Associates, Atlanta, Georgia

O'Brien, J. and Tyne, A. (1981) *The Principle of Normalisation: A Foundation for Effective Service*, Campaign for Mentally Handicapped People, London

Open University (1986) *Mental Handicap: Patterns for Living*, DHSS with MENCAP, London

Raynes, N. (1986) Approaches to the measurement of care. In *Evaluating Quality of Care (Proceedings of a Conference held at Holme Pierre point, Nottingham)* (eds J. Beswick, T. Zadik and D. Felce), British Institute of Mental Handicap, Kidderminster

Schachter, M., Rice, J., Cormier, H., Christensen, P. and James, N. (1978) A process for individual programme planning based on the adaptive behaviour scale. *Mental Retardation*, **16**, 259–263

Throne, J., Hand, R., Hupka, M., Lankford, W., Luther, K., McLennan, S. and Watson, J. (1977) Unified programming procedures for the mentally retarded. *Mental Retardation*, **15**, 14–17

6

Communication

6.1 Augmentative and alternative systems of communication

Jois Stansfield

Augmentative and alternative systems of communication have been increasingly used in the past decade to enhance the communication skills of people with severe learning difficulties. Augmentative systems are introduced to increase communicative competence from a baseline where the client has some existing skills (perhaps vocalizations which are unintelligible), or is considered to have the potential to develop spoken language (such as babies with Down's syndrome). Alternative systems are seen as a substitute for spoken language. It must be stressed, however, that many systems may first be introduced as an alternative system but subsequently become augmentative as language skills emerge.

Before specific systems are discussed, a number of issues must be addressed.

Client-centred considerations

Cognitive level

Much of the literature in the field has taken account of cognitive skills when discussing the introduction of an augmentative system. Romski and Sevcik (1988) stated that augmentative systems should only be considered if the client was at or above sensori-motor stage V; several other authors discuss the necessity for object permanence to have developed, although there is inconclusive evidence that this is related to successful progress in learning a technique (Reichle and Karlan, 1985). Some augmentative systems do require specific cognitive levels of functioning. These will be discussed below.

Verbal skills

A number of authors (Sailor *et al.*, 1980; Owens and House, 1984) imply that a speech programme must have been tried and failed before augmentative techniques are introduced. In the light of findings that augmentative techniques facilitate vocal communication (Harris and Vanderheiden, 1980) and because there is no evidence that the use of such techniques adversely affects verbal communication development (Daniloff *et al.*, 1982) it would appear appropriate to introduce augmentative techniques without waiting for protracted failure in therapy.

Physical skills

The client's physical skills must be considered in introducing any augmentative system of communication. Clients without physical impairment can be introduced to dynamic or static techniques equally successfully, all other considerations being equal. Visually impaired clients, however, may find static display difficult to perceive, while physically handicapped individuals may have difficulties in producing signs, particularly those that are asymmetrical or involve crossing the midline of the body. As with speech, one does not always expect total accuracy in signing, but the potential level of intelligibility is a consideration in introducing signing.

The increased availability of technological aids has resulted in a similar increase in the number of severely physically impaired individuals able to utilize systems of augmentative communication. While detailed discussion of the range of hard- and software available is beyond the remit of this chapter, readers are referred to Enderby (1987) for further information.

Motivation

The client's motivation to communicate in any mode must be taken into consideration when introducing an augmentative system. Not all people with severe difficulties perceive a need to communicate in any form, and this is particularly the case with the most profoundly disabled individuals (Jones and Cregan, 1986). No intentional communication will develop in the absence of motivation.

For more able people, speech is the most socially acceptable form of human communication. Augmentative techniques tend to be more conspicuous than verbal communication and as such can be less acceptable to some clients than attempting to speak. AAC systems are also invariably slower than the normal flow of speech. In addition, they may be rejected because of inappropriate vocabulary or the choice of a particular technical aid (Shane, 1986).

Communication needs

Shane (1986) listed a number of goals when introducing augmentative communication techniques. These include promoting greater participation, promoting interpersonal and social interaction, reducing frustration, enhancing language development and organizing language processing. Kraat (1985) specified the profound differences in the way communication is perceived by verbal and non-verbal communicators, and focuses attention on the pragmatic aspects of communication from the client's viewpoint. Light (1988) specified the necessity for 'active co-construction of a message' by communicative partners, so that feedback is given as it is throughout normal verbal communications. Each writer stresses that the use of augmentative communication by definition, disrupts the normal pace of turn-taking. It does, however, enhance the client's ability to communicate, so long as the system is recognized and understood in the client's normal environment.

Support of carers

No communicative system will succeed unless those people who spend most time with the client use the system. This is common to speech, signed or symbol communication. Disadvantages of augmentative communication, and the perceptions of carers must be thoroughly discussed, if possible also involving the client, and agreement reached on the introduction and use of a technique, for any work to be successful (Jones and Cregan, 1986). As stated above, it is rare for carers to use the sign or symbol systems as a first language, and therefore continued support of the carers, including practice in use of the system, is central to the successful use of a system.

System-centred considerations

Mode of transmission

There are two modes into which AAC systems may be divided, dynamic and static systems. Manual systems are dynamic, involving movement, although individual signs may be held static, and they can be shaped by the partner in communication. Symbol systems are static. Symbols are presented in two-dimensional or three-dimensional form which cannot then be changed.

Each of these modes can benefit a large number of clients, and most recently, discussion has moved from choice of mode, to promoting a use of sign and symbol systems to mutually support language learning (Reichle and Karlan, 1985). This is justified by reference to experiments in normal development, where, for instance, word plus gesture can be used to indicate two ideas prior to two-verbal words. Some augmentative techniques (e.g. BSL Makaton) now combine formal sign and symbol intervention.

Iconicity

Iconicity is the strength of association between the form of the sign or symbol, and what it represents. In spoken language the comparison is onomatopoeia (e.g., 'cuckoo', 'splash'). Very few spoken words sound exactly like the item they represent. Augmentative techniques tend to have a higher level of iconicity but none have more than about 50% of the vocabulary which is absolutely clear to the naïve observer.

Iconicity can be viewed in terms of transparency, translucency and abstraction.

Transparency is the level where the meaning of a sign or symbol can be guessed by a naïve observer.

Translucency is when there is a relationship between the sign or symbol and its meaning, that can be understood once it has been explained.

In *abstract* signs or symbols there is no apparent relationship between them and the meaning they convey.

Hurlbert *et al.* (1982) found that iconic symbols were learned approximately four times as quickly as their equivalent Blissymbols and were retained longer, by physically handicapped adolescents. Orlansky and Bonvillian (1984), however, found that less than 40% of the first signs learned by deaf 10–18-month-old infants were iconic, and suggested caution in assuming iconicity to be the primary factor in sign learning.

Iconicity is a subjective experience. For example, a sign such as the BSL-Makaton sign for 'man' may have no translucency for a child who knows no bearded man.

Vocabulary

Availability of vocabulary is an issue in deciding upon a particular system. Many mentally handicapped clients will have a limited vocabulary requirement, but it is essential that a particular scheme is extensive enough to meet the clients' needs (Jones and Cregan, 1986). The majority of systems available have either an extensive vocabulary (BSL, which as a living language, is constantly extending and changing, and Paget-German Sign System PGSS) or a method of extending a basic vocabulary (clients can move beyond the 300 word Makaton vocabulary, and Amerind allows agglutination of signals to create new meanings). Symbol systems are perhaps less flexible but clients can move on to the written word once the entire vocabulary is known. In addition, personal strategies in communication can enhance the meaning through novel combinations of words, as in spoken language, thus ensuring flexibility of expression.

Correspondence with spoken language

When augmentative and alternative systems are introduced, the potential communicative setting of the client must be considered. The majority of people with mental handicaps will be living with verbal communicators, and as such, the closer their form of communication is in terms of grammatical construction and word order, the more meaningful will be any communicative interaction. Various systems have advantages in this respect. Signed English and PGSS are designed to follow syntactic and morphological grammatical constraints of English, while Blissymbols are organized in a visual left-to-right order which enables some correspondence to English word order. Most other systems are at a less sophisticated grammatical level.

The systems

There is a wide variety of systems of augmentative communication available (Table 6.1). The list below gives examples of each type of system.

Dynamic systems

Finger spelling

In Britain a two-handed system is most commonly used, while in the USA there is a one-handed system. One sign is used for each letter of the alphabet. It is rarely used in isolation but can occasionally supplement another form of signing with the learning disordered client group.

Table 6.1 Overview of characteristics of the most widely available ACC systems

	Client-centred considerations			System-centred considerations			
	Minimum cognitive skills	Verbal skills	Physical skills	Mode	Ionicity	Available vocabulary	Support for speech
Finger spelling	High	High	High	Dynamic	Zero	Equivalent to written English	Equivalent to written English
Signed English: PGSS	Low; amount of input can be varied according to clients needs	Low	High	Dynamic	Very low	3000 words plus	Equivalent word order to English regularizes irregular grammatical forms
SE	As above	Low	Moderate	Dynamic	Low	1500 formal signs plus availability of BSL vocabulary	Equivalent word order to English
Native sign language: ASL BSL	Moderate–high Input can be varied according to clients needs	Low	Moderate–high	Dynamic	Low	Extensive – there are a number of specific hand shapes using as basis of vocabulary	Very limited. There is no precise sign-word or grammatical match
Key-word signing: Makaton vocabulary	Low	Low	Moderate	Dynamic	Low	350 words	Some-same word order of English but no grammatical markers

Signal system:						
Amer-Ind	Low	Moderate–high depending upon complexity of signal	Dynamic	Moderate	236 words	Limited – can use English word order but this is not essential
Written word	High	Low–high depending upon method of transmission, (written, typed, etc.)	Static	Zero	Equivalent to spoken word	Equivalent to spoken word
Ideographs and pictographs:						
Premack system NONSLIP	Low	Moderate (manipulating small three-dimensional symbols)	Static	Zero (intentionally designed to be abstract)	Very limited	Very limited. Can be used in English word order
Blissymbolics	Moderate–high depending on level aimed at	Low	Static	Low	2000 words	Arranged to correspond partly to English word order
Rebus	Low	Low	Static	Moderate	Approximately 2000 rebuses	
Picture Boards	Low	Low	Static	High	Limited to concrete concepts	Zero

Signed English

There are two major British systems and several American systems which share very similar characteristics.

(a) Paget Gorman sign system (PGSS) (British)

This is an artificially designed language (Paget *et al.*, 1968) which aims to be an almost exact translation of English. There is one sign for each morpheme (unit of meaning) and irregularities of English are removed, e.g.:

$$\left.\begin{array}{l} \text{shop}+\text{ s} \\[1em] \text{sheep } + \text{ s} \end{array}\right\} \text{ both use two signs to indicate plurality.}$$

Signs are concept based, with a root and branch system, but the system is not widely known and rarely used with this client group.

(b) BSL signed English (SE)

Originally developed in the USA in the 1970s SE has been established in Britain using the BSL vocabulary but following English word order and adding sign-markers to indicate changes in syntax (Jones and Cregan, 1986). SE has a direct correspondence with English, and can be used as a supplement to the Makaton vocabulary, thus having a considerable potential for the mentally handicapped client.

(c) American systems

- Linguistics of Visual English (Love).
- Manual English.
- Seeing Essential English (SEE).
- Signing Exact English (SEE).
- Signed English (SINGLISH).

Each of these is a system of signed English, using different signs but having the same characteristics as the British systems.

Native sign languages

(a) American Sign Language (ASL),
(b) British Sign Language (BSL)

These were developed and are used by the native deaf populations of the USA and Britain, and the deaf populations of many other countries also have their own sign language.

ASL and BSL have very similar motor and cognitive characteristics, because they are natural and not artificial languages (Miles, 1988). ASL tends to have many signs using both hands performing mirrored gestures, while BSL has more one-handed signs. Each language varies through a continuum, from using signs, a few finger spellings, limited lip movements, vocalizations, and a great deal of facial expression to 'total communication' where all modalities are used as fully as possible. There is also a 'pidgin' form of signing, using just key concept signs and facial expression. Natural signing is not a poor and ungrammatical attempt to translate verbal language. Sign languages have their own intrinsic grammars, using changes of speed, size of gesture, and direction to express grammatical distinctions (Miles, 1988), but these do not easily translate into English. They should generally be regarded as different, and not inferior in terms of the semantic and syntactic information they carry.

Key word signing

The Makaton vocabulary

Makaton is a language programme, derived from the signs in BSL (above) but following the word ordering of English (Walker and Armfield, 1981). Key words are signed, always accompanied by grammatical spoken English. Facial expression and body language is used to increase intelligibility (Walker, 1986). Originally designed specifically for deaf mentally handicapped people, it is the most common introduction to signing used with mentally handicapped people (with or without hearing handicap) in Britain (Kiernan *et al.*, 1982). It is becoming accepted in other parts of the world, using the signs from the native sign languages.

There is an excellent support system for Makaton, with frequent national and local workshops enabling carers and professionals to maintain and enhance their skills in the use of the vocabulary.

Signal system

Amer-Ind

Developed from American Indian Hand Talk (Skelly, 1979), Amer-Ind is a gesture system of signals. Each gesture represents a single concept, which can be translated into its verbal equivalent. Strings of gestures can be used to form sentences, and agglutination of two or more gestures can produce new ideas. It operates at a concrete level, with no true grammatical rules. Skelly claims high iconicity (80%), and although other studies have suggested it to be closer to 40% iconic (Kiernan *et al.*, 1982) this is still higher than most other systems, which may increase its acceptability to carers.

Static systems

Written word

This is of limited value as a first line of communication for most mentally handicapped people. Those who can read and write can, almost without exception, also communicate verbally and therefore do not require an alternative system of communication. The rare exception is generally a person originally of normal intelligence who is suffering progressive physical and mental deterioration for some reason. In such a case, the written word may be used in some form temporarily, if, for instance, the speech musculature fails before intellectual deterioration becomes too severe.

The written word can be transmitted using traditional pencil and paper, the printed page, and increasingly through the use of a wide variety of high-technology equipment, when funds can be found (Turner, 1986).

Ideographs and pictographs

These use either mobile or static two-dimensional or three-dimensional displays of symbols to represent different concepts or ideas.

(a) Premack system (USA)   This was originally designed to teach language skills to chimpanzees and although there is no evidence that a neurologically intact

chimpanzee is comparable with a neurologically deficient (mentally handicapped) human (Carrier, 1977), the same behaviour modification techniques are used to teach symbolic using the three-dimensional colour-coded symbols, which can then be combined to produce limited grammatical structures (Deich and Hodges, 1977).

(b) Non-speech language initiation programme (non-SLIP) (USA)   This was developed from the Premack system, using three-dimensional colour coded plastic chips to teach tactics for functional communication (Carrier, 1977).

Neither of these systems is easily accessible and they are unnecessarily complex. It is not felt that their use can be justified purely as a form of augmenting communication.

(c) Blissymbolics (Canada)   A system originally designed (Bliss, 1966) as a form of written Esperanto, this has since been developed for use mainly with physically handicapped people. Some of the symbols are pictographic but the majority ideographic (abstract). It is widely used in Britain, and is also used in many other countries. Grammatical word ordering is attempted, and the basic vocabulary taught follows a normal developmental pattern. Symbols have logical roots, and several symbols can be combined to produce new words (Hehner, 1980).

Bliss does require a higher cognitive level of functioning than many of the other systems if it is to be used to the full, but some symbols can be introduced to less able people who can recognize two-dimensional images as meaningful.

(d) Rebus and Makaton symbols   Any pictographic system uses Rebuses but in the past few years a formalization of available Rebuses has been published (Van Oosterom and Devereux, 1985) developed from the Peabody Rebus Reading Program (Woodcock *et al.*, 1979) and associated with the Makaton vocabulary.

More Rebuses are iconic than Blissymbolics or the written word, and as such they are becoming increasingly popular as a method of augmenting verbal communication with people with cognitive deficits.

Picture systems
Picture and photo-boards are produced by a number of commercial firms, although it is often more suitable to design one individually for a particular patient using appropriate vocabulary. They are useful for those people not able to communicate by the higher symbolic functions of writing or symbol systems.

Conclusion

Augmentative techniques have got obvious limitations compared with normal communication:

1. Spoken language is more adaptable and socially acceptable.
2. Alternative systems are conspicuous.
3. Sign and symbol languages tend to cut off the user from the general population as very few people will use them as a first language.
4. Alternative systems may be seen by some people as proof that the patient will not talk, despite a great deal of evidence to the contrary.

5. In common with verbal communication development, comprehension of signs and symbols precedes expressive use, and this can cause patients, parents, care-staff, etc., to become discouraged because they expect too much of the system.

The development and increased sophistication of use of systems of augmentative and alternative communication has, however, made a major difference to the lives of many with mental handicaps, enabling an increased ability to communicate with others.

References

Blackstone, S.E. (ed.) (1986) *Augmentative Communication: An Introduction*, American Speech-Language-Hearing Association, Rockville

Bliss, C. (1966) *Semantography*, Blissymbolics, Sydney, Australia

Carrier, J.K. (1977) Application of a non-speech language system with the severely language handicapped. In *Communication Assessment and Intervention Strategies* (ed. Lloyd, L.L.), University Park Press, London

Daniloff, J., Noll, J., Fristoe, M. and Lloyd, L. (1982) Gesture recognition in patients with aphasia. *Journal of Speech and Hearing Disorders*, **47**, 43–49

Deich, R.F. and Hodges, P.M. (1977) *Language Without Speech*, Souvenir Press, London

Enderby, P. (1987) *Assistive Communication Aids for the Speech Impaired*, Churchill Livingstone, Edinburgh

Hargie, O. (ed.) (1986) *A Handbook of Communication Skills*, Croom Helm, London

Harris, D. and Vanderheiden, G.G. (1980) Enhancing the development of communicative interaction. In *Non-speech Language and Communication. Analysis and Intervention* (ed. Schiefelbusch, R.L.), University Park Press, Baltimore

Hehner, B. (1980) *Blissymbolics for Use*, Blissymbolics Communication Institute

Hurlburt, B.I., Iwata, B.A. and Green, J.D. (1982) Non-vocal language acquisition in adolescents with severe physical disabilities: Blissymbol versus iconic stimulus formats. *Journal of Applied Behavioural Analysis*, **15**, 241–258

Jones, P.G. and Cregan, A. (1986) *Sign and Symbol Communication for Mentally Handicapped People*, Croom Helm, London

Kiernan, C., Reid, B. and Jones, L. (1982) *Signs and Symbols. Use of Non-vocal Communication Systems*, Heinemann Educational Books, London

Kraat, A.W. (1985) *Communication Interaction between Aided and Natural Speakers*, Canadian Rehabilitation Council for the Disabled

Light, J. (1988) Interaction involving individuals using augmentative and alternative systems: state of the art and future directions. *Augmentative and Alternative Communication*, **4**, 66–82

Miles, D. (1988) *British Sign Language*, BBC Books, London

Owens, R.E. and House, L.I. (1984) Decision making processes in augmentative communication. *JSHD*, **49**, 287–292

Paget, R., Gorman, P. and Paget, G. (1986) *A Systematic Sign Language*, Royal National Institute for the Deaf, London

Reichle, J. and Karlan, G. (1985) The selection of an augmentative system in communication intervention: a critique of decision rules. *Journal of the Association for the Severely Handicapped*, **10**, 146–156

Romski, M.A. and Sevcik, R.A. (1988) Augmentative and alternative communication systems. Considerations for individuals with severe intellectual disabilities. *Augmentative and Alternative Communication*, **4**, 83–93

Rozelle, R.M., Druckman, D. and Baxter, J. (1986) Nonverbal communication. In *A Handbook of Communication Skills* (ed. Hargie, O). Croom Helm, London, pp. 59–94

Sailor, W., Guess, D., Geetz, L., Schuler, A., Utley, B. and Baldwin, M. (1980) Language and severely handicapped persons. Deciding what to teach to whom. In *Methods of Instruction for Severely*

Handicapped Students (eds Sailor, W., Wilcox, B. and Brown, L.) Paul H. Brooks, Baltimore, pp. 71–108

Shane, H.C. (1986) Goals and uses. In *Augmentative communication: An Introduction* (ed. Blackstone, S.E.) American S.L.H. Association

Silverman, F.H. (1980) *Communication for the Speechless*, Prentice Hall, Englewood Cliffs, NJ

Skelly, M. (1979) *Amer-Ind Gestural Code*, Elsevier, Amsterdam

Turner, G. (1986) Funding VOCAS for the low-functioning. *Communication Outlook*, **8.2**, 12–14, 27

Van Oosterom, J. and Devereux, K. (1985) *Learning with Rebuses*, LDA, Wisbech

Walker, M. (1986) *Line Drawings for the Revised Makaton Vocabulary*, MVDP, Camberley

Walker, M. and Armfield, A. (1981) What is the Makaton vocabulary? *Special education: forward trends*, **8.3**, 19–20

Woodcock, R.W., Clark, C.R. and Davies, C.O. (1969) *Teachers Guide: The Peasbody Reading Program*, American Guidance System, Minnesota

6.2 Communication and behaviour disorders

Bill Fraser

Finding meaning in disturbance

If we were to do a comprehensive inventory of behaviour problems it would seem endless, ranging from problems of verbal aggression to physical attacks and from irritating behaviours such as teeth grinding to unacceptable sexual deviance. To make sense out of the list. Leudar, Fraser and Jeeves (1984) prepared such an inventory and factor analysed the problem behaviours in people with mental handicaps. Factors could then be used as headings under which to classify challenging behaviours. These factors are virtually identical in most scales. Most prominent are aggression, stereotype behaviours, antisocial conduct, self-mutilating behaviours, mood disturbances and withdrawn behaviours. These category headings cover most of the behavioural problems of mental handicap. It is to be noted that these behaviours are not usually directly related to physical or mental illness. It is nonetheless essential to conduct a physical examination for undetected pain, a neurological assessment for epilepsy, etc., and also a mental assessment to exclude the effects of medication, depression or psychosis.

The starting point is a search for environmental causes and maintenance factors; then consider the developmental stage of the person and whether the behaviour represents a 'frozen' stage of development; and particularly communication deficits. Such deficits reflect perhaps poor room management of the training centre in which the person works, poor skills at 'reading' the handicapped person's unclear and blurred messages, or simply communicatively insensitive staff, and also the communicative faults which the mentally handicapped person himself may have in expressing his intentions and feelings about the predicament that he may be temporarily or permanently in. (For milestones of language development see Appendix 1).

The literature on dual diagnosis, i.e. the study of psychopathology and emotional disturbance in the mentally retarded, is now expanding. These studies raise the question of how much communication failure interferes with reported incidence of mental illness in the handicapped, uses of instrumentation, diagnosis and treatment.

The pragmatics of language

Psycholinguistics in the 1960s was bogged down as regards practical applications by its concentration on theoretical aspects such as syntax (the organization of sentences). The 1970s saw the emergence of pragmatics as a useful approach to the understanding of mentally handicapped people's behaviour. Pragmatics involves the management of communication – its 'housekeeping' such activities as tactfulness, taking turns and speech acts such as requesting and exclaiming. The autistic person has specific pragmatic deficits. A Pragmatics approach stresses that understanding language does not simply consist of knowing the meanings of words and sentences but also involves interpreting what is said (this may include inferring the speaker's intentions and beliefs) against a background of what the communicators know, and assume they know about each other.

Communication requires that people construct models of each other's (in this case mentally handicapped persons) knowledge, beliefs and actions. Leudar and Fraser (1985) have argued that many emotional problems are associated with communication problems of individuals, and Leudar has carried out a series of studies which highlighted the importance of the communication environment in contributing to the causes of and the maintenance of emotional disturbance.

Three concerns of contemporary linguistics (to be more precise, pragmatics) are relevant here: *intentionality*, *conventionality* and *face*. Most current models of pragmatics theory are based on the fact that human communication is *intentional*. That is to say, meanings of utterances and dialogues are not necessarily the same as what the sentence says; and correct *grammatical* speech is not essential for conveying the communicator's intentions. However, the mentally handicapped are poor at conveying their intentions because of language delay, speech impediments, dysarthria, lack of social skills and sometimes dysphasia; and if their intentions are not understood then 'learned helplessness' develops, fluency decreases yet further and withdrawal can result.

Even amongst mentally handicapped people who seem to make sense, often they fail to get their meaning over. Like Duncan, when he's asked why he stopped going to Adult Training Centre Duncan replies, 'Well, really, they carry on with all the noise. . . Ann's really not well. . . They don't let you go on holiday.'

Instead of telling the interviewer of his suspension from the Centre, he starts talking about one of the background factors, that he was trying to protect a girlfriend from a stressful situation and was misunderstood; and launches then into an entirely different topic: why, because of a lack of his own funds, he couldn't go on holiday. That was no doubt a contributory factor to his general feeling of irritation but one has to fit together, as Kernan and Sabsay say, his explanations and digressions 'like a jigsaw puzzle with some of the bits missing'.

Jim thinks very slowly, largely as a result of the anticonvulsant medication he is on, but also because of his mental handicap, so he gets two steps behind quickly in what he is talking about compared with what has been asked; so at the checkout counter in the supermarket, he gets confused and irritable and eventually aggressive.

Janet usually gets so far behind in the conversation that she withdraws and just gives up.

Similarly, Timmy. Psychiatrist (seeing him standing disconsolately in the corridor): 'How are you doing, Timmy?'

Timmy: 'Am seb rup.' (I'm fed up.)

Psychiatrist: 'Jolly good.'

Meanings are inferred on the assumption that speakers adhere to communicative *conventions* (e.g. the maxim to provide the optimum amount of information necessary in discourse). Leudar and Fraser (1985) have shown that withdrawn mentally handicapped people violate a maxim of conversation by being too economical in utterances because they have learned to be helpless as a deliberate strategy.

Maxims of conversation include trying to ensure what you say is true; be polite and cooperative in interactions; be tactful; make your contribution as informative as is required but no more so; avoid ambiguity; be orderly and be relevant.

Mentally retarded individuals are not only limited in the topics they can choose to discuss, they often fail to display interest in other people's topics; they also make false claims to accomplishments (don't many of us?).

Robert is autistic. At some point in any conversation he breaks in with his favourite topic: 'Grannie died on Wednesday', which is a showstopper. This plus constant questioning is simply an attempt to cooperate in conversation.

Shirley at the local fete sees a group of Army cadets about to play in the band. She mingles amongst them, talking immoderately about her sexual feelings and about her private life.

The third pragmatic concern is *face*. Positive face is the need for an individual to be appreciated by his or her communicative partners. Leudar points out that in some types of dialogue the duty of participants to consider other participants' face is 'suspended'; for example, one normally is apologetic when pointing to another's error but a teacher, e.g. a gym teacher, will not necessarily do so when correcting a pupil. Usually one apologizes for an imposition but a sergeant major doesn't apologize to a private.

Johnny often stands on the edge of groups of staff and is ignored. When he does try to break into the conversation, he's elbowed out again. One can see the humiliation on his face.

It is clear, as Leudar points out, that the face of mentally handicapped people 'is consistently under attack. . . politeness is rarely used to maintain their face'. Thus the mentally handicapped person has more opportunities than the person of normal intelligence to be irritated, exasperated and humiliated.

All behaviour is communicative

Leudar's studies have shown that several maxims of conversation may not be in power to the same extent for conversations in which the mentally handicapped person participates. Mentally handicapped individuals are reported to be more often difficult to make out what they say, and what they say is said to be less likely to be true, relevant and coherent, and the information they convey often insufficient, less relevant and less direct.

Leudar (1988) also investigated the relationship between behaviour disturbance and the communicative background using the Behaviour Disturbance Scale (Leudar, Fraser and Jeeves, 1984) which measures aggression, conduct disorder, mood disturbance, self-injury, stereotyping and withdrawness. The aim here was to investigate whether each aspect of behaviour disturbance is associated with changes in communicative conventions. The scores for each of the dimensions of disturbance was correlated with the handicapped person's Communicative Style Score. This is derived from the Communicative Style Scale (CSS) which measures the impressions of individuals' communicative actions on his or her social environment. Leudar found a strong relationship between behaviour disturbance and communicative problems on the CSS. Violations of communicative cooperativeness are particularly characteristic of aggressive individuals. Leudar and Fraser (1985) argue that behaviour disturbances should not only be seen from the point of view of their causes but also understood as communication problems. Each dimension of behaviour disturbance is associated with a distinct pattern of violations of communicative conventions. All behaviour has a functional message.

Aggression and self-aggression in the profoundly handicapped

Most studies of self-injurious behaviours in the past were based on hospital populations. Prevalence rates of around 15% amongst whom 2% were most severe, were found and recent studies in the community have shown that most self-injurious behaviour is untreated.

Organic factors play a part, e.g. in Lesch–Nyhan syndrome which affects only males, there is a genetic enzyme fault. The consequence is a high uric acid in the blood. Not all Lesch–Nyhan victims are severely mentally handicapped. The self-mutilation begins around 4 months of age, and those who acquire language describe the torment of their compulsive biting of lips (we all know how irresistible it is to 'worry' a loose and painful tooth!). Lesch-Nyhan victims also comment on how comforting it is to have some form of physical restraint. The cause of Lesch–Nyhan mutilating is unclear. It is not the presence of a high level of uric acid that is the irritant, and the pathology and maintenance may be similar to self-injurious behaviour in other handicapped people, and include a communicative function.

Although only 6% of self-injurious behaviour could be directly attributable by Leudar to the problems of communication, Carr and Durand (1985) have shown that the training of 'special request signs' can reduce the likelihood of non-verbal (e.g. self-mutilative) behaviour which was previously being used by a mentally handicapped child as aberrant communication. Carr and Durand present evidence that problems such as self-injury and aggression and tantrums fall into two broad classes: escape behaviours, controlled by negative reinforcement processes, and attention-seeking behaviours, controlled by positive reinforcement processes. They also theorize that such behaviours are primitive forms of non-verbal communication. MacLean and Snyder-MacLean (1987) have shown that those profoundly mentally handicapped subjects using the more primitive forms of signalling, including direct actions on object or people and/or gestures with objects, employ predominantly imperatives (e.g. 'do this').

In fact such subjects *never* produce a communicative act intended to act as a declarative (i.e. to direct the attention of the other person to some interesting object or event). Less severely handicapped people, even if they cannot actually speak, produce a relatively high rate of declarative type communicative acts, greetings, etc. Many idiosyncratic responses in the more profoundly handicapped seem to serve communicative functions, including slapping at tables, clapping and flapping, as part of a general excitation state. Other behaviours that can be a sign of intent but are not clearly intentionally communicative, include tantrums and self-injurious acts like hand-biting and head-hitting. This means that all idiosyncratic acts, stereotyped behaviours and mannerisms should be examined for possible communicative significance.

Carr and Durand suggested treatments: escape-motivated behaviour could possibly be helped by teaching the handicapped person to emit a verbal response, such as 'help me' or 'I don't understand', whenever confronted with a difficult task. Attention-seeking behaviour could possibly be dealt with by teaching the handicapped person to emit a verbal response such as 'Am I doing okay?' Of course, most of these people cannot actually produce such words so that much simpler signals must be employed such as tapping to mean 'I can't cope with this – I must "escape"'. Confirmation of this concept of escape and attention signals comes from study of aggression in toddlers when one child hits another with an open hand and the other child typically breaks off the interaction, suggesting the aggression means 'leave me alone'. Conversely, hitting another toddler with a teddy bear suggests 'do you want to play?', i.e. attention seeking. Furthermore, the often observed wish to remain in restraint of a self-mutilating mentally handicapped person, suggests that the restraining garment or bandages may be a 'safety' *signal*, i.e. a stimulus that signals the absence of an aversive stimulus, and supports Carr and Durand's escape hypothesis that whenever the mentally handicapped person who self-abuses is provided with a reliable safety cue, escape behaviours should decrease in frequency.

In addition to teaching alternative communications, e.g. tapping 'help' signing, other function-related alternatives such as ear-muffs or Sony headsets may enable autistic people whose aberrant behaviour is often a signal of overload from highly stimulating environments, to screen out excessive environmental input.

Antecedent interventions are the best way of reducing aberrant communicative functions. This means decreasing the stress of demands to what the handicapped person can cope with, and using simpler less stressful kinds of teaching methods. Donellan *et al.* (1984) have created an observation tool for analysing the communicative functions in behaviour. This lists functions – requests for attention, negations and protests, and declarations of the need to escape from boredom, pain, etc. – against a range of behavioural phenomena including aggression, hysteria, screaming, etc. The person's ability to use communication in everyday situations and the communicative environment's sensitivity can be assessed by the Communication Assessment Profile (CASP) (von der Gaag, 1988).

A functional analysis of multiple aberrant responses is possible by time sampling handicapped people who show challenging behaviour in their everyday and analogue environments, e.g. alone; social disapproval; academic demand; and unstructured play (Iwata *et al.*, 1982; Sturmey *et al.*, 1988). This may shed light on which of the strange behaviours are related to which settings and stresses, and help to alert staff to what the mentally handicapped person is attempting to communicate.

The most basic antecedent intervention is a communicative one – movement therapy. This is based on research into development of early communication which acknowledges the infant as an active partner in his communication with others. Mothers are seen to act on the spontaneous actions of their babies as if they were meaningful, communicating in a way that follows the turn-taking of normal verbal conversation. Through such encounters, babies come to realize that their actions have effects on others. By similarly examining the spontaneous actions of profoundly mentally handicapped people, the caregiver can learn about the profoundly handicapped person's intentions and enable him to become an active partner in communication, albeit of a primitive non-verbal nature (see Section 6.3).

The expression of grief

Robert was profoundly handicapped, unable to speak or to walk. He shared a room with Leonard. They seemed to have much contact with each other. Leonard died suddenly, and Robert's sleep patterns after a few weeks became increasingly disturbed. He became more agitated. He had a massive gastric bleed and died.

Parents and caregivers find it difficult to talk about death to mentally handicapped people. They fear it might add to their upset to go to the effort to explain in simple terms that a brother, father or mother has died and will not return. In the case of the severely and profoundly handicapped, even if the caregiver is willing, the comprehension of the severely mentally handicapped person may not be sufficient or may not be present at all.

The profoundly handicapped person nevertheless will be able to detect change in the environment, the stress in his caregivers, and a puzzling, frightening atmosphere.

At the time of a family death, it is common for the mentally handicapped person to be sent away, to go to a relative (often not a close one), to return home to find the father, mother, brother or Gran gone away, and then to be told that they will not return. The handicapped person will have been excluded, as he has from so many celebrations and ceremonies, whether it is bar mitzvah, coming of age, entering high school, passing 'A' levels and other initiation rights of adults; and now attendance at a funeral is barred. Sireling and Hollins in their video 'The Last Taboo', point out that worries about the handicapped person's understanding and attempts to protect them from grief are not a sufficient reason for denying them the right to a normal healthy grief reaction. As the mentally handicapped person may have lived with elderly parents in particularly close and narrow relationship, excessive grief reactions can be expected. The communication of grief to the severely and profoundly mentally handicapped may take the same forms as people of normal intelligence – a period of withdrawal, lower appetite, crying; or may appear as refusal to eat, massive weight loss, agitation, or going walkabout – a hazardous wandering – soiling or smearing or, in the case of the person with severe social impairment, apparent indifference.

Furthermore, caregivers should not consider as insensitive the mentally handicapped person who is indifferent when told that relatives, who have seldom visited him over the last years, have died. This is more an indictment of the system which causes such separations. It is important that carers understand the normal healthy grief reaction and how it can manifest itself in people who have a mental handicap. It is important that carers know a sequence of breaking bad news to mentally handicapped people, and encourage them to grieve. It is important that they remember to commemorate with the handicapped person the death, and in the later stages of grief, enable its resolution, helping the handicapped person through photographs and taking them to visit crematorium or cemetery to place the loved one and his or her own life in context. Such are amongst the most skilled communications that carers can make.

References

Carr, E. and Durand, V. (1985) In *Theoretical Issues in Behaviour Therapy* (eds Reiss, S. and Bootzin, R.), Academic Press, New York, pp. 219–253

Donnellan, A.N., Mirenda, T., Mesaros, R. and Fassbender, L. (1984) Analysing the communicative functions of aberrant behaviour. *Journal of the Association of Persons with Severe Handicaps*, **9**, 201–212

Iwata, B.A., Dorsey, M.F., Slifer, K.J., Bauman, K.E. and Richman, C.S. (1982) Toward a functional analysis of self-injury. *Analysis and Intervention in Developmental Disabilities*, **2**, 3–21

Kernan, K. and Sabsay, S. (1988) Communication in social interactions. Aspects of an ethnography of communication of mildly mentally handicapped adults. In *Language and Communication in Mentally Handicapped People* (eds Beveridge, M., Conti-Ramsden, G. and Leudar, I.), Chapman and Hall, London, pp. 229–253

Leudar, I. (1988) Communicative environments for mentally handicapped people. In *Language and Communication in Mentally Handicapped People* (eds Beveridge, M., Conti-Ramsden, G. and Leudar, I.), Chapman and Hall, London, pp. 274–299

Leudar, I., Fraser, W. and Jeeves, M. (1984) Behaviour disturbance and mental handicap: typology and longitudinal trends. *Psychological Medicine*, **14**, 923–935

Leudar, I. and Fraser, W. (1985) How to keep quiet: some withdrawal strategies in mentally handicapped adults. *Journal of Mental Deficiency Research*, **29**, 315–330

Leudar, I., Fraser, W. and Jeeves, M.A. (1981) Social familiarity and communication in Down syndrome. *Journal of Mental Deficiency Research*, **25**, 133–142

Leudar, I., Fraser, W. and Jeeves, M.A. (1987) Theoretical problems and practical solutions to behaviour disorders in retarded people. *Health Bulletin*, **45**, 347–355

Sireling, L. and Hollins, S. (1985) *The Last Taboo*. A video programme on mental handicap and death. Department of Psychiatry, St. George's Hospital Medical School, London

Sturmey, P., Carlson, A., Crisp, A. and Newton, J.I. (1988) The functional analysis of aberrant responses. A refinement and extension of Iwata *et al*'s (1982) methodology. *Journal of Mental Deficiency Research*, **32**, 31–46

van der Gaag (1988) *The Communication Assessment Profile (CASP)*, Speech Profiles Ltd.

McLean, J. and, L. Snyder-McLean (1987) Form and function of communicative behaviour among persons with severe developmental disabilities. *Australia and New Zealand Journal of Developmental Disabilities*, **13**, 83–98

6.3 Communicating through movement and posture

Bronwen Burford

The purpose of non-verbal behaviour

Non-verbal behaviour plays a part in communication from birth and throughout life. Although when we talk to someone we are usually much more aware of what we are saying than what we are doing, our movements and postures play a major part in the conversation. We communicate, intentionally or otherwise, through our gestures, postures, facial expressions, the amount of space we keep between ourselves and others, the ways in which we touch or react to being touched, the looks we give or avoid and our general body movements. Non-verbal behaviour accompanies, complements and modifies what we are saying and plays a part in all human interactions (Mayo and Henley, 1981).

Of course, not all non-verbal behaviour is deliberate and intended to communicate. People are often unaware of the movements and expressions they are using, but these nevertheless give us information. We should always remember, however, that whereas *observation* can be accurate and objective, the *interpretation* of what we see, especially when we are personally involved, is subjective and influenced by our own attitudes and feelings. It should also be taken into account that non-verbal behaviour does not occur in a vacuum. We need to take note of the situation in which it is occurring and the relationship between those who are interacting before we can make sense of what we see.

Association with speech

Non-verbal behaviour becomes mutually communicative when the non-verbal behaviours have the same meaning for all who are participating (Weiner *et al.*, 1972). The meaning of the facial expressions and gestures used by one person will be similarly interpreted by another, e.g. that a smile is friendly, that a hand waved is a greeting or farewell.

Some elements of non-verbal behaviour are more closely associated with speech than others. They help the interaction to run smoothly and add meaning to what is being said. The pattern of looking at and away from a person when you are speaking helps to allocate listener and speaker roles and is one of the signals that tells you when it is your turn to speak.

Speech is also accompanied by gestures called emblems and illustrators which emphasize and embellish what is being said and can fill in for words (Ekman, 1977). Emblems have a very precise meaning, e.g. a head nod means 'yes'. Illustrators are also closely linked with speech, but are less specific – the person creates a drawing in the air as he or she is speaking. Some people with Down's syndrome develop complex gestures to describe and indicate what they cannot express through speech (Leuder, 1981).

However, non-verbal behaviour is not solely associated with speech. For example, movements called body manipulators, such as scratching, playing with your fingers, rubbing one foot against the other, are also part of non-verbal behaviour, but do not enhance or illustrate speech, and often occur when the person is alone as well (Ekman, 1977). Someone who uses a lot of these movements is often regarded as nervous and tense by others.

Movements have meaning

Our body movements are not random and meaningless. They have communicative value which tells something about our moods, emotions and attitudes (Key, 1980). Leuder (1981) observed people with Down's syndrome during interactions with a stranger and with someone they knew and found that they moved less and in a more restricted way with a stranger, kept a greater distance and held a neutral orientation or one that was turned away from the other person and often adopted a closed posture by bringing a hand across their chest. In this way their body movements and postures reflected their social relationship with their conversation partner.

It is through their interactions that people are able to express and share their feelings with others and to form relationships. The experiences people have during their interactions can have an effect on their inner lives, deeply affecting how they feel about themselves (Condon, 1980). Emotional communication forms a large part of human communication (Buck, 1984) and the non-verbal aspects seem to be more important in interpersonal relationships than the spoken language (Danziger, 1976).

'Wrong' non-verbal communication causes problems

As long as communication is going well we are less likely to pay much attention to the non-verbal part. However, when something goes wrong with this it can cause surprise, misunderstanding and distress. For example, eye contact has a powerful effect on us which we probably do not appreciate until it is absent for some reason. Fraiberg (1974) describes how blind 2- and 3-month-old babies can mislead parents into thinking that they are not attending. They show apparent avoidance because they incline their heads in order to improve listening, instead of seeking eye contact the way sighted babies do. She also noted that she did not talk to the blind babies in her studies as she did to the sighted babies. She suggests that the reason for this is because young, blind babies do not give the responses such as smiles and facial focusing that sighted babies do – responses that adults find so rewarding. Mothers report that they begin to develop affectionate feelings when their babies begin to make eye contact with them (Haviland and Malatesta, 1981). However, eye contact is not a prerequisite for successful communication. Parents do develop good communication with children who are blind and with sighted children who avoid looking at other people.

Those to whom we cannot 'get through' because their non-verbal behaviour is 'odd' have broken the unwritten rules about how to use non-verbal communication (Mayo and Henley, 1981) – rules that are often difficult for people who are mentally handicapped to fully understand. Someone's non-verbal behaviour might go against the rules because it is exaggerated or too restricted, or a response is given at the wrong time, a pause is too long, or a reply comes too quickly. Such problems do not arise only with people who are mentally handicapped. There are many differences in the way people of different cultures use postures, movements, facial expressions and eye contact and this can cause difficulties for strangers.

The power of non-verbal rules

Researchers do not fully agree on the extent to which non-verbal behaviour is innate or learned from the culture in which the individual lives. Most believe that both play a part and that humans learn how to use a system of communication which has deep biological roots (Buck, 1982). Cross-cultural comparisons do show that some patterns of behaviour occur universally and in the same social context and are similarly interpreted by the participants (Eibl-Eibesfeldt, 1972). One example is the eyebrow flash, which is a rapid raising of the eyebrows. This is said to exist in all cultures and signals a readiness for interpersonal contact. Similarly, smiling is seen as expressing a friendly intention, although there are cultural variations about how and when to smile. There are many such variations in non-verbal behaviour, e.g. the meaning of gestures or the use of eye contact, and some are very clearly linked with correct social behaviour within a culture.

Posture

Postures serve different purposes in different communities, although within a community they will have the same style and meaning (Key, 1975). Britain does not have strict rules about postural behaviour, but in some cultures, e.g. among the Balinese, posture can be an indicator of status and is part of social etiquette. Friends of equal status may assume a similar posture when they are communicating, whereas those of unequal social status may have to assume different postures according to the rules of their culture.

Closeness and touching

While postural behaviour does not feature prominently in social etiquette in Britain, there are two behaviours associated with intimacy that do play an important part – close physical proximity and touching. There are considerable differences in the distance people keep from each other when they are talking which can have a powerful effect on how well or badly the communication goes. Hall (1959) has studied the use of space in everyday conversations. He describes how people from South America stand close to each other during conversations – a closeness that people in Britain would see as intimate. When two people from cultures with different rules about this social spacing speak to each other they continually adjust the space between them to keep the 'normal' distance. Obviously this can lead to misunderstandings about the 'cold' or 'overbearing' behaviour of the other.

Touch plays a crucial role in healthy development. However, people differ markedly in how they react to and interpret being touched and in the degree of comfort they feel when someone touches them (Major, 1981). The rules of the culture will have some effect. In cultures where physical contact is used frequently during everyday conversations it is seen as simply another channel of communication. In Britain there is infrequent physical contact during interactions, especially in public.

Given the power that cultural and social rules have in communication, it is very important that a person who is mentally handicapped is helped to gain some understanding and awareness of these rules as far as he or she is able. Shanley (1986) describes how the first encounter that new staff have with residents in institutions for people who are mentally handicapped can result in 'culture shock'. They are propelled into a world that breaks many of the rules about touching, looking at and being close to other people, making it difficult for the newcomer to know how to respond. Many of these behaviours are threatening or very intimate in our society, but do not carry the same meanings within the institution (Shanley, 1986).

Unfortunately, because we in Britain do not touch people very much and keep quite a distance between ourselves in everyday communication, our culture causes problems for the many people who are mentally handicapped who like to touch more and get closer than the rules permit. The possible serious misunderstandings that can arise from breaking these rules, especially for men who are mentally handicapped, and the hostility and lack of acceptance such behaviour might engender means that any approach aimed at helping a person who is mentally handicapped to integrate with his or her community must pay attention to this aspect. However, it should not be forgotten these problems have, in part, been created by the rules of our culture and there should also be opportunities that allow the person who is mentally handicapped to express his or her spontaneity and warmth in an appropriate way.

Difficulty being near others

Not all people who are mentally handicapped enjoy physical contact. Some find being near other people distressing and frightening, and will move away when someone gets too close and often use body movements and postures as protective barriers. Many people who closely guard their personal space in this way can be helped to lessen their fear and find some degree of interpersonal contact tolerable and pleasurable. A person who can at least tolerate other people near him or her and make limited contact without upset is obviously going to have fewer distressing moments. One way of helping someone to feel easier about people being near is to begin by simply being as close as they can comfortably tolerate, sitting, standing or being on the floor beside him or her.

Gradually the distance can be decreased as tolerance develops and perhaps some gentle physical contact introduced. Often it helps to speak only quietly or not at all in this situation. There is no need to try to get the person to DO something, because he or she is already DOING something, i.e. sharing the same space with another person. Sharing is as much a part of interpersonal communication as doing something more obviously active.

Sharing

Interpersonal sharing is a part of ordinary communication. Stern (1985) has a category for analysing mother–infant interactions which he has called 'interpersonal communion', referring to the mother 'sharing' or 'being with' the baby. During interpersonal communion the mother is not trying to influence or change what the baby is doing. Rather, she is participating with and sharing in the baby's experience without attempting to alter his or her behaviour. The mother reflects and empathizes with the baby's affective state rather than imitating what he or she is doing.

There are many lessons to be learned from the development of early interactions between non-handicapped babies and their parents, particularly in relation to people with profound mental and multiple handicaps.

The development of early communication

In 1902, before the age of film and video made detailed and accurate observation of interactions possible, Cooley wrote that young children closely watched the movements of others and because of this the children soon saw a connection between what they did and the changes this brought about in other people's movements. Cooley noted how the child recognized that he or she had some influence over these movements and described how a 6-month-old baby might attempt to attract attention by using his or her actions, such as wriggling or stretching out arms, constantly watching the adult's movements for the desired effect (Cooley, 1902).

Research has since confirmed Cooley's observations that babies play an active part in their communication with adults and it is believed that they are born able to communicate (Newson, 1979; Bullowa, 1975). By the time a baby is 6 months old he or she will have developed skills for coping with social interaction (Stern, 1977), having mastered the cues and conventions for initiating, responding to and ending interactions. During interactions the adult responds to the baby's spontaneous actions and sounds, commenting and expanding on them in a conversational style. These daily conversations help the baby to realize that what he or she is doing has meaning and can have an effect on other people. The exchanges are very repetitive and this gives the babies an opportunity to practise their part in them and become able and active participants in interactions (Schaffer, 1977).

The development of language is related to the baby's ability to participate in interactions during the first year of life (Bruner, 1974) and this places the acquisition of language within a social setting (Schaffer, 1977). Babies also form their first relationships through non-verbal interactions and through these relationships begin to learn about the world around them (Bullowa, 1979). Therefore, these early exchanges are important in laying the foundation for the development of interpersonal relationships (Stern, 1985).

Communicating with people with profound mental and multiple handicaps

Adults use what the baby is able to do to make interpersonal contact with him or her, thereby responding appropriately to the baby's level of development and ability to participate. This seems a good overall strategy in helping people with a mental handicap to further develop the ways in which they communicate with other people – building on what the person can already do, however limited, rather than trying only to fill in gaps. Sternberg and Owens (1985) adapted procedures described by Van Dijk (1965) for use with deaf/blind students to establish pre-language signalling behaviour with students who were profoundly mentally handicapped. In these procedures the adult responded to any kind of movement produced by the students as if it were communicative, teaching them that their movements could affect, influence and change another person's behaviour.

Building interactions around actions and sounds

Children with profound mental and multiple handicaps who have not developed language and are unable to use a manual system of signing can become active partners in communication through the caregivers (parents or residential staff) creating a dialogue around his or her movements, facial expressions and vocalizations.

The following example shows how a caregiver helped communication in this way. A young child with profound multiple handicaps had very restricted body movements and was slower than normal in the time he took to respond to others. His caregiver discovered that he consistently responded with the same tiny movements when she patted, stroked and played with his hand, but that the gap between her doing this and the child's response was long. She responded to his looks, facial expressions and finger movements, treating them as words, and gave him time to take his turn. In this way the child was able to participate in interactions with her.

Some people with profound mental handicap clearly enjoy certain forms of movement play, such as being bounced vigorously or having their feet patted and, through many games based on what they enjoy, come to anticipate what will happen next. There are many ways in which they might show this anticipation, such as lifting a foot to have it patted again or raising their arms because they want the bouncing to continue. Some of these personal signals are more obscure, e.g. holding the body in a certain position, slightly inclining the head, or responding with tiny movements as in the previous example. By acting on these movements in a consistent way the adult can help the person with profound handicap to become aware that his or her actions can have an effect on others and that as well as responding, he or she can initiate and direct what will happen. It does seem that once a person has gained this awareness it is robust and can be generalized to other people and other situations. The person may lose interest in the original activities but still retains the knowledge that what he or she does can influence other people and will apply this knowledge to new interests.

Movement therapy

Movement therapy aims to develop communicative interactions with people with profound handicaps. Many of the methods used show striking similarities to the patterns of communication normally found in the earliest stages of development. Therapists who practise this form of movement therapy often work with the caregiver and person with profound handicaps together, so that the communication which is developed is part and parcel of their everyday life. It is important to remember that an interaction needs more than one person – it is *inter*action and what one person does will affect the other. The way in which the caregiver moves and speaks has as much of an effect on the interaction as the actions of the person who is handicapped.

Action cycles

Caregivers use many contact movements like tapping, patting and stroking during interactions. In a study of interactions between caregivers and children and young adults with profound handicaps, analysis of such actions – action cycles – showed that different caregivers all performed them at similar rates for similar communicative purposes (Burford, 1988). Although they used them much less frequently, the people with profound handicaps were also seen to use the same actions at similar rates during communication. Analysis of interactions between Scottish and Nigerian mothers and their non-handicapped babies revealed similar actions being performed at identical rates (Burford, 1988). This suggests that these rates play a very important role in communication and also that they probably have a biological basis.

The importance of timing in interactions

As well as deliberate actions such as patting and stroking, people use many spontaneous and less well-defined movements when they are communicating. The rates at which a person performs his or her movements and the ways in which he or she coordinates them with the movements and speech of the other person are crucial to the success of the communication.

This coordination is seen from the time of birth. Condon (1979) found that babies who were only 20 minutes old synchronized their movements with human speech, but not with regular, inanimate sounds. It is difficult to imagine how babies could learn to do this in such a short time and it is likely that this synchronization is an innate capacity.

The existence of a common timing for communicative movements, present from birth and unaffected by cultural influences, is supported by the findings of extensive research in many countries. Babies can respond to the communication movements of adults and initiate many such movements themselves (Bullowa, 1979). The rhythms and patterns of these movements are found in all human social interaction and are believed to be innate (Newson and Newson, 1975). Mothers are seen to establish a tempo suited to maintain the baby's attention and involvement (Stern, 1985). Microanalysis of interactions reveals that mother and infant coordinate with each other with a timing precise to a fraction of a second (Trevarthen, 1984). When the mother's response is interrupted, causing a disruption in her timing with what the baby is doing, babies show immediate distress (Murray and Trevarthen, 1984).

Condon (1979) noted how, in adult communication, a person's body movements were in precise synchrony with his or her speech and that the listener also moved in synchrony with the speech. Interactional synchrony has been observed in all normal human interactions, including those of non-literate cultures (Gordon, 1968). When adults talk to each other their movements coordinate with each other in a way that looks like a dance going to and fro (Kendon, 1970). A person is literally out-of-step with others if he or she cannot coordinate his or her movements with theirs. 'Out-of-sync' timing has an adverse effect immediately on the communication and ultimately on the development of relationships. It has been found that children with a wide range of learning difficulties do not respond to human speech with the same timing as is usually observed in non-handicapped children and that this difficulty increases with the severity of the child's condition (Condon, 1979; 1980).

However, although it is difficult, people do manage to develop some form of communication with those whose timing is disrupted in some way. The key to this success probably lies in the way in which the non-handicapped person fits in with what the person who is handicapped is doing, all the time coping with and adapting to the pauses that seem to go on forever, the response that takes ages to surface, the jerky movements that distract his or her attention, the words or movements that interrupt his or her turn. In this way the difficulties caused by a person's inability to coordinate his or her movements with others can be overridden and effective interpersonal contact can be established.

Summary

Non-verbal behaviour is present in all human interactions at all ages and in all cultures. It accompanies and complements speech and expresses moods and feelings. Cultures vary in their use of non-verbal behaviour and the importance of its 'correctness' makes it vital that people with a mental handicap are helped to assimilate the cultural rules as much as they can. The development of early communication provides helpful guidance for establishing and developing interactions with people with profound handicaps. One important aspect in all communication is timing. If timing is disrupted it has adverse effects, which can be minimized by other people adapting to the movements and timing of the person who is handicapped.

References

Buck, R. (1982) Spontaneous and symbolic nonverbal behaviour and the ontogeny of communication. In *Development of Nonverbal Behavior in Children* (ed. Feldman, R.S.). Springer-Verlag, New York

Buck, R. (1984) *The Communication of Emotion*. The Guildford Press, New York & London

Bruner, J. (1974) From communication to language – a psychological perspective. *Cognition*, **3**, 255–287

Bullowa, M. (1979) Prelinguistic communication: a field for scientific research. In *Before Speech: The Beginnings of Interpersonal Communication* (ed. Bullowa, M.). Cambridge University Press, Cambridge

Bullowa, M. (1975) When infant and adult communicate how do they synchronise their behaviors? In *Organisation of Behavior in Face-to-Face Interaction* (eds Kendon, A., Harris, R. and Key, M.). Mouton Publishers, The Hague

Burford, B. (1988) Action cycles: rhythmic actions for engagement with children and young adults with profound mental handicap. *European Journal of Special Needs Education*, **3**, No. 4, 189–206

Condon, W.S. (1968) Linguistic–kinesic research and dance therapy. *American Dance Association Proceedings*, 21–44

Condon, W.S. (1979) Neonatal entrainment and enculturation. In *Before Speech: The Beginnings of Interpersonal Communication* (ed. Bullowa, M.). Cambridge University Press, Cambridge

Condon, W.S. (1980) The relationship of interactional synchrony to cognitive and emotional processes. In *The Relationship of Verbal and Nonverbal Communication* (ed. Key, M.R.). Mouton Publishers, The Hague

Cooley, C. Horton (1902) Looking-Glass Self. In *Symbolic Interaction – a reader in social psychology* (eds Manis, J.G. and Meltzer, B.N.). Allyn and Bacon, Inc., Boston

Danziger, K. (1976) *Interpersonal Communication*. Pergamon Press Inc., Oxford

Eibl-Eibesfeldt, I. (1972) Similarities and differences between cultures in expressive movements. In *Nonverbal Communication* (ed. Hinde, R.A.). Cambridge University Press, Cambridge

Ekman, P. (1977) Biological and cultural contributions to body and facial movement. In *The Anthropology of the Body* (ed. Blacking, J.). Academic Press, London

Fraiberg, S. (1974) Blind infants and their mothers: an examination of the sign system. In *The Effect of the Infant on its Caregiver* (eds Lewis, M. and Rosenblum, L.A.). Wiley, New York

Hall, E.T. (1959) *The Silent Language*. Doubleday and Company, Inc., New York

Haviland, J.J. and Malatesta, C.Z. (1981) The development of sex differences in nonverbal signals: fallacies, facts and fantasies. In *Gender and Nonverbal Behavior* (eds Mayo, C. and Henley, N.). Springer-Verlag, New York

Kendon, A. (1970) Movement coordination in Dance Therapy and Conversation. Proceedings of Workshop in Dance Therapy: Its Research Potentials, pp. 64–69. Committee on Research in Dance, New York

Key, M.R. (1975) *Paralanguage and Kinesics*. The Scarecrow Press, Metuchen, NJ

Key, M.R. (ed.) (1980) *The Relationship of Verbal and Nonverbal Communication*. Mouton Publishers, The Hague

Leuder, I. (1981) Strategic communication in mental retardation. In *Communicating with Normal and Retarded Children* (eds Fraser, W.I. and Grieve, R.). John Wright and Sons Ltd, Bristol

Major, B. (1981) Gender patterns in touching. In *Gender and Nonverbal Behaviour* (eds Mayo, C. and Henley, N.). Springer-Verlag, New York

Mayo, C. and Henley, N.M. (1981) Nonverbal behaviours: barrier or agent for sex role change. In *Gender and Nonverbal Behavior*. (eds Mayo, C. and Henley, N.), Springer-Verlag, New York

Murray, L. and Trevarthen, C. (1984) Emotional regulation of interactions between two-month-olds and their mothers. In *Social Perception in Infants* (eds Field, T. and Fox, N.). Ablex, Norwood, NJ

Newson, J. (1979) The growth of shared understandings between infant and caregiver. In *Before Speech: The Beginnings of Interpersonal Communication* (ed. M. Bullowa). Cambridge University Press, Cambridge

Newson, J. and Newson, E. (1975) Intersubjectivity and the transmission of culture. *Bulletin of the British Psychological Society*, **28**, 437–46

Schaffer, H.R. (1977) Early interactive development. In *Studies in Mother–Infant Interaction* (ed. Schaffer, H.R.). Academic Press, London

Shanley, E. (ed.) (1986) *Mental Handicap: A Handbook of Care*. Churchill Livingstone, Edinburgh

Stern, D. (1977) *The First Relationship: Infant and Mother*. Fontana/Open Books, London

Stern, D. (1985) *The Interpersonal World of the Infant*. Basic Books, Inc., New York

Sternberg, L. and Owens, A. (1985) Establishing pre-language signalling behavior with profoundly mentally handicapped students: a preliminary investigation. *Journal of Mental Deficiency Research*, **29**

Trevarthen, C. (1984) How control of movement develops. In *Human Motor Actions – Bernstein Reassessed* (ed. Whiting, H.T.A.). Elsevier Science Publishers B.V., Amsterdam

Wiener, M., Devoe, S., Rubinow, S. and Geller, J. (1972) Nonverbal behaviour and nonverbal communication. *Psychological Review*, **79**, 185–214

Van Dijk, J. (1965) Motor development in the education of deaf-blind children. *Proceedings of the Conference on the Deaf-Blind, Refnes, Denmark*. Perkins School for the Blind, Boston

7

Managing difficult behaviours

7.1 Understanding behaviour disturbance

Peter Baker

Those involved in the care or teaching of children and adults with *learning disabilities* will undoubtedly come across individuals who exhibit disturbed behaviour. There is evidence that this group have a higher incidence of behaviour problems than the general population. Some authors have claimed that as many as 50–60% of people who have learning difficulties are likely also to present with a significant behaviour disorder.

What is behaviour disturbance?

A wide range of behaviours have traditionally been classified as disturbed. Two examples might indicate the extent of this range.

J.B. is a 39-year-old moderately handicapped man living in a staffed house in the community. Staff at the house and in his Training Centre have complained about his inappropriate speech. Typically he will greet them with one of his favourite phrases, e.g. bacon and eggs, new shoes. He will frequently repeat himself during conversations and change the subject inappropriately. It was claimed this severely affected his quality of life resulting in him being ostracized by those he lives and works with.

V.B. is a 20-year-old severely handicapped young man. He has lived in a hospital since he was 5 years old. He is currently living in sparsely furnished locked ward in a Mental Handicap Hospital. He has been labelled as extremely aggressive. He frequently attacks those around him, either biting, slapping or scratching. There is an added risk as he carries hepatitis B. Ward staff claim there is no pattern for his attacks, he will even strike out at those whom he appears to like and are engaging him in his favourite activities.

The term behaviour disturbance lacks specificity, covers a wide variety of behaviours and it tells us little about the actual behaviour and little about its causes. When the term is applied, perhaps it is more likely to tell us one of three things:

1. We do not understand why the person is behaving in this fashion.
2. The person's behaviour affects the smooth running of their environment.

3. The person's behaviour has violated the rules regarding the norms of conduct of their particular subculture.

The knowledge of these factors and the more recent changes in philosophy have led professionals in the field of mental handicap to examine the label behaviour disturbance. This examination has in turn led to the adoption of the term 'Challenging Behaviour'.

The basis for this change in terminology is that the previously used terms 'disturbed' or 'problem' imply that the difficulty lies within the individual. The term 'challenging behaviour' shifts the emphasis away from the individual to those who are providing a service for them.

Whilst applauding the sentiments behind this switch of labels, the term 'challenging behaviour' raises several problems and concerns:

1. There is even greater loss of specificity of description for those in teaching and caring. Many behaviours present a challenge ranging from the child who cannot dress themselves through to the adult who exhibits dangerous assultative behaviour.
2. The term challenging may imply that an individual is being deliberately provocative towards us.
3. Re-labelling a problem creates a false impression of having done something about it.
4. Re-labelling a problem creates a false impression of having understood it.
5. The labelling process itself forces us to think about people who exhibit such behaviour as an homogeneous group. This tempts us to think of blanket solutions, e.g. special units, specific techniques, etc. This detracts from planning around individuals.

For these reasons I will not use the term challenging behaviour but will refer to the general term behaviour disturbance with all the difficulties incumbent in that term. I will be an advocate for an approach based on the understanding of individuals.

However, before accepting that a particular individual is exhibiting disturbed behaviour, it should be considered very carefully for whom is this behaviour a problem. If the answer is that it disrupts the smooth running of an institution, then before pursuing the idea of that person being the problem, serious questions should be asked regarding the flexibility of the system the person is living in.

Why do we need to understand?

Faced with what can often seem to be overwhelming problems, carers and teachers understandably seek urgent answers to the questions of what can we do with these problems. The technology of behaviour modification has enjoyed the reputation of being able to offer the answers. Unfortunately there has been a tendency to use this technology in a cookbook fashion, with intervention strategies offered for particular problems without recourse to any understanding of why the individual is behaving in this fashion. This has undoubtedly led to a high rate of failure in practice and a subsequent disillusionment with the technology.

Describing the behaviour

Often people who exhibit difficult behaviours have a tendency to be labelled according to that behaviour: violent, aggressive, scratcher, head banger, self-injurious, etc. The unfortunate effect of this labelling is that the person's identity gets lost, including all the positive things about them.

We also tend to label people with reference to internal states; a person who overeats might be labelled greedy; a person who bangs on the walls and shouts, angry; a person who refuses to get out of bed, lazy. These references to internal states have their associated problems.

1. The first is it creates a false impression of understanding why the behaviour is occurring. We might then be satisfied with our explanation that the individual who will not get up is lazy, missing the fact that he is having problems at work and is attempting to avoid them by not getting up.
2. The second problem is that this form of labelling is imprecise. We cannot see laziness or anger, but can only guess that this is the internal state that is making the person behave in this manner. Thus if two people independently observed a person red in the face and jumping up and down, one might say the person is angry, the other excited, thus offering two completely different explanations for the same behaviour, neither of which tells us anything about the cause.
3. The third problem is that once applied, labels tend to stick and everything that person does is interpreted in the light of that label. Every time the greedy person eats, it is because of greediness and not hunger. Every time the lazy person refuses to do something it is due to laziness rather than the suitability or lack of suitability of the task. Every time the angry person asserts themselves they are perceived as angry rather than having a legitimate need that is somehow being denied.

An important first step in understanding why an individual is exhibiting a difficult behaviour is therefore to describe the actual behaviour in very precise, i.e. observable, objective and measurable terms. Thus at this stage we will throw out the guesswork and not describe the behaviour with reference to internal states that we cannot see, but say precisely what the person does, how often they do it and to what severity. Therefore, 'James played up' will not be an acceptable description of the behaviour, but, 'James shouted and ran about the room upsetting furniture and pinching the teacher for 5 minutes', would be acceptable.

Looking for the cause

Once the behaviour has been precisely described the next step is to look at the relationship of that behaviour to the individual's environment. A behavioural approach rests on the assumption that any behaviour is determined by what happens before it and what happens after it.

This approach has various names, including applied behavioural analysis, functional analysis, all of which simply describe the process where the observer will seek to make clear the following:

1. *Antecedents* – The settings in which the behaviour occurs and the specific trigger within that setting.

2. *Behaviour* – What the person actually does, how often and to what severity.
3. *Consequences* – What happens immediately after the behaviour.
This can easily be remembered as the *A B C* of understanding behaviour.

Consequences

What happens after the behaviour occurs determines the likelihood of that behaviour being repeated. If the individual perceives the consequences of their behaviour as good or to their advantage, they are likely to behave in that way again. Alternatively, if they perceive the consequences as bad or adversive, they are less likely to repeat the behaviour. This is a simple law which lies at the foundation of the behavioural approach.

An important point to which we will return later is that it is the individual's perception of the consequences as good or bad that is important, not ours. You might find the idea of touching or smelling faeces repulsive, but the individual who indulges in such behaviour might well find these sensations pleasant and thus is likely to continue to indulge in such behaviours.

Consequences of behaviours are classified as either reinforcers or punishment.

Reinforcement

Any consequence that makes the behaviour more likely to occur is called a reinforcer. Just as when we reinforce concrete by the setting of iron girders it becomes strengthened, so when we reinforce behaviour it also becomes strengthened. There are two types of reinforcement. Positive and negative.

Positive reinforcement occurs when an individual's behaviour is followed by something they see as pleasant. For example, a trainee in an Adult Training Centre enjoyed the attention of staff. He had learnt that if he picked fights with other trainees this resulted in him receiving a lot of attention from staff. Thus something this individual saw as pleasant, staff attention, follows the behaviour of fighting. Therefore fighting is positively reinforced and is more likely to occur in the future.

Negative reinforcement occurs when an individual behaviour is followed by the termination of something seen as unpleasant, e.g. a child who does not like going into shops will become disruptive whenever his mother takes him into a shop, resulting in her making a hurried exit. Thus something this child sees as unpleasant, being in a shop, is removed following his descriptive behaviour. This behaviour is negatively reinforced and is likely to re-occur in the future.

Obviously exactly the same consequences rarely follow a behaviour every time. Such consistency is an unusual occurrence in the real world. When a gambler plays a fruit machine he is not rewarded every time he puts money in but receives a reward now and again, yet he continues to put money in the machine. This is called *intermittent reinforcement* and is a common occurrence. Reinforcement does not have to follow a behaviour every time it occurs for that behaviour to persist. In fact, if a behaviour is rewarded intermittently, or every now and again, it is more difficult to get rid of. If we rig a fruit machine so that it no longer pays out, the gambler will continue to play the machine; he does not expect a reward every time thus it will take a long time for him to realize that the rewards are not forthcoming. If we compare him with a person buying a drink from a machine, they would only need to experience lack of reward, i.e. no drink, once for them to stop the behaviour of putting money into the machine.

Punishment
This occurs when something the individual perceives as unpleasant follows their behaviour. When a behaviour is punished, in this sense, it is less likely to occur, e.g. when a child touches a hot fire, this behaviour is followed by something the child is likely to see as unpleasant – pain. Thus the behaviour is punished and unlikely to occur again.

Many people confuse negative reinforcement with punishment. The simple way to differentiate is that negative reinforcement leads to behaviour increasing in frequency. Punishment leads to a decrease in frequency.

When considering the consequences of an individual's disturbed behaviour we are attempting to discover the possible reinforcers of that behaviour. In other words what are the gains that person receives? It is important that we do not only look for consequences we might consider pleasant. A reinforcer for that individual might well be something we would find unpleasant. We should also be looking for something the person sees as unpleasant stopping as a result of their behaviour as it may well be negatively reinforced. Finally, remember that the consequence need not occur every time for it to be important in the causation of the behaviour.

Antecedents

An individual rarely exhibits disturbed behaviour at all times. If we try to understand why a behaviour occurs, identifying what happens prior to the occurrence of that behaviour that is different from that which happens when the behaviour does not occur, might help us. This we will refer to as the antecedents.

When considering antecedents we should look at two differents levels of analysis. The broader settings within which the behaviour occurs, and the more specific triggers within those settings.

Broad settings
The broad settings in which behaviour occurs can be viewed as factors that are internal or external. These types of experiences are often couched in vague terms but do have some common meaning. *External factors* would include tension and conflict between people in the individual's environment, creating conditions where disturbed behaviour is likely to occur. Periods of change and upheaval might leave the individual unsettled, this might include moving away from home, or changing from school to a more adult setting. Bereavement also increases the likelihood of descriptive behaviour.

General levels of stimulation within the person's environment might well be affecting behaviour. An under-stimulating environment with few meaningful activities or interaction might predispose to disturbed behaviour. Similarly, an environment with too much stimulation – i.e. noise, movement etc. – might equally precipitate disturbed behaviour.

These types of factor are generally seen by all people as stressful. In a person with limited comprehension and impaired ability to articulate their feelings, the stressful aspects of these experiences are likely to be compounded. It must never be assumed that individuals with a mental handicap are impervious to the effects of these life events.

Internal factors that would influence an individual's behaviour would include states such as fatigue, hunger, thirst and pain. The incidence of psychiatric illness in individuals with a mental handicap is a matter of some debate; however, few people would deny that people with a mental handicap are at least as susceptible to psychiatric illness as the general population. An individual with a mental handicap who is suffering from some form of psychiatric illness would display a change in their behaviour. With psychosis this would probably be disturbed behaviour.

Specific triggers
We have stated that a behaviour is more likely to occur if it is followed by consequences that the individual perceives to be pleasant (positive reinforcement), or the removal of something they perceive to be unpleasant (negative reinforcement). The trigger or stimuli would be an event in that person's environment that would signal that the positive reinforcer was available or that the adversive event was going to occur, from which usually the individual would attempt to escape. Once the individual has observed the trigger, the disturbed behaviour would result. An example would be a child who self-injures in order to avoid work at school. In the past she has learnt that if she hits her head at school she will receive attention from the teacher (positive reinforcement). She has also learnt that the teacher will no longer continue to make demands on her, thus something she sees as unpleasant is removed (negative reinforcement). In this situation where self-injurious behaviour is both negatively and positively reinforced in school, it is likely that the incidence of this behaviour would be higher within this environment. We would observe that the broad setting of the school was an important antecedent factor. As it is one particular teacher who provided the reinforcement, it is likely that she will be the trigger. In this scenario, we would predict that the incidence of self-injurious behaviour would be generally higher at school and it would increase further in frequency in the presence of the particular teacher.

How do we find the causes?

It is necessary to observe the individual directly to obtain information regarding the actual nature of the behaviour disturbance and the potential antecedents and consequences. The methods available include paper and pencil techniques, filming and taping. Event recorders and micro-computers may add a degree of accuracy, reliability and sophistication to the basic data which can be gathered using pencil and paper techniques. The format of this is illustrated in Table 7.1. The need to use concrete behavioural description is important. If the targeted behaviour was hair pulling, to describe the antecedents as 'became upset' and the consequence as 'eventually calmed him down' would be almost worthless. To be useful, information such as 'requested to complete reading work' and 'cuddled him and removed the work' would need to be gathered.

Summary

The term disturbed behaviour covers a wide variety of behaviours. Its use is determined by many factors including the actual behaviour, our degree of understanding and the expectation of a particular subculture. It is necessary to understand the cause of disturbed behaviour within an individual to provide an effective management programme.

Table 7.1 Behaviour observation chart

Antecedents: What occurred immediately prior to the behaviour	Behaviour: Describe behaviour in full	Consequences: What occurred immediately after the behaviour

Using a behavioural analytical approach we can attempt to understand why the behaviour occurs. Part of this approach is to describe the behaviour in concrete unambiguous terms. The approach rests on the assumption that the behaviour is determined by what happens before and after it occurs. Therefore, for a full understanding, we need to be aware of the antecedents, the broad settings in which the behaviour appears and the specific triggers immediately prior to the behaviour as well as the consequences for the individual of the behaviour. Direct observation of the individual is required to elucidate these factors.

7.2   A behavioural approach to management of behaviour disturbance

Peter Baker

As stressed in the previous section the perception of carers that a certain individual exhibits disturbed behaviour is not wholly influenced by that individual's actual behaviour. Therefore before considering any intervention, the question 'for whom is the behaviour a problem?' needs to be addressed. If the answer is that it is genuinely a problem for the individual exhibiting the behaviour, in as much as it severely restricts their development or their quality of life, then a behavioural intervention is clearly needed. Indeed it would be unethical not to attempt to reduce these problem behaviours.

We have established that people's behaviours are determined largely by the reaction of their environment to that behaviour. The behaviours have a meaning in as much as they achieve important results for that person. Therefore a knowledge and understanding of the results the particular behaviour achieves will allow us to manipulate the triggers or consequences of the disturbed behaviour in order to make its recurrence less likely. A knowledge of the function of a particular behaviour will also enable us to select a skill or alternative behaviour which, if taught, will achieve the same important result that the disturbed behaviour achieves.

Altering antecedents

A knowledge of what typically occurs prior to the disturbed behaviour will enable us to effect the likelihood of the recurrence of that behaviour. This can be achieved by either eliminating the antecedents or altering their meaning for the particular individual. As we did in the previous section we will look both at the broad settings in which the behaviour occurs and the specific triggers that precede the behaviour.

Altering broad settings

External or environmental factors will always need to be altered at some level. Questions of under- or over-stimulation are of particular relevance, especially in institutional settings. Altering the amount of meaningful activities and interactions within a setting will have a direct effect on the recipients. However, it should be remembered that it is the individual's perception of the pleasantness of the stimulation that determines their response. There is a possibility that some people, especially those made vulnerable by physical or sensory handicaps, might perceive a sudden increase in levels of stimulation as threatening. If this is the case, a gradual introduction of higher levels of stimulation coupled with reassurance is required.

Tension and conflict in an environment are likely to make the occurrence of disturbed behaviour more likely, but is more difficult to prescribe solutions for. Professional counselling may be required if this occurs in the family. In professional settings effective management and staff support are necessary.

As mentioned in the previous section, coping with times of change is difficult for all of us but is arguably more so in somebody with limited ability to understand and express themselves. In planned change a gradual approach with support and genuine consultation with the individual should be made available. In unplanned change such as bereavement, counselling should be provided, along with access to those things that help all of us come to terms with the death of a close person, e.g. attending the funeral, visiting the grave, keeping photographs, etc. In the past these activities have commonly been denied to people with a mental handicap. This is usually so as not to upset the person unnecessarily. These activities and rituals ordinarily serve the function of enabling the process of acceptance of the death of loved ones. It can be argued that in someone with limited comprehension and ability to communicate they are even more important.

Internal states precipitating disturbed behaviour will need to be remediated. Sleep problems causing tiredness ought to be addressed by either changing those environmental factors contributing to the difficulty of sleeping, or the prescription of medication. Thirst and hunger need to be detected and remediated, as will pain or psychiatric illness which would again perhaps require medication.

Altering specific triggers

A trigger or stimuli signals to the person that a reward is available or that something bad is going to happen (in turn leading to escape behaviour). If we therefore decide to intervene at this point in the chain we should either make sure the trigger does not occur or try to alter the person's perception of the meaning of the trigger and associated reinforcers.

If the behaviour has a highly specific trigger, removal of that trigger will result in a decrease in the associated behaviour. In our example of the teacher who provides positive and negative reinforcement for the child's self-injurious behaviour, the removal of that particular teacher will result in a decrease in the associated self-injury. This type of approach may well create problems and is perhaps, at best, a short-term solution. The teacher may well be the only one available, therefore the removal would mean the child receives no teaching. In addition it is unlikely that the teacher alone is the specific trigger and the actual environment of the classroom and the school have become triggers in themselves. In this case removal of the teacher would not result in a decrease in disturbed behaviour if the child continues to be taught in the same environment. The phenomena of disturbed behaviour being specific to one environment is quite common. Parents will often observe that their child behaves quite differently at school than they do at home.

In many cases it is not always possible to remove specific triggers as they are often necessary for the individual's quality of life and development. When disturbed behaviour is clearly communicating that the individual finds the presence of the carer/teacher aversive, i.e. they are telling us to go away, we cannot simply remove the demands that are being made. In these cases the triggers meaning for the individual needs to be changed. This can be done by altering the consequences (to be discussed later) of the behaviour or by trying to get the trigger associated with more pleasant events. In the example of our self-injurious child we might encourage the teacher to provide, in addition to her demands to complete school work, demands to engage in activities the child likes, e.g. eating sweets, going on outings. This would have the effect of weakening the association of the teacher with only aversive events. In practice these new associations will take time to occur and if attempted should continue for a long enough period for the new associations to be made.

Some individuals may have difficulties in differentiating between when demands are being made and when they are not. This confusion would result in high frequency of escape motivated behaviour, i.e. behaviour that communicates that the individual wants the demands to go away. In such cases the introduction of a *safety signal* might serve to decrease the frequency of the disturbed behaviour. A safety signal is something in the environment that would consistently signal that an aversive event is absent. An example might be a severely handicapped adult who exhibits severely self-injurious behaviour at bath times, clearly communicating that she found the experience of the bath aversive. Unfortunately this behaviour occurs at other times, and appears also to be triggered by the presence of staff. It was thought there might have been some confusion in this lady as to whether the staff were going to offer a bath or not. The incidents of self-injurious behaviour at times other than bathing is decreased by staff wearing plastic aprons only when approaching the individual at bath times and not at others. Thus the absence of plastic aprons became a safety signal that the staff were not going to put her in the bath. Thus avoiding the necessity for her to indulge in the self-injurious behaviour.

Altering consequences

A frequently occurring behaviour is usually followed by consequences that the person sees as advantageous; these are called reinforcers. If these reinforcers are no longer made available the behaviour will be less likely to occur. This process or procedure is called *extinction*; just as when we extinguish a fire it dies, extinction refers to the behaviour dying.

If a behaviour is being positively reinforced by attention, for example, removing the attention will result in the behaviour decreasing. If the teacher stopped cuddling our self-injurious child each time she hit her head, this behaviour would be likely to extinguish. Other examples might include: stop giving the child who cries at night a drink to calm them; the adult who throws their dinner is no longer rewarded by others cleaning up.

Some behaviours are maintained not by outside reinforcers but by the sensations they create. For example, 'eye gouging' will produce a 'flash' sensation in the eye for the person who engages in this; people might enjoy the noise that banging against reverberating objects makes; an individual who smears faeces might enjoy the texture and the smell. The process of cutting out the reward from these behaviours is called *sensory extinction*. Not all of these examples would be amenable to this procedure, but in the example of head banging a pillow could be placed between the head and the reverberating object, thus eliminating the rewarding sensation of the noise. We could endeavour to mask the smell of faeces with a smell the individual might consider to be noxious.

A procedure commonly used to alter the consequences of disturbed behaviour is *time-out*. Unfortunately time-out is often confused with seclusion. Time-out should provide a positive learning experience whereas seclusion is just a punishment. Time-out is the short form of 'time-out from positive reinforcement'. The procedure usually involves the removal of the individual from the environment in which the disturbed behaviour occurs. This environment, it is assumed, contains positive reinforcers of that behaviour. The person is removed for a set minimum period of time, and is reintroduced after that minimum period of time has elapsed, providing they behave appropriately. There are other variants that might include removing yourself from the individual exhibiting the disturbed behaviour by either turning away or actually leaving the room. To use time-out properly it is essential to understand the causes of the behaviour. When an individual is exhibiting disturbed behaviour to escape from demand situations, it will obviously be wrong to use time-out, as this will be reinforcing the disturbed behaviour by allowing the individual to escape from the demands. The following points are guidelines for the use of time-out:

1. Time-out should be based on an understanding of the cause of the targeted behaviour.
2. Time-out should be short (2–5 minutes) to be maximally effective.
3. The period should be specified in advance.
4. The individual should be unobtrusively observed if placed in a separate room.
5. The release from time-out should occur at the end of the pre-determined length of time, providing the individual is behaving appropriately. In other words, release has to be earned by good behaviour.
6. A maximum length of time in time-out should be determined in advance.
7. Records of length of time and those responsible should be kept in order to prevent abuse of the procedure.

When utilizing an extinction programme the phenomena known as *extinction-burst* should be expected. In an extinction programme the disturbed behaviour is no longer reinforced, the individual will consequently feel that they have not tried hard enough, leading to an increase in severity and frequency of the disturbed behaviour. This increase will, in an effective programme, eventually fall as the realization that the reinforcers are no longer available sets in. If this is expected the programme is less likely to be abandoned at this point, when it is assumed that it hasn't worked.

For an extinction programme to be maximally effective consistency is essential. Consistency in this case refers to everybody withholding the reinforcement at all times. If this is not the case the disturbed behaviour will become intermittently reinforced and therefore more resistant to extinction.

Punishment

Punishment is a way of altering the consequence of behaviour, in as much as an aversive consequence is applied in order to counteract the reinforcer. Serious ethical considerations are raised in the use of punishment for people who are vulnerable to being perceived as devalued. The application of punishment is based upon dominance and power; this can result in subservience and helplessness in the recipients. Punishment will also hinder the promotion of independence and the promotion of a positive image of people with a mental handicap as valued citizens. Punishment also suffers from not providing the opportunities for the individual to learn new skills.

When *time-out* is not based upon removal of the specific reinforcers for a behaviour this is technically a punishment. Positive reinforcers in this case is a less specific term and refers to things in the environment the person likes. Time-out in this sense refers to the systematic removal of some or all of these things.

Response-cost has generally been used within token economies. This is a procedure where individuals are given tokens to reward appropriate behaviours. These tokens can in turn be exchanged for reinforcers, e.g. sweets, outings, etc. Response-cost is the action of taking tokens away following disturbed behaviour. It is also used as a system of fining, where individuals are not given money that they would have otherwise earned. Research has indicated that this procedure is only effective when the individual has few tokens or money and/or little opportunity to earn more.

Over-correction is a procedure developed to add an educational aspect to punishment. It generally involves two separate procedures, restitution and positive practice. The restitution phase refers to the returning of the situation to a vastly improved state and positive practice requires the individual to practise appropriate behaviours where he usually misbehaves. For example, a child with night-time wetting may be required to strip and re-make their bed (restitution) and practise getting out of bed, going to the toilet, sitting, flushing the toilet and washing their hands, several times (positive practice).

Restraint may be used to decrease disturbed behaviour. This may involve degrees of restriction of movement from the whole body to one small part. Similar rules should be applied to that suggested for time-out.

Aversion therapy is a well-known treatment although its use is limited. It involves the introduction of physically noxious stimulation immediately following the maladaptive behaviour. A large number of stimuli have been used, ranging from unpleasant mouthwashes through to electric shocks.

All of these punishment procedures raise serious ethical concerns. Treatment of choice should always be the more constructive approaches outlined in this section. A technique that uses the infliction of pain and discomfort needs a clear justification. The only imaginable circumstances for its use might be for those behaviours that are life threatening.

Skills teaching approaches

A skills teaching approach would look to teaching or building up new skills which if performed would make the occurrence of the disturbed behaviour less likely. This approach can also be referred to as *Differential Reinforcement of Other Behaviours (DRO)*; this approach varies in the specificity of the replacement behaviours to be reinforced. A general skills teaching environment may be set up where it is hoped that providing independent living skills will somehow lead to a reduction in disturbed behaviour. More specifically, skills or behaviours that are incompatible with the disturbed behaviours might be reinforced. Examples might be rewarding a child that screams for talking normally; he cannot scream and talk normally at the same time. Rewarding somebody who bangs their head for holding their hands by their side – two incompatible behaviours. The teaching of relaxation techniques have been used in behaviours that are thought to have an anxiety element. The assumption here is that the individual cannot be anxious and relaxed at the same time. In many cases a DRO programme can quite simply be reinforcing the individual for not behaving in a disturbed fashion. An example might be providing a child with a reward at the end of each day in which they do not have a temper tantrum.

A more sophisticated use of a DRO would be to base the skill to be taught on the analysis of the communicative intent of the behaviour. In other words, we would try to give the individual a more appropriate way of communicating the message that they communicate through their disturbed behaviour. For example, WG is a profoundly multiply handicapped adult living in a hospital ward. He has no speech, but actively tries to communicate. He is a person who likes routine; when this is disrupted he will try to inform those around him of what he requires. If they do not comply immediately he will have quite severe temper tantrums, often harming himself by overturning his wheelchair. The disturbed behaviour communicates that routine has not been adhered to and this should be rectified. A programme was devised using a communication board whereby he could point to the photographs and drawings which made his intentions more clear. This resulted in a subsequent reduction in the frequency of tantrums.

Summary and conclusion

By basing an intervention for disturbed behaviour on an understanding of why the behaviour occurs we have access to options that do not rely upon the infliction of degrading experiences on those who we choose to help. Traditionally, a behavioural approach has concentrated only on the manipulation of consequences and the application of punishment. This is now neither justified nor necessary.

7.3 The intensive treatment service

Ann M. Green and Bill Fraser

The Centre for Human Policy at the University of Syracuse provides several principles common to the best practices for people with challenging behaviours (University of Syracuse Centre for Human Policy, 1986):

1. An absolute commitment to community integration.
2. Problem behaviours are not seen as part of a person but as caused by interaction of all the elements present in the environment in which the behaviours are exhibited. All people do things for a reason: behaviour has a meaning for the person exhibiting it. It is the task of service providers to try to understand this meaning.
3. Persons feel more secure with fewer people to relate to, and in smaller residential settings have a greater sense of control over their lives.
4. The best practices are often to be found in the smallest agencies where everyone continues to be directly involved with the people being served.
5. Generally people with challenging behaviours should not be gathered together in large numbers: people who already show challenging behaviours may learn new ones; and the staff have to spend time controlling the group rather than any individual. (However, to put a person with severe challenging behaviour with other disabled people who may not show such problems, also creates ethical problems.)
6. The place where a person with a handicap lives is first and foremost a home and a human service setting only second. The home and the programmes should be structured to the needs of the person and not vice versa.
7. Flexibility is required in human services. The more policy, union rules and procedures there are the less sensitive may be the approach. This is particularly important for short-term crisis relief.
8. Intervention should be positive. The idea of 'extinguishing' the problem behaviour when it has an important communicative function is unacceptable. It is vital to consider rather developing socially valued behaviours which are either incompatible with undesirable behaviour or make the problem behaviour unnecessary.
9. There ought to be an open-door policy which places no impediment in the way of relationships with families, friends and neighbours, or in the use of generic services.
10. There has to be an effective array of services to support the carer and the person with challenging behaviour: this may include a 24-hour on-call community team, homemaker aids, respite and small enough caseloads to

ensure that managers (i.e. social workers, psychologists, teachers and nurses) have real involvement where the problems are.
11. The direct service provider is not simply a personal attendant but is involved in planning and facilitating community integration, so that there is a 'bottom up' planning system and professional consultants are supportive rather than hierarchical and 'top down' in their approach.

These basic tenets have been elaborated by Blunden and Allen (1987): 'to enable the person eventually to take control of his or her own life, not to take that control away'. Blunden and Allen also see no quick and easy solutions. There has to be investment in staffing services, and the timescales for programmes are lengthy.

Challenging behaviours often develop over many years and there may be a complex range of causal and maintaining factors. Knowledge of why a behaviour started years ago may not be much help in deciding what to do now. It is much more important to understand the present situation, even imperfectly. Blunden and Allen emphasize how important it is, particularly with people with communication problems, to try to feel oneself into their predicament.

Service design

Blunden and Allen address the problem of where can a person with challenging behaviour stay, and particularly the case for and against Intensive Treatment Units – from which, according to the name, people will be returned 'treated' after a short stay. They list the points for such a special Unit:

1. The Unit provides a very controlled environment.
2. The Unit has the capacity to contain episodes of very challenging behaviour; for physical or medical restraint without causing disturbances to others; and conversely, allows the individual to be taken off medication and perhaps have anticonvulsants changed, with less risk.
3. Staff obtain particular expertise in assessing and dealing with difficult behaviours.
4. The environment can be customized to deal with extremely hazardous behaviours such as pica, swallowing the contents of ashtrays, going on to main roads, etc.
5. The Unit can be a resource centre to which all the services of the area can turn for help and advice.

Blunden and Allen also itemize difficulties that the establishment of special Units creates:

1. Removing individuals to an alternative Unit for treatment makes little sense if they then go back to the previous setting which has not modified what may be the causal or maintaining factors in the behaviour disturbances; thus, as special Units usually work in semi-isolation, it is important that they have an outreach team. (In fact, there ought to be more emphasis on the outreach team than on the base service.)
2. Labelling as 'ex-special Unit client' might occur.
3. An atypical environment exists in the special units and because of the high tension, staff may have to be reactive in dealing with problem behaviours rather than pro-active.

4. The number of people who require such a specialist Unit is likely to be very small. (We have no accurate estimate of the prevalence of extreme behaviour disturbances that require a highly specialized Unit. This varies with the threshold for tolerance of services. One place per 100000 is one common guess in the UK.) Thus the Unit is potentially quite a distance from the family and community that the person with a mental handicap has come from.
5. A centralized Unit tends by its very existence to lower the threshold of tolerance of other services and may prevent the development of more widespread locally based skills.
6. A Unit will be used by some as a place of first resort.
7. It is accepted that most severe challenging behaviours are the products of years of spiralling circles of failed communication and ineffective interventions, that such people may have become very chronically disabled, and that the prospect for improvement, even in the long term, may be limited. Short-stay intensive treatment services then are likely to become repositories for people with extreme behaviour and 'silt up'.
8. Staff in specialized Units may come to be considered either élitist or conversely may become isolated and demoralized.

It remains our view at present that the case for these Units is unproved but in the absence of an alternative, it is at least a start in addressing the problem of challenging behaviour. To maximize success services have to be provided on a time-limited basis with a clear multi-disciplinary individual plan for the treatment and subsequent maintenance care on the severely disturbed person.

There are a number of alternative service designs which may augment, complement or replace challenging behaviour services based on specialized Units:

1. Specialist teams whose primary responsibility is the development of new services for people with challenging behaviour, e.g. the specialist development team of the South East Thames Health Authority and University of Kent.
2. Specialist teams whose primary function is to support people with challenging behaviour in existing local services. These focus on providing intensive support for individuals in the course of their normal daily lives.
3. The attachment of specialist staff to existing community support teams, e.g. Community Mental Handicap Teams.
4. Establishing posts, e.g. project officers, with a specific brief for enhancing the ability of existing services to cope with people with challenging behaviour.
5. Establishing a 'flying squad' of expert local staff to cope with crises.

Again the problems inherent in the arguments for and against Intensive Treatment Units to some extent apply also to alternative strategies. Although such services could undoubtedly cope with all but those people whose behaviour presents a danger to themselves or others, the question is 'at what cost?' Society at present may not be prepared to accept the very considerable cost of care and support in the community of even a small number of such individuals. Moreover, the service system also has to take account of the wide range of threshold of tolerance for stress of caregivers. Our current view is that an integrated service, combining the advantages of a specialized unit with the flexibility of an outreach community service presents a useful way forward.

Service delivery

An Intensive Treatment Unit must involve care and treatment planning systems which fit the nursing process with staff members being allocated the responsibility of coordinating delivery of care to one or two individuals from admission through to discharge. Unit staff may subdivide into small management-of-care teams providing nursing care for the group of two or three clients. Each team will usually be coordinated by a Charge Nurse in consultation with a psychologist, and will devise individual care programmes for their group of clients. The Coordinator/Nurse in Charge ensures that residents have relevant, appropriate and achievable goals set; that the measurement of progress is clearly recorded; and that staff are trained to approach each client as someone who requires to be educated in order that the deficits in their repertoire are removed or reduced and their general social and personal skills are increased or enhanced.

Clients therefore cease to be 'problems' to be coped with and become *people* who present a challenge and an opportunity for change and development. The skills, however meagre, that each person with a handicap has must be built on. The Charge Nurse certainly must employ 'room management' procedures to ensure that the signals and repertoires of every person with a mental handicap are noticed, facilitated and enhanced. The psychologist, doctor and charge nurses require to inculcate a team attitude which positively supports the management of change and promotes the ability of team members to produce individually tailored treatment programmes with clear goal plans.

The whole team implements the programmes, records observations and results, suggests changes and documents effectiveness. Care teams will review and evaluate programmes of care and treatment on a weekly basis. Wherever possible, psychotropic medication can be stopped on admission and the effects closely monitored. It is particularly important that night staff are fully involved in planning, programmes and recording, as many daytime problems are a reflection of sleep apnoea, nocturnal agitation and fits.

Recording may involve listing and describing interactions between staff and residents; noting seizure frequencies and mood changes; and detailing aspects of behaviour disturbances as labelled in checklists (see elsewhere) and customized charts. When an individual leaves his usual place of residence, whether he comes from his home or a hospital, it is vital to consider his rights, and these may well best be protected by detention under the Mental Health Act. This is particularly important if treatments may involve short periods of *de facto* detention, e.g. restraint or Time Out.

Individuals within Intensive Treatment Unit settings require structured daily routines incorporating therapeutic input from a wide range of therapists and services both inside and outside the Unit. Each client should have a full timetable schedule of activities and appropriate therapies. Each therapy session should consist of a period of structured activity geared to the individual's needs and attention span and allow time for recording observations.

Individual programmes may include Occupational Therapy, Movement Therapy, Arts and Craft, Education, Physiotherapy, Speech Therapy, Play Therapy, Use of Computers, and Music Therapy as available. Other activities may include soft play, aquatherapy, trampolines, transport for excursions, horseriding for the disabled, etc.

Thus an Intensive Treatment Unit provides a structured environment in which clients can be observed and assessed under conditions which could not be met elsewhere, and their behaviour and communications clearly documented, recorded and various interventions tried and compared. The person can be provided with individual multi-disciplinary action plans (e.g. I.P.P. system for long- and short-term goals) and with an increased range of therapeutic and recreational activities both in hospital and in the local community. Difficulties encountered in the commissioning and running of an Intensive Treatment Unit most fundamentally tend to centre around staff attitudes, orientation and training. Often staff may come from a forensic, adult psychiatric or mental handicap hospital background and find it difficult to move to a developmental approach. The setting (e.g. the hospital or hostel) from which the client originally came may not share the developmental attitude; it may be reluctant to readmit clients on completion of treatment; and staff may be sceptical whether change will be maintained, and this may be a reasonable doubt if there have been no radical changes to their original environment in which problem behaviours occurred. It may be difficult to obtain alternative placements for clients leaving the Unit as their reputations go before them. There are problems also of maintaining a treatment programme because many therapists work 9 to 5, five days a week.

It is in this context that an integrated outreach team supporting the client and the staff of the community setting may be a crucial factor in skill transfer and the maintenance of behaviour change.

Monitoring and evaluation

Programmes of intensive treatment require consistent and systematic implementation, detailed monitoring and regular evaluation to maximize effectiveness and minimize the period of time during which clients are removed from their normal lifestyles and settings.

Referring settings need to identify priority areas of concern; state the individual problems and needs; and carry out basic frequency counts of behaviour disturbances (e.g. head-banging, physical aggression) prior to admission to an Intensive Treatment Unit.

Basic observation checklists can be drawn up and used both before and during treatment in the Unit. Once a client is in the Unit, these checklists can be monitored and collated on a daily basis; and information can be summarized for discussion at clinical team meetings on a weekly and monthly basis. Computer and video equipment may be used to facilitate the collection of information and encourage reliable record-keeping. On discharge, staff from the referring setting together with the Outreach Team should continue to monitor behaviour for say, 2–4 weeks, and then one week out of four for a further 6 months.

Where the causes of behaviour disturbance are hard to fathom, functional analysis of multiple aberrant responses is possible by time-sampling handicapped people who show challenging behaviour in analogue settings, e.g. observing the person with a mental handicap alone, in unstructured play and under academic demand; and this may shed light on what is triggering, for example, breath-holding or head-banging (see Communicative Functions). Hand-held recorders, e.g. the Psion Organiser, lap-top computers such as the EPSON or the Amstrad p.p.c. 640, can be used to collect data in real time, or form portable video units for on-ward behaviour recording. The hand-held computer and the portable p.p.c. can both download onto larger IBM computers and vice versa.

It is important that programme and service evaluations focus on process and outcome. Service design and delivery should be linked with a system of evaluation which has clearly defined measures. In the context of the Intensive Treatment Unit that the present authors were instrumental in setting up, Cheseldine (unpublished observations) offered the following approach during the first year of operation:

1. Change in the individual – detailed behavioural observations which show changes in problem behaviours; changes to the adaptive behaviours repertoire; the relationship between different aspects in an individual's behaviour, e.g. epileptic seizures, changes in medication, requests to perform tasks, and number of aggressive outbursts; and identification of the function of behaviours in its context, e.g. does the frequency of the behaviour alter in context of demand, no stimulation and overstimulation?
2. Changed behaviour in the base setting from which the person came (e.g. a group home, hospital ward) – when the client is removed, what changes in quality of life, adaptive skills and behaviour of the other residents occur?
3. Length of stay and place of discharge.
4. Behaviour on return to referring ward or setting – behaviours are largely environmentally controlled both for initial cause and subsequent maintenance and improvement in Intensive Treatment Units such as we describe may be simply due to an overall improvement in the quality of life.
5. Measures of the comparative effectiveness of specific forms of interventions – interventions need to be consistently applied and constantly monitored, and a combination of intervention techniques will have an effect in building new skills to reduce opportunities for frustration.
6. Reduction in medication – psychotropic drugs, as distinct from anticonvulsants, are usually correlated with the severity of the behaviour problems. Reduction in total medication can therefore be used as a measure of outcome.

A prerequisite for good practice and skilled performance is that the Unit is run by staff who have experience and training established by workshops and guided practice as described by Cullen (1987).

It is important that staff know how to measure the contingency sensitivity of the environments that the client inhabits and will inhabit, that is, the extent to which the person with a mental handicap receives responses that are contingent on the person's own actions, and is given opportunities to respond contingently to the actions of others. We know from special education that children with profound and multiple learning difficulties may often receive no response to their actions. Client engagement can be measured by a modified form of P.L.A. check (Rusley and Cataldo, 1972) developed by Ware and Evans (1987). The resettlement of a client involves 'ecoanalysing' of the place he is living in after discharge and recognition that 'minor' staff changes in terms of different personalities may make massive climatic changes for the person with a mental handicap. An extremely overactive individual, used to plenty of space, resettled in a tiny terraced house with pool staff caregivers is not uncommon.

Services to offenders

Whenever an Intensive Treatment Service starts, there will be many enquiries as to whether mentally impaired offenders can be managed. The mentally impaired offender requires a different type of service. Firstly, he (much more likely than a she) is probably a potential danger to society and may be subject to the Mental Health Act. Secondly he is likely to be mildly mentally retarded and extremely disdainful of contact with the more severely retarded – he wishes to 'pass' as normal. Thirdly, the nursing, medical and psychological techniques are more closely tied to the forensic and probation services than to the developmental and educational services.

The treatment techniques may include further education (e.g. social skills training), group therapy, anger management by assertiveness training, and (more controversially) Novaco methods (which involves the subject in keeping a diary of antecedents and perceptions of the violent incidents).

The offences are likely to be sexual (reaction to unavailability of normal and desired sexual activities), arson (an angry reaction of unassertive individuals) and violent (often a reaction to name-calling, frustration and humiliation). For every offence where charges are pressed, there are likely to be five where the victims or authorities have not proceeded. In a catchment of a million people, there is a need for at least 10 medium secure treatment places for offenders with mental handicaps. There is still debate as to whether such units should be incorporated in Regional Secure Units, or in mental illness hospitals in a specialized unit; or in a residential care mental handicap service.

References

Blunden, R. and Allen, D. (ed.) (1987) *Facing the Challenge. An Ordinary Life for People with Learning Difficulties and Challenging Behaviours*, Kings Fund, London

Cullen, C. (1987) Nurse training and institutional constraints. In *Staff Training in Mental Handicap* (eds Hogg, J. and Mitler, P.), London, Croom Helm

University of Syracuse Centre for Human Policy (1986) *TASH Newsletter*, July

Ware, J. and Evans, P. (1987) Room management is not enough. *British Journal of Special Education*, 1478–1480

8

The management of epilepsy

Eric Fischbacher

Introduction

The care of the mentally handicapped demands close attention to the problems of epilepsy. Precise figures are difficult to come by, but the incidence increases with the severity of the mental and physical handicap. In the wards of an institution caring for the severely and profoundly handicapped it is likely that at least one-third of the residents will suffer from epilepsy.

The occurrence of epilepsy varies considerably in the various syndromes associated with mental handicap. The myoclonic epilepsies of early childhood are usually associated with severe mental retardation in later life, the majority showing brain damage or malformation. The Lennox–Gastaut syndrome with its multiple seizure types and chaotic EEG appearances is almost always associated with cerebral defects and restricted mental function. Epilepsy is common in tuberous sclerosis and in the various forms of cerebral palsy, causing partial seizures of focal origin where the damage is localized to the motor cortex. It occurs in about one third of patients with phenylketonuria and similar metabolic disorders.

The problems of diagnosis and treatment of epilepsy in the mentally handicapped are compounded by the difficulties they have in communicating: in addition EEG recordings are in general more difficult to obtain and may be distorted by movement artefacts.

Prodromal symptoms or an aura may pass unnoticed by carers and inability to describe feelings and sensations may make the diagnosis of temporal lobe epilepsy more elusive. The mentally handicapped child may be quite unable to convey to caring staff his discomfort, or misery, caused by the side-effects or toxicity of anticonvulsant drugs, and runs the risk of receiving additional medication for a 'behavioural problem'. Intelligent observation and recording are the most important requisites for the proper management of epilepsy in the mentally handicapped.

Causation

Epilepsy can be separated into two main categories – primary or idiopathic epilepsy, and secondary, or symptomatic epilepsy. The distinction is simply between those in which no cause can be found for the seizures, and those in which a probable aetiological factor is discovered. Such factors can be divided into three categories, according to whether they exert their effect prior to birth, around the time of confinement, or in early infancy.

Prenatal factors include the effects of X-rays and of teratogenic drugs. Virus infections such as rubella, cytomegalovirus and toxoplasmosis can cause cerebral abnormalities which give rise to seizures. Genetic defects may also be associated with the development of epilepsy. Around the time of birth obstetric complications may lead to anoxia and physical trauma to the soft cranium, and again epilepsy may result. Post-natal factors include metabolic disturbance such as hypoglycaemia and hypocalcaemia and infections such as meningitis and encephalitis. Accidental injury may result in a subdural haematoma, and of course one must also keep in mind the possibility of non-accidental injury. Vascular abnormalities such as aneurysm or arterio-venous malformation may lead to haemorrhage, and so to damage to brain substance, and brain tumours can signal their presence at any stage of their growth by causing a seizure.

In addition to the underlying aetiology it would appear that some kind of trigger is necessary to provoke a seizure. In photosensitive epilepsy seizures are caused by flickering light within a certain range of frequency, and 20–50 Hz flicker in a malfunctioning TV set is distinctly epileptogenic. Sufferers from this condition should stay at least 4 m from the set, and should cover one eye when changing channels, as the trigger is dependent on stereoscopic vision. A lighted lamp placed on the TV may be helpful, even in daytime.

In other kinds of epilepsy the trigger is less specific. Emotional stress or excitement, or sudden noise may precipitate a seizure, and infections, metabolic disturbances or fluctuating hormone levels in the menstrual cycle may become triggering influences. Some drugs, notably the phenothiazines, will reduce the seizure threshold, making the individual more vulnerable to seizures, and on occasion the withdrawal of drugs or of alcohol may lead to convulsions.

Investigation

It is of the utmost importance that a correct diagnosis be made in patients who are apparently suffering from epileptiform events. Some neurologists report that up to 25% of new referrals to epilepsy clinics do not in fact suffer from epilepsy. To make the diagnosis of epilepsy erroneously and to commence long-term therapy is a clinical and social catastrophe, and true epilepsy must be distinguished from such conditions as benign paroxysmal vertigo, breath-holding attacks, syncope of various causations, and from manifestations of psychiatric disturbance.

The diagnosis will be based largely on a careful history involving a precise eye-witness account of the events preceding the 'fit' and a detailed description of the sequence of the incident itself and of subsequent events until the patient has fully recovered. There are, however, certain investigations which may help with the diagnosis and with identification of the underlying cause. Routine blood and urine testing should be done, and a chest X-ray, as part of a general search for systemic disease.

The EEG is a necessary investigation, and may be conclusive in the search for a diagnosis. It may also indicate the presence of generalized epileptic activity, or pin-point the location of an active epileptic focus. 'Spike and wave' forms at the slow rate of 3 per second may be seen, or intermittent spikes. The interpretation of electroencephalograms is a highly specialized area and not within the scope of this book.

However, an EEG recording made between seizures may be perfectly normal, and such a negative recording is of minimal significance. To make certain of the diagnosis it may be necessary to obtain prolonged continuous recordings or even to use special techniques to place electrodes in closer proximity to the brain (e.g. sphenoidal or depth electrodes).

There are also a growing number of sophisticated imaging techniques available to visualize the brain in great detail – the CAT and PET scans, and magnetic resonance imaging are current examples. Cerebral angiograms will provide information about the cerebral arteries, and where infection is suspected lumbar puncture may be indicated.

It cannot, however, be emphasized too strongly that the diagnosis of epilepsy is largely a clinical one, resting upon a very close observation of the patient's 'turns', and not solely upon the results of laboratory and other investigative procedures.

Classification of seizures

The latest classification to be generally adopted is that produced by the International League Against Epilepsy in the early 1980s. Others continue to be devised and to find varying degrees of support, but this one appears to be widely supported in publications over the past decade. It distinguishes broadly between generalized seizures which are more or less symmetrical, with no evidence of focal onset; and partial seizures which start by activation of a group of neurones in one part of the brain. It also acknowledges that some seizures will not fit either of these categories. An abbreviated summary of the classification is given in Table 8.1.

Generalized seizures

Absence seizures
Known in previous classifications as *petit mal*, they consist of brief periods of unawareness, of abrupt onset and recovery, occurring mainly in children and young adults. School lessons may be repeatedly interrupted by these events, which are not always immediately recognized. When attacks occur during EEG recording, 3 Hz 'spike and wave' patterns will be seen. Such seizures do not usually cause falls or muscle activity, but occasionally there may be slight twitching of the face or limb muscles.

Tonic–clonic seizures
These are the classical *grand-mal* seizures, following a typical pattern which warrants detailed description as follows.

Prodromal period – The seizure may be preceded by vague symptoms lasting as long as 24 hours, or even longer, which to the experienced nurse may indicate the imminence of a seizure.

Aura – As the seizure commences the patient may be aware of some physical or psychological sensation, often highly unpleasant, which heralds the onset, and may cry out or show sudden distress or alarm before being engulfed in the seizure itself. The occurrence of an aura suggests a focal origin, preceding the origin of the generalized seizure.

Table 8.1 Classification of seizures

---

1. Partial seizures:

   A. Simple partial seizures (consciousness not impaired)
   B. Complex partial seizures (consciousness impaired) (Both of these types may present with motor, sensory, autonomic or psychic symptoms.)
   C. Partial seizures, secondarily generalized

2. Generalized seizures:

   A. Absence seizures
   B. Myoclonic seizures
   C. Clonic seizures
   D. Tonic seizures
   E. Tonic–clonic seizures
   F. Atonic seizures

3. Unclassified seizures

Based upon the International Classification approved by the International League Against Epilepsy.

Tonic phase – The patient becomes rapidly unconscious. Extensive strong muscle contraction leads to clamping of the jaws, constriction of respiratory movement and consequent cyanosis, and tightening of abdominal muscles which may contribute to urinary and perhaps faecal incontinence. This phase lasts around 1/2–1 minute.

Clonic phase – Lasting usually around 1–2 minutes this phase consists of clonic or repetitive jerking movements of the head and limbs, often some frothing at the mouth, and some gasping attempts at breathing.

After the convulsion has subsided there is a phase of unconsciousness, of variable duration, followed frequently by sleep. The fit may be followed by a period of confusion, known as *post-ictal automatism*, and transient weakness of a limb or limbs may occur – *Todd's paralysis* – particularly if the attack has commenced focally.

Occasionally the clonic phase will be followed immediately by another tonic phase, and the cycle repeat itself in a continuous convulsive state known as *status epilepticus*. This is a serious medical emergency, can lead to brain damage, and can be life threatening. It calls for very urgent treatment.

Myoclonic seizures

These consist of sudden spasmodic contractions of muscle and are commonest in infants – infantile spasms. The sudden extension of arms and flexion at the waist inspired the term 'salaam attacks' and they may occur singly or as multiple events.

Tonic or clonic seizures

These are major generalized seizures in which either the tonic phase or the clonic phase is absent.

Atonic or akinetic seizures

Also known as *drop attacks*, sudden total loss of consciousness and postural control leads to a precipitous fall, and almost immediate return to full consciousness. Injury frequently occurs to the head and face. Occasionally the period of unconsciousness is so brief that it causes only a momentary drooping of the body.

Generalized seizures are generated by a stimulus commencing deep in the centre of the brain, and spreading symmetrically to all areas, producing symmetrical and generalized effects.

Partial seizures

Partial seizures are generated locally in the brain, and the effects will depend on the part of the brain affected. If the stimulus commences in the motor cortex the effect will be seen in the movement of muscle groups normally controlled by these motor neurones. The stimulus may spread from the source, and result in the progressive involvement of successive muscle groups, and may ultimately proceed to trigger a generalized seizure.

If the problem arises in an area not responsible for motor control, the seizure will be of a sensory or psychological nature. Temporal lobe epilepsy is characterized by an internal experience similar to a dream or nightmare, with a host of sensations including sight, hearing, smell, taste, and others, and is frequently accompanied by chewing movements of the mouth and tongue and stereotypic movements of the hands and head. These are sometimes known as psychomotor seizures. Speech and thought difficulties, numbness and tingling, are some of the effects of partial sensory seizures.

Partial seizures can therefore be classified as *motor* or *sensory*, and depending on whether consciousness is clouded, as *simple* or *complex*. A simple partial motor seizure will be one in which, for example, a limb shows continuous jerking movement, but the patient is fully conscious and aware.

Unclassified seizures

The presence of this category indicates that there are seizures that do not appear to fit into the classification described, and a precise description of the series of events in the course of a seizure may be of much greater value than a diagnostic label.

Status epilepticus

This situation has been described already in the section on tonic–clonic seizures. It can also occur in all other types of seizure. For example, continuous absence seizure activity can persist for long periods, and is known as *non-convulsive status*. The same term could be used for a dream-like state produced by prolonged partial sensory activity. These other forms of continuous epileptic activity do not appear to be as harmful or dangerous as tonic–clonic status, but need to be recognized and treated.

Therapeutic management

In the treatment of a chronic and persistent condition many differing approaches may be suggested. Special diets and nutritional supplements and exclusions have been tried, the best known being the ketogenic diet – an attempt to induce a continuing state of ketosis. This diet is extremely unpleasant, and not strikingly effective. Patients with sufficient intellectual capacity may learn 'feedback' techniques to help delay or minimize seizures, but this approach is confined to a small minority of individuals, and few with mental handicap can master the methods.

Surgical treatment has been available for a very small minority of people with epilepsy. In the light of progress in defining the precise location of causative lesions, and improvement in neurosurgical technique, more of the cases resistant to anticonvulsants may well come to operation in the future.

The mainstay of treatment, however, is anticonvulsant medication. Once the diagnosis is firmly established most individuals suffering from epilepsy will require long-term control with appropriate drug therapy. Because of the long-term aspect, it is extremely important that the correct drugs should be prescribed, and the minimum number of drugs should be used to control seizures. Prior to the availability of blood levels of anticonvulsants, one drug tended to be added to another in the attempt to control seizures, until the patient was taking four or five drugs concurrently. Now that drug levels can readily be obtained the aim is to use the smallest number of drugs possible, and to prescribe these in dosage sufficient to control seizures without toxic side-effects.

It has been shown that most new cases of epilepsy not associated with major neurological abnormality can be controlled by one drug. In the field of mental handicap more severe and intractable forms of epilepsy are likely to be met with, and more than one anticonvulsant drug may be required in such cases. It should also be borne in mind that the addition of drugs to the treatment regimen may not in the long run improve the seizure rate greatly, but may add the additional burden of drug side-effects. Some of the psychiatric features of the so-called 'epileptic personality' are now considered to be due to the untoward effect of long-term drug therapy.

The frequency of dosage of anticonvulsants is of some importance. Those drugs that have a long 'half-life' (a term from the science of pharmacokinetics, referring to the time a drug remains in the blood stream after a single dose) may only require to be given once daily, and while more frequent dosage is unlikely to be harmful, a single daily dose regimen is more convenient for patients self-medicating, and may assist compliance, whereas a more frequent dosage scheme may result in omission due to inconvenience or forgetfulness.

The main anticonvulsant drugs in current use are:

Carbamazepine	Nitrazepam
Sodium valproate	Clobazam
Phenytoin	Primidone
Ethosuximide	Phenobarbitone
Clonazepam	Diazepam

Carbamazepine was originally developed for the treatment of trigeminal neuralgia, and subsequently found to have anti-epileptic activity. It is particularly effective in the partial epilepsies, but is also a good choice for generalized tonic–clonic seizures. Its value in absence seizures has not been established.

Its shorter half-life requires it to be given two or three times daily, and it should be introduced slowly, building up the dose over 3–4 weeks to avoid nausea or dizziness. Side-effects are not prominent, although acute allergic rashes appear occasionally, and high dosage can cause drowsiness and ataxia.

Sodium valproate is of value in all forms of epilepsy, and is perhaps currently the drug of choice in absence seizures. Its value in treatment of the partial epilepsies is less clear. The enteric-coated form of tablet has largely eliminated gastric intolerance, and syrup, slow release and intravenous formulations make it a versatile medication. Occasional side-effects include mild alopecia which is reversible, weight gain, and a very small number of cases of liver toxicity have been reported in children under the age of 2 years. It should rarely be used in this group of patients.

Phenytoin is a well-established and effective drug for most forms of epilepsy. The main difficulty in its use is the maintenance of a dose level which will be effective, while at the same time avoiding toxic side-effects. Metabolism of the drug readily becomes saturated, leading to sudden escalation in blood levels, and this problem can be exacerbated by changes in other medication given concomitantly. Particular attention must be given to checking of blood levels.

A once daily dosage schedule should be adequate. The toxic effects of dosages that are too great consist of nausea and vomiting, ataxia, excessive salivation, nystagmus in some cases, and increased seizure frequency. Nurses and other carers need to be watchful for these signs. More chronic side-effects include hypertrophy of gums, and a subtle change in facial appearance which makes it particularly inappropriate for the treatment of girls and young women. It may interfere with cognitive function and alertness.

Ethosuximide – The main use of this drug is in typical absence seizures with the classical 'spike and wave' EEG pattern, as an alternative to sodium valproate. Its long half-life indicates a once daily dosage if appropriate, and as with other drugs it should be introduced slowly to avoid early side-effects.

Clonazepam, nitrazepam and clobazam are all benzodiazepine derivatives, the first two being used largely in the treatment of young people suffering from the myoclonic epilepsies of childhood. The last is used as an adjunct to other anticonvulsants and is rarely adequate on its own. The benzodiazepines tend to be sedative, depending on dosage, and also present a special problem of bronchorrhoea for physically handicapped children who are particularly susceptible to respiratory infections.

Phenobarbitone has held a prime place in the treatment of epilepsy for many years and is an extremely effective anticonvulsant. Despite its effectiveness and relative cheapness it has lost its dominant place in the treatment of epilepsy in view of increasing awareness of its unacceptable side-effects, particularly hyperactivity, behaviour disorders and impaired learning ability in children, and its tendency to depression and over-sedation in adults.

Primidone is broken down in the body to phenobarbitone, and phenylethylmalonamide. Its main action would appear to be largely that of phenobarbitone, and carries the same disabilities.

Other drugs or variants of those above are also used in treatment, and new drugs such as lamotrigine and vigabatrin are undergoing clinical trials at the time of writing. Others are under development. Special situations call for the use of other drugs, such as ACTH in the treatment of myoclonic epilepsy of infancy.

A number of other drugs are used in the control of status epilepticus. Diazepam by the intravenous route has been used for many years to abort or to treat this condition. Since this drug is of no value for this purpose by the oral or intramuscular route, it has become common practice to instil the solution by the rectal route, where its absorption is said to be almost as rapid and complete as by the i.v. route. It may be given by syringe, or by a special plastic-nozzle pack, in children and also in adults. Since it can be administered by nurses it provides a rapid anticonvulsant effect when status threatens.

Paraldehyde intramuscularly is a safe alternative, and intravenous preparations of clonazepam, lorazepam, chlormethiozole, phenytoin, sodium valproate and phenobarbitone may all be considered in the treatment of status epilepticus, though some are best monitored in an intensive care unit.

General points

Folate deficiency sometimes occurs in patients taking anticonvulsants. Folate levels should be checked annually, and if low, cautious replacement therapy instituted. Folic acid is considered to be epileptogenic in the usual therapeutic doses, and a small dose given twice weekly seems safer. It has been suggested by some that replacement therapy is indicated only if there is evidence of haematological or neurological effects of the deficiency, or if learning capacity in children appears to be affected.

Deficiency of vitamin D may also occur in long-term anticonvulsant therapy. The more severely handicapped may be less exposed to sunlight and the insidious development of metabolic bone disease may be missed. The prophylactic use of vitamin D has not been recommended but blood levels of calcium, phosphate and alkaline phosphatase should be checked from time to time, and X-rays of bone structure carried out if suspicion arises.

Frequent occurrence of seizures which cause repeated injury may be an indication for some form of protective headgear. Further efforts are needed to design models which will be comfortable, functional and presentable.

As regards work and leisure it will be tempting for the conscientious carer to provide safeguards against injury, but such safeguards are inevitably confining and can be a serious barrier to the individual's enjoyment of a reasonable lifestyle. Some balance must be found between the obvious risks of injury and the experience of a free and happy life. Where seizures are well controlled few restrictions need be imposed.

In the area of mental handicap the issue of driving may not often arise, but it is important to remember that a person suffering from epilepsy who has been free of daytime seizures for a period of 2 years is not debarred from holding a driving licence. This kind of enlightened legislation accepts a certain degree of risk, and in the care of the mentally handicapped who suffers from epilepsy a certain degree of risk must also be accepted in order to permit a reasonable quality of living.

Carer management

The carer is in a unique position to make a major contribution to the care and treatment of epilepsy in the mentally handicapped. He or she may be present at the onset, during its development, and after the seizure is over, and detailed observations will enable a precise diagnosis to be made and the correct treatment regimen selected.

Questions a nurse or other carer may be able to answer include the following: Was there any precipitating factor such as previous malaise or a fall, or perhaps a sudden fright? Immediately prior to the onset of the seizure was there any warning, such as a cry? In the case of a tonic–clonic seizure, how long was the tonic phase, and was there cyanosis or incontinence? Did the seizure have a focal onset, and during the clonic phase which parts of the body were moving? How long did this last, and was the person injured, and did he vomit? How deeply unconscious was he during the phase of muscular relaxation and was there any evidence of post-ictal automatism or Todd's paralysis?

Precise answers to these questions will be of much more value than a general statement such as 'tonic–clonic seizure, good recovery'. Description of a seizure event in terms of its length and associated movements and loss of postural tone, or a description of a psychomotor attack in as precise terms as possible, will be most helpful in planning treatment. Facial expressions, grimaces and gestures may indicate seizure activity, or may simply convey the discomfort or anxiety being experienced during a partial seizure.

During the seizure itself there is little indication for active intervention other than to protect the patient from injury, making sure that he is in the position least likely to lead to airway obstruction, especially should he vomit. The traditional advice to place a padded object between the teeth to prevent injury to the tongue is liable to lead to severe dental injury, and is therefore not now advised. Emergency treatment such as diazepam rectally will be given according to instructions and should the seizures recur or proceed to status epilepticus immediate medical advice must be sought. Continuous convulsion can lead to serious cerebral injury.

Carefully kept charts of the occurrence of seizures can be of great value, and bar-graphs showing the number of seizures per week and the current drug therapy can assist greatly in monitoring epilepsy. Computer software is available which will help in this area.

Conclusion

Many mentally handicapped individuals suffer from epilepsy, and the additional disability makes life more difficult. Every effort must be made to control seizures, while avoiding the burden of drug side-effects. Support and encouragement will be especially needed by those who carry this dual handicap.

9
The assessment and delivery of health care

9.1 Physical health

Eric Fischbacher

A Report on Services for the Mentally Handicapped in Scotland (*A Better Life – 1979*) looks on mental handicap as '85% outwith the concern of doctors'. At one time a great deal of the planning and provision of care and training of the mentally handicapped was provided by doctors and nurses, but over recent years the burden has rightly been shouldered by multidisciplinary teams, including ancillary medical services such as physiotherapy. Psychology, speech therapy, occupational therapy, music and movement therapies, art therapy, social services, and others have increased their contribution toward the welfare of the handicapped. Educational services have also become more specialized, and have a major input into the group approach.

Medical care, however, remains an essential element. Paediatric neurologists and geneticists make their contribution at an early stage, and thereafter there is the day-to-day physical care which is one of the main concerns of this book.

Beange (1986) made the point:

'It is my contention that developmentally disabled people are basically a population with many unmet health needs, and that these needs must be met with a wise application of the medical model. I wish to argue that compared to the average, people with developmental disabilities are beset with multiple physical problems; that their life expectancy is low; that they have remediable disabilities, which are not being recognised or treated; that they are not being referred for remedial and preventive health services, and that because of this, they are functioning below their ability and will continue to do so until proper provision is made for their care, with due regard to the best principles of medical science.'

The Apostle Paul makes the point that 'if one member suffers, all the members suffer' and there is little doubt that if the body is uncomfortable the mind will be affected. A behavioural problem may well be a form of protest against the neglect

132

of a physical problem, and successful treatment of the former will require prior and proper attention to the latter.

General health care

General principles of hygiene and health care are important for all of us, and many need to be reminded of them. Many handicapped people have a childlike unawareness of these principles, and may need some guidance or even close direction and supervision.

Cleanliness

Washing and bathing or showering daily is a necessity for those liable to incontinence, and beneficial for anyone. Skin folds and crevices can harbour skin pathogens which are responsible for the common furuncle, and the more major abscesses and cellulitis. Fingernails can hold the ova of threadworms, a recurring problem even in the smallest institution – the normal family.

Regular bathing with clean water and cotton wool will help control blepharitis, common in Down's syndrome, and external nares may have to have crusts removed during the common cold. The external ear may have to be cleaned, but the external canal should not be invaded. If wax is causing deafness, arrangements can be made for ear lavage to be carried out.

Diet

The importance of an adequate and well-balanced diet need hardly be emphasized, and the inclusion of fresh food needs to be encouraged. Many who have attended cookery classes, and learned well, resort to tins when left to their own devices. Obesity is a frequent result of personal choice in diet, and can be a serious threat to health. In most situations the advice of a dietitian can be obtained.

Exercise

Many mentally handicapped people have a history of restriction of physical exercise, because of institutional residence, limited opportunity at home, or restricted physical range. All forms and degrees of movement need to be encouraged, from change of position in a wheelchair to sports for the disabled. Inertia is a threat to good health.

Constipation

Concern about bowel movement can range from complete disregard to total obsession. Deficient bowel tone, a defect in some forms of physical handicap, can be responsible for minor discomfort to complete obstruction requiring surgical action for its relief. The addition of roughage and encouragement of physical exercise are preferable to the use of laxatives, but medication may be necessary in some cases. Medical advice should be sought about the type of medication most appropriate, since some proprietary preparations are inappropriate and even harmful.

Common medical problems

The following comprise some of the common medical conditions met with over a period of precisely 10 years in an institution for the mentally handicapped. The list cannot be comprehensive, as people in this category are liable to any of the conditions to which we are all vulnerable.

Infections

This is the largest category of common conditions. Respiratory infections by viruses and other pathogens result in the common cold, influenza, sinusitis, bronchitis and pneumonia in its various forms. Urinary tract infections are common in women, and especially in the elderly, and can be difficult to eliminate. The skin is surprisingly vulnerable to infection, and furunculosis, superficial abscesses, and cellulitis are all seen frequently. Secondary infection occurs in injuries, which can be self-inflicted or accidental. Conjunctivitis and blepharitis affect the eyes, and acute and chronic infections of the external and middle ear are common. A persistent and often foul-smelling discharge from one nostril can be the clue to a foreign body lodged at a higher level.

Disturbance of body function

Normal body function can be disturbed, and symptoms develop, without any disease process being present. Stomach and bowel upsets can occur, usually as a result of intolerance of food, and vomiting or diarrhoea are not always indicators of infection. Loss of appetite and weight can have many causes other than a physical disease process, and these include emotional distress, drug side-effects, and mental illness, particularly depression.

Menstrual problems

Dysmenorrhoea can be a distressing discomfort but simple analgesics are usually appropriate – they should be made available. Prolonged and heavy menstrual bleeding can lead to severe anaemia and the extent of blood loss may not be reported to carers. One woman described her bleeding cervical polyp as 'my secret', and only a severe anaemia brought the secret to light.

Toothache

Regular dental care will prevent tooth decay, but toothache can be a hidden cause of distress and behavioural problems in a severely handicapped individual who has difficulty in communicating. It should always be considered when unexplained crying or general upset is observed. A general anaesthetic may be necessary to permit an adequate examination of the mouth, and such a requirement should not deny a handicapped person the dental attention he needs.

Deficiencies

Iron deficiency anaemia and its less common but equally important relation pernicious anaemia, can be insidious, and lead to considerable disability and weakness before being unearthed. For this reason, in hospital, annual blood tests are carried out, especially in the elderly. These conditions are readily remedied once they are detected. Similarly failing thyroid function needs to be watched for, especially likely in the elderly, in Down's syndrome, and associated with treatment with certain drugs such as lithium.

Diabetes mellitus needs special knowledge, and the training normally given to the patient will need to be taken in many cases by the carer. In any setting where there is a diabetic, some member of staff should take a special interest in the condition, and be prepared to advise and guide, and see to it that emergency items such as glucose and glucagon are to hand.

Vitamin deficiencies are uncommon, but where care is poor, or individuals are caring for themselves dietary inadequacy can lead to serious depletion of necessary vitamins, and to consequent health problems.

Special medical problems of the mentally handicapped

Some problems beset the mentally handicapped more than the rest of the population.

Cerebral palsy

The more severe forms of cerebral palsy are often associated with physical immobility and deformity, and subsequent contractures which make toiletting awkward, and cleansing and general care of the skin more difficult. Chafing and consequent breakdown of the integrity of the skin can progress to areas of skin loss and damage to deeper tissues, down to bone. Chronic infection adds its local effects and eventually septicaemia can be life threatening. Prevention is the only satisfactory solution, and techniques include careful hygiene, avoidance of continuous pressure on vulnerable areas by frequent change of position, and appropriate padding and support. Many types of aids are available – special wheelchairs, water-beds, and special types of mattress. The physiotherapist has special skills in this area and should be consulted.

Perhaps because of immobility and chest deformities, the person with cerebral palsy is more liable to respiratory infections of a more serious degree. Epilepsy is common, and often severe, and the benzodiazepine anticonvulsants sometimes used, particularly in the younger patient, increase bronchial secretions and compound the danger to the respiratory system.

Epilepsy

Epilepsy, in addition to the discomfort and direct cerebral impact of seizures, brings with it a number of hazards. Injuries are not uncommon, and it is important to check thoroughly for the integrity of the skeletal system, when a fit has caused a fall. It is a good rule that the severely handicapped who have difficulty in communicating their needs should, in privacy and warmth, be stripped completely and carefully examined for signs of bone or internal injury.

Anticonvulsants are, without exception, capable of inducing unwanted side-effects, and at times frank toxicity. Patients taking phenytoin particularly need to be watched for the appearance of ataxia, anorexia and hypersalivation, indicating overdosage. The mentally handicapped may have difficulty in indicating to carers the less obvious side-effects of dizziness and nausea which some experience on anticonvulsant treatment. Chronic underfunctioning, drowsiness, diminished appetite, and other effects, can result from over-medication.

The emotional, psychological and stigmatizing effects of this condition receive a great deal of attention amongst non-handicapped groups, but it is perhaps forgotten that the same problems are faced by the handicapped, who add these additional burdens to their already heavy load. They also need support, encouragement and reassurance. Much more detail about this extremely common and important condition is given in Chapter 8.

Injuries

Injuries can occur as a result of several factors. Damage to the motor areas of the brain may result in clumsiness, or frank incoordination leading to considerable difficulties with standing and walking. Stumbling over obstructions and falling cause injury, and such injuries can be quite severe: fractures of the skull with cerebral injury, or fractures of large bones – in particular fracture of the femur in the more elderly. Epilepsy adds its quota, and where there is aggression associated with behaviour disturbance or mental illness mutual injury can occur in a group.

Since a surprising tolerance to pain is noted in some mentally handicapped individuals, and communication difficulties can conceal the area of hurt, a full examination is mandatory.

Hiatus hernia

Incompetence of the cardiac end of the stomach, or frank herniation through the diaphragm is not uncommon in the handicapped, particularly those who suffer from cerebral palsy. These changes lead to gastric discomfort, heartburn and bouts of regurgitation of food. Slight blood loss from the site of oesophageal irritation can lead to progressive anaemia.

Cardiac problems

In some cases where brain damage has occurred, leading to mental handicap, damage has also been sustained to other organs. Syndromes such as Down's and the rubella virus can interfere with the normal development of the heart, and appropriate treatment will be required for the consequent long-term results. Severe chest deformity can also compromise cardiac function, and of course the elderly may show the signs of an ageing cardiovascular system.

Eyes

Cataracts occur in a number of syndromes, and can also occur in association with some drugs ('star cataracts'). It is important that a watch be kept on these cases, in order that appropriate treatment can be instituted at the right time, avoiding unnecessary visual restriction.

Keratoconus is a condition not uncommon in Down's syndrome. The cornea becomes thinned, and the anterior chamber pressure causes a forward bulging or coning. Referral to an ophthalmologist is urgent when this is observed, as rupture of the cornea can occur.

Special efforts must be made to ascertain the integrity of the sight of those handicapped people who are unable to convey that information for themselves. The provision of spectacles will occasionally quite radically change a lifestyle. Specialist advice is available from various agencies caring for the blind, and registration will automatically lead to a range of services which may improve the quality of life of the blind considerably.

Ears

Some of the mentally handicapped appear to have a high threshold to pain. For this reason examination during pyrexial illness where the cause is not otherwise clear, should include a look at the ear-drums. Neglect of acute otitis media has left not a few with recurrent and chronic suppurative otitis media, a condition requiring specialized treatment.

Deafness can be overlooked, and where the question arises, it requires specialized assessment. The provision of a hearing aid may be a great boon to someone already disadvantaged in other ways, and societies for the deaf can make a major contribution in this area.

Skin

Seborrhoeic dermatitis is common in Down's syndrome, especially around the mouth and face, and around the eyelids. It may benefit from simple treatments, and prolonged use of fluorinated steroid preparations should be avoided, as they can cause permanent skin damage. Psoriasis is not uncommon, and needs energetic treatment intermittently.

Skin reactions to drugs can be a problem, occasionally being extremely severe. Sensitivity to ammoniacal urine, and to incontinence pads can lead to an extensive atopic dermatitis requiring careful preventive measures, and treatment.

In the institution scabies can spread within wards, especially where towels, facecloths are shared. Attention to individual hygiene practice, and appropriate skin treatment will control these outbreaks. Itching due to eczema and other irritating skin conditions can provoke scratching which may be so uncontrolled as to lead to severe damage to the skin. Protective dressings or clothing may be advisable, as well as treatment for the underlying condition.

Hepatitis

These infections are considered to be more common in long-stay hospitals than in the general population and carriers of the virus are usually sought and identified. Three types are characterized as 'A', 'B' and 'Non-A,non-B'. The first is usually a moderate infection with good recovery, the others often in a more severe category. Immunization against hepatitis B is now readily available for staff and for others thought to be at risk of infection.

Over-medication

People with a mental handicap may require medication for a number of separate clinical problems. Medication may be appropriate at a particular time, but should not be continued longer than absolutely necessary. Carers should ensure that medication be reviewed by the general practitioner, and if necessary the psychiatrist or other specialist responsible for the original prescription. Great benefit has resulted from review of medication in institutions, with removal of drugs not essential, and the reduction of dosage where possible. 'Drug holidays' are useful, and will often demonstrate that certain drugs were not exerting any significant beneficial effect. Regular review of chronic conditions is important for health and well-being.

Who supplies the medical care?

At present medical care is supplied by hospital specialists in the Mental Handicap field, in wards and through out-patient clinics. Where clients are living at home or in community facilities, they are cared for in the main by general practitioners. As more and more of the mentally handicapped leave hospitals and large residential institutions, and settle in hostels and small group homes, the main burden of care is moving to the general practitioner services, many of which are already finding a flood of mentally ill, mentally handicapped and elderly folk moving from hospital to community, placing a severe strain on resources.

As large numbers of the mentally handicapped move into the community, will the general practitioner have the expertise and time to meet all their special medical needs?

Dr Beange (1986) again:

'It is said that developmentally disabled clients should obtain their medical care from generic services – i.e. the friendly neighbourhood GP. I have never been able to see the logic in the argument that generalists can give all the physical care, while at the same time more and more specialists are needed to deliver behavioural and educational services.'

It does seem that doctors with extensive experience of the medical problems of the mentally handicapped will still have a role to play, in the specialized institutions so long as they continue to function, and through clinics and domiciliary consultation in the community. At present paediatricians who care for children with mental and physical handicap fulfil this kind of role, and in some areas clinics are being set up to provide for adults with a developmental disability. At such clinics basic advice will be given in respect of epilepsy, the problems of cerebral palsy, and psychiatric and behavioural difficulties. Referral to other specialties – orthopaedics, ophthalmology, etc., can be made from there, close liaison being maintained with the general practitioner.

How and when do we obtain this service?

(This section is relevant to the UK in 1990.)

Make an appointment with the GP

A normal appointment can be made, that is, whenever time is available, for such minor events as skin rashes, various aches and pains and minor injuries. Anorexia, insomnia, weight loss and such symptoms may have significance but not urgency, and the same applies to increasing seizure frequency in epilepsy. It is sometimes useful to explain the problem to the receptionist, who will often try to arrange an appointment appropriately.

An early or urgent appointment can be made for sudden severe symptoms such as acute and severe abdominal pain, possible fractures where the patient can be transported to the surgery, or minor injuries which might require stitching. In some areas direct transport to the Accident and Emergency Unit of the local hospital may be appropriate – the GP will advise on that point. A clear message, such as 'she needs to see a doctor today. . .' will be helpful, and the doctor will decide what steps have to be taken to deal with the emergency.

Ask the GP to visit

Where the patient is unable to walk or be helped to the doctor's surgery, and is clearly quite unwell and in need of medical attention, a request may be made for a home visit. Again, a clear message such as 'please ask the doctor to call...' is helpful, with an explanation of the problem. The doctor will make the decision as to what action is to be taken. House call requests that are not really necessary put extra burden on the GP services, and will result in a loss of mutual confidence, so important for the doctor–patient relationship.

Specialist consultation

The general practitioner will normally suggest referral to a specialist where that is indicated. The handicapped will from time to time require special help in the areas of orthopaedics, dermatology, neurology, and psychiatry, and indeed in any of the specialties available to the normal population. It is important to ensure that the services available to others are made fully available to this vulnerable group of people.

The mental handicap specialist

The mental handicap specialist continues to be available in the local specialist hospital, and it is expected that his or her services will continue to be made available in the community setting. In some areas developmental disability clinics are being set up, to provide overall care for the handicapped, and the general practitioner and others will be able to arrange referral there.

Community mental handicap teams are already functioning in most areas, and these include the services of the community nurse, physiotherapist, social worker, psychologist and specialist doctor and may involve other personnel who are involved with this client group.

Reference

Beange, H. (1986) The medical model revisited. *Australia and New Zealand Journal of Developmental Disabilities*, **12**, No. 1, 3–7

9.2 Nursing care of the profoundly handicapped

David Keith

Since the last edition of this textbook, there obviously have not been significant changes in the physical nursing care of the mentally handicapped person but there have been many changes in the philosophy of care which obviously have had an overall effect on nurses' delivery of care.

The reason for such a change in the image of mental handicap nursing has a great deal to do with the 1982 Modular Scheme of training. The new syllabus aims to cater for the modern nurse caring for the mentally handicapped emphasizing the changes that society is making towards meeting the needs and the rights of the mentally handicapped. Nurses themselves have questioned their attitudes towards the handicapped and are now very positive and self-critical.

I will be writing about the total nursing care of the profoundly mentally handicapped person, average mental age 4 months, in the context of a Health Authority Special Care dwelling.

The nurse's role as a provider of physical nursing care

Society has a confusing picture of the role of the mental handicap nurse. The word 'nurse' paints a picture in many people's minds of looking after people in their sick beds. The nurse looking after the mentally handicapped person has many varied and multi-functional roles. The many roles of the nurse in this chapter include: The Educator, The Therapist, The Advocate, The Substitute Parent.

The profoundly mentally handicapped person is often not ill but has many common health problems due to the extent of their handicap.

The Nursing Process, which must be mentioned whenever the subject of nursing care is delivered, is an essential framework of care, giving the nurse a better understanding of residents' needs, and a way of setting the highest standards of care.

Some common health problems affecting profoundly mentally handicapped people are illustrated in the following example.

John – age 20 years. Assessment

Problem	Plan
Pneumonia Upper respiratory tract infections	Postural drainage Antibiotic treatment. Care when feeding. Never let John's head fall back. Use suction to remove excess secretion
Neurological damage, epilepsy	Monitoring of epilepsy by regular blood checks. Correct First Aid. Observing and records fits. Reporting and caring
Skin problems, pressure sores	Daily baths. Washing and drying of resident very carefully. Inspect skin closely. Application of barrier cream. Regular changes of John's position
Prone to constipation	1. *Diet* – Ensuring that resident has a balanced diet. Encouragement with fluids. The importance of dietary fibre should increase the bulk of stool. 2. *Exercise* – The changing in positioning and general exercise and fresh air will help the resident 3. *Medication* – Unfortunately many profoundly mentally handicapped people require suppositories and evacuant enemas. Oral laxatives and stool softener drugs such as Duphalac (lactulose).
Prone to incontinence of urine and faeces	It is important to ensure that the incontinent person is checked on a regular basis and to make sure that the person is changed immediately when wet. It is important that the skin is cleaned and dried. Application of barrier creams. Use of incontinent items – nappies. Macrodoms if required. Observation must be taken by the nurse of any unusual strong smell which may indicate a urinary tract infection. Any abnormality of faeces are noted.

Problem	Plan
Prone to dental problems due to poor oral clearance and enamel deficiencies	Oral hygiene. Many profoundly handicapped people breathe through their mouths. This often causes dryness to the mouth and can lead to infection and general tooth decay. Correct diet to ensure that meals are not too sugary. Regular toothbrushing after meals and attention to keeping the mouth clean and moist throughout the day. Regular appointments with the dentist.
Orthopaedic problems: hip dislocation, scoliosis, contracture	Ensure good position seek advice from physiotherapist. Provide a variety of positions so that the individual does not become progressively stiffer. *Side lying* – John should be positioned in the side lying position so as to prevent him from pushing his head backwards and arching his backwards. It also keeps the shoulders forwards and allows the arms to come into the midline position, his hands are brought forward and together into a functional position for play. This position encourages symmetry and can involve John in social activities within group work with other residents who are positioned likewise.
Orthopaedic problems: hip dislocations, scoliosis, contractures	*Prone position* – John can be positioned in prone and this position enables John to straighten his back, hips and knees. It encourages John's head control – position a mirror in front of John who enjoys looking at himself in the mirror or using a squeaky toy encourages John to lift his head. This again is a symmetrical position which prevents John from going into a wind-swept position. This position is great for play – prone wedges can be positioned in a group and this encourages communication between the people using them. *Prone standing frames* This helps John to be in a symmetrical position. It keeps his hips in joint and encourages John to push on his arms and lift up his head. It improves John's circulation, breathing and digestion. It is a good position for John to play

The nurse frequently encounters problems owing to the severity of the brain damage of the mentally handicapped person.

The nurse not only has to learn correct techniques of feeding but also to ensure that the individual is receiving enough nutritional intake. The nurse should be aware of the normal development of feeding from infancy.

The nurse helping people to eat and drink

1. Discover individual likes and dislikes. Record likes and dislikes in care plan.
2. Make sure food is not too cold or hot.
   The correct use of microwaves and hot plates are very useful for this purpose.
3. Sit down in front of the person and talk to the individual. It is important care staff concentrate on what they are doing.
4. Nurses should become familiar with techniques in feeding individuals with:
   (a) Hypersensitivity.
   (b) Bite reflex.
   (c) Tongue thrust.
   (d) Sucking reflex problems.
   (e) Exaggerated gag reflex.
   (f) Tight jaws and lips.

Position for feeding and drinking when head control is achieved

1. Table and chair designed at correct height for the person.
   Seek advice from the physiotherapy department.
2. Person is sitting upright.
3. Hips should be flexed.
4. Bottom should be well back on the chair.
5. Leaning slightly forward with elbows on table if possible.
6. Slumping forward and back can be avoided by the person wearing an H strap or harness to ensure that their shoulders are fixed straight while positioned in wheelchair.
7. Feet should be flat.

When head and trunk control is absent it is advisable for the nurse to seek advice and information from the physiotherapist and occupational therapy department. Special cushions and wedges can be used to ensure an upright position. What must not be done is to tilt the head backwards known as gravity feeding.

This is a dangerous practice as the person is likely to gag or choke on the food. This can cause inhalation pneumonia and consequent death among profoundly mentally handicapped people.

Steps in feeding a profoundly mentally handicapped person

1. Place a small amount of food on the spoon. A plastic unbreakable spoon when dealing with a person who has exaggerated bite reflex.
2. Food is pulled from the spoon by closed lips rather than scraped off by top teeth.
3. Don't rush food.
4. Use special cups, i.e. 'Doidy' cups.

5. Consider potential for self-feeding.
6. Processed food better served separately.
7. Correct environment and atmosphere important.

Drinking

1. The head must not be tipped back, remember this opens the airways.
2. The cup rests between the lips, not teeth.
3. Encourage a closed mouth and lips round the cup edge.
4. Give drinks one gulp at a time.

Positioning

The nurse has a vital role in understanding and ensuring good techniques of positioning. It is, therefore, vitally important that the nurse works in partnership with the physiotherapist. Through good communication misunderstandings between nursing staff and physiotherapy can be avoided. This is achieved by means of house meetings, case conferences, videos, wall-charts, timetables, information packs, and frequent information discussions.

These occasions are used, among other things, by nurses to demonstrate the value of having time to cuddle and play with residents without them using any equipment and for therapists to demonstrate the necessity of using equipment and orthotics for most of the time.

The physiotherapist will advise on the different types of positions. To prevent deformity it is not enough just to position someone and then to leave him in that position for hours. If the person is kept moving from one position to another he is less likely to become deformed.

Aids and appliances

Nurses should become familiar with special equipment to help multiply handicapped people lead a more normal life:

- AFO (Ankle Foot Orthosis).
- Plastazoa spinal jackets.
- Ritchie bars.
- Prone lying wedges.
- Side-lying wedges.
- Walking frames.
- Hydrotherapy and Jacuzzi facility.
- Specially adapted chairs.
- Tommy trolleys.
- Vibration equipment.
- Tri pillows.
- Tables.
- Wedges.

It is important to offer a variety of positionings throughout the day so that the resident does not become progressively stiffer and more deformed.

The nurse as a provider of play, recreation, stimulation and social outlet

The nurse has to adopt a positive and imaginative approach towards what the handicapped person is capable of doing. Not dwelling on what they can't do. The nurse has an important role in providing a stimulating and learning environment. However, many people who visit special care dwellings for the most handicapped people are often apprehensive and adopt a negative attitude. It is not as easy a task in any way trying to stimulate an individual who shows no interest or awareness that you are even there. The resident who sits quietly and appears in a world of his own is very little trouble to those who care for him. He does not have the natural curiosity to explore the environment around him and does not show any signs of likes or dislikes. He sits quietly and there is a temptation for staff to leave him. He is not able to move to lift his head, he is blind and is completely dependent on staff for all his daily living needs. He cannot grasp objects due to the degree of deformity of his hands. As well as having a pronounced asymmetrical tonic neck reflex (ATNR) (in ATNR when one arm is flexed the other one is extended and the head turns towards the extended arm).

This particular resident needs help and constant stimulation if they are to become more aware of themself and the world around him. Individuals such as the child described can develop to their full potential but what is needed is a commitment from nurses who shouldn't see education and stimulation as something that is carried out only by therapists or school teachers in a different building. Nurses/care staff need to work in partnership with teachers and therapists and each individual should be assessed. A well thought out structured plan should be implemented and reviewed on a regular basis. In saying that play should be fun and is often spontaneous it needn't have an end result. It is important for nurses not to feel shy and inhibited. Nurses need to realize that play and stimulation is natural. The baby/child learns about the world around him by sucking, hearing and seeing, smelling, touching. Unfortunately the profoundly mentally handicapped person is so handicapped that they require all these different stimuli to be introduced into their world. Play/stimulation shouldn't be seen as separate activity from daily living. Mealtimes and dressing and bathing are activities that can involve staff playing and getting involved in games and generally making the activity fun.

Nurses should seek advice from teachers, therapists, play centres/therapists, toy libraries on play aspects and ways of providing stimulation. Many firms who specialize in toys for the handicapped will demonstrate their toys to staff. However, it would be important to involve the resident in the demonstration of the toy as a lot of money can be spent on equipment and toys that don't best suit the individual needs.

It is important that the profoundly mentally handicapped person is positioned in such a way so that they have the potential to learn. It would be a wasted exercise if a child was positioned in a standing frame facing a blank wall or in side lying position without anything in their arms or any stimulation provided around them.

Education programme for Graham

Graham is 19 years of age.

He has left school and the special care house where he now lives is trying to carry on where school finished.

Requirement	Nursing action
Graham required a good deal of stimulation and involvement	1. Referral to play therapist 2. Referral to play centre 3. Advice from Graham's teacher 4. Referral to neighbourhood Therapy Centre 5. Indicate Graham's likes/dislikes

Programme of activities in unit

1. *Water play* – Jacuzzi. In the house there is a Jacuzzi which gives Graham a lot of stimulation through the buoyancy and massaging effect. Graham smiles a lot and shows a great deal of pleasure. We have noticed that just prior to use, putting Graham into the Jacuzzi. He is beginning to smile and makes pleasant noises. He is beginning to anticipate pleasure which is an important aspect of learning.
2. *Hydrotherapy* – Graham has two sessions in the Physiotherapy Department. The facility enables Graham to move about in water. It helps Graham to relax. Some examples of other residents who use the facility:
   Jim kicks his legs and only needs a little support under his back. Alan kicks vigorously and sometimes floats alone.
3. *Prone position* – Playing with toys in paddling-pool.
   Graham enjoys this activity but requires staff to move his hands to feel the water and hear noise that can be made. Susan will play for ages in this position.
   Bathtime: fill up water in a bottle and let the water fall on skin of child or on water.
   Filling up coloured bottles of water improves visual stimuli.
4. *Finger painting* – Graham is positioned at table cut-out for his wheelchair and is presented with paper and finger paint. The member of staff encourages Graham to feel and move the paint around the surface of the paper. Presenting a variety of colours it isn't obvious in any way if Graham enjoys this activity but we have noticed he is making more random movements.
5. *Other activities* – Battery operated toys are converted so that they can be operated with prompt by Graham. Mobiles are particularly useful for encouraging visual stimulation as well as encouraging some of the residents to reach and touch.
   Within the home there is a music class in which one of the teachers plays the piano and we sing with the residents. We try to involve the child in the tempo and movement of the music and we have a general theme which we work into the songs. In the past we had songs about the sea and the children were involved with the school staff and nurses in designing pictures and dressing-up around the theme.

Tactile stimuli/aromatherapy/olfactory stimulation

The use of different oils/lotions can have a relaxing effect when massaged on Graham's back when he is in the prone position. Within the ward we have various toning and massaging (electrical) machines that are purchased by the general public to relieve tension and strain. Graham due to the fact that he is often quite stiff and tense responds well to being massaged – these sessions can be even more effective with quiet music to evoke a relaxing and calm atmosphere. Graham also responds well to the foot spa which massages his feet. As well as the foot massager which he clearly enjoys.

The different oils/lotions can also help the olfactory stimulation of Graham. Some oils can have a strong and pleasant effect. We are trying to initiate cause and effect which we take for granted. Graham's responses are obviously very slow but giving him the opportunity to experience different tastes and smells. Enlightens him and gives him more experiences.

Various oils and lotions can have a very calming and therapeutic effect and used in conjunction with shiatso the whole exercise can be very effective.

Social outings and events

It is very important for Graham as well as the other residents within the special care house to be involved in activities and events outside. To plan ahead, to celebrate birthdays by having parties or going out for a meal. Always buying a birthday present. Within the unit we have had regular holidays and weekend trips. Events connected with food. For example, we had an Indian Day where we all dressed-up around the theme as well as cooking the food in the unit so that some of the residents could experience the different smells and tastes.

We purchased a vehicle out of a fund raising project which enables us to take the residents out on a regular basis. The feeling of involving the residents in everything is important. It is easy for people to say that when we are doing cooking with the residents we are actually doing it, but within the whole experience we encourage Graham to experience the different smells/tastes of what we are cooking. Some of the residents with prompt (physical) are able to stir the contents in the basin.

9.3 Dental health

Karen Allen

Healthy teeth and gums are important for the mentally handicapped person's overall health and well-being. They are needed to improve feeding, aid speech development and maintain an attractive appearance. For some the mouth may even be needed for use as an accessory limb.

Tooth decay and gum disease are caused by the sticky film of plaque which builds up on our teeth all the time. If not removed daily it may harden to become dental calculus or tartar which can cause further gum disease. Tartar must be removed by a dentist or dental hygienist as it cannot be brushed away.

Generally mentally handicapped people have a similar level of tooth decay to that of their non-handicapped peers. In contrast the amount of gum disease is much greater and is most commonly due to poor oral hygiene. Severe gum disease is a particular problem for the person with Down's syndrome, the lower front teeth can be severely affected and are frequently lost early in life, posing both functional and aesthetic problems.

The mentally handicapped person may have additional problems which predispose them to increased levels of disease.

Dental facial abormalities

Malocclusion occurs more often in the handicapped, the teeth being irregularly arranged in the jaws. This causes food debris and plaque to accumulate more quickly and increases the difficulty of plaque removal during tooth brushing.

Malocclusion is commonly found in people with cerebral palsy and is thought to be caused by abnormal muscle behaviour. In the profoundly mentally handicapped person the persistence of the infantile swallowing behaviour pattern causes the upper teeth to become proclined, due to the forward position of the tongue in contact with the lower lip.

Teeth and oral structures

Delays in tooth formation and eruption patterns are more frequently seen in the mentally handicapped person. In Down's syndrome some permanent teeth may fail to develop and the first teeth may have to last a lifetime.

Mouth-breathing

There may be an increased tendency to mouth-breathe especially in the profoundly handicapped. This causes the lips and tongue to become dry and fissured. Small sips of water and Vaseline applied to the lips regularly can help to reduce this effect. Mouthbreathing can also increase the risk of tooth decay and halitosis (bad breath).

The non-functional mouth

Limited tongue, lip and cheek function in many profoundly handicapped people can lead to an excessive plaque build up and gross calculus formation. This increases the likelihood of gum disease, especially in the areas towards the back of the mouth where access for tooth brushing can be most difficult.

Bruxism

Tooth grinding is another common occurrence in the profoundly mentally handicapped and can cause excessive wear on the teeth. An unexpected increase in the amount or frequency of grinding may indicate the presence of dental pain and a dentist's opinion should be sought.

Epilepsy

Epilepsy is often treated with phenytoin (Epanutin). In approximately 50% of patients, a marked chronic hyperplasia of the gums can occur. The gums may become so grossly enlarged that they mask the teeth beneath, making plaque control extremely difficult. The hyperplasia is the cause of a reaction of the gum to an irritant such as plaque and it is rarely seen in those patients who maintain good oral hygiene.

The aims of dental care for the mentally handicapped person should be to ensure complete dental health, through the assessment and development of a comprehensive preventive and treatment programme, to begin as early in life as possible. In this way both tooth decay and gum disease and their treatment can be reduced to a minimum and the child's future behaviour pattern can be shaped.

Prevention

Diet

Avoid sugar right from the start so that your child does not get a taste for sweet things. Remember it is the pattern of food and drink consumption that is important, as frequent and prolonged intakes of items containing sugar leads to multiple and prolonged periods of acid attack of the tooth's enamel surface. Sugar-containing foods and drinks should be restricted to meal times.

The long-term use of syrupy medicines in children can lead to tooth decay. Medicines contain sugar to encourage children to take them but some medicines are available in sugar-free forms. Your doctor can advise you and can prescribe this whenever possible. If a child is on long-term medication containing syrups, extra care should be taken to ensure the teeth are cleaned after giving the medicine.

Oral hygiene

It is gum disease, in particular the daily control of dental plaque which represents the greatest difficulty for many mentally handicapped people. Shaw (1983) did, however, demonstrate that even severely mentally handicapped children could be instructed in oral hygiene and could carry out tooth brushing procedures for themselves. The individual should always be encouraged to participate and whenever possible become responsive for their own oral hygiene care. As many mentally handicapped people may never be motivated to carry out oral hygiene procedures spontaneously, success is ultimately dependent on the involvement and supervision by parents and staff, at home, at school, on the wards or later in Adult Training Centre as part of the individual's personal hygiene programme.

Brushing (Figure 9.1–9.9)

The carer assisting with brushing must have control of the mentally handicapped person's head and body, have adequate light and maximum visibility. The position will vary according to the person's handicap, size and cooperation. Whatever position is chosen, it is important that the handicapped person feels as relaxed as possible. This may be aided by brushing at the same time every day, at a time when the person will be at their most receptive. It is better to brush thoroughly and properly once a day at this time, than several times a day and not effectively. Further relaxation can be achieved by maintaining some kind of physical contact, e.g. stroking the face or talking in a low, calm voice.

A good position for tooth brushing is to stand or sit behind the person, whilst supporting the head and opening the mouth with your free hand. Bean-bags or a chair with a head-rest are also good supports and may help the person feel relaxed and secure. If the person has uncontrolled movements or is uncooperative, it may be easier to do the brushing with the help of another carer who can hold the arms and/or the legs.

The toothbrush of choice should have a small head and flexible nylon bristles. It should allow the user to reach all tooth surfaces and gum margins easily. Toothbrushes should be replaced at regular intervals, the time interval varying with each individual, but may be approximately every 2–3 months. Modifications of toothbrushes can be made where arm, hand or finger movements are limited. Bending the handle can be helpful and can be done by gently heating the handle in very hot water (Figure 9.9). The dentist or dental hygienist can help to select the correct tooth brush for each individual.

The chosen toothbrushing technique is not as important, providing it removes all plaque. A suggested method is to ensure that the bristles are angled towards the gum margin and the teeth are brushed two or three at a time, in a circular or 'mini scrub' motion. By gently pulling the cheek to the side and ensuring that the person does not open their mouth too widely, the teeth at the back of the mouth should be easily accessible (Figures 9.4–9.6).

In a similar manner the teeth and gums at the front of the mouth are easily visible when the lips are gently but firmly retracted as shown (Figures 9.5–9.7). Care should be taken to ensure that all surfaces of the teeth and gums are brushed. Disclosing tablets and solution can be used to stain plaque on the teeth and can provide a quick check on the effectiveness of toothbrushing.

In exceptional circumstances the profoundly mentally handicapped person may be unable to tolerate toothbrushing. In this case chlorhexidine mouthwash, an effective plaque inhibiter, may be applied to the teeth and gums using a foam tipped stick. Dental advice should be sought before routine use of chlorohexidine, however, as regular use leads to staining of the teeth.

Fluoride

Fluoride is particularly beneficial for the teeth. The regular use of a fluoride toothpaste can substantially reduce tooth decay. In the absence of water fluoridation, the child whose medical, physical or mentally handicapping condition places them at risk from tooth decay or its treatment should be given fluoride supplements (BASCD, 1988).

Dental assessment

Prevention is the key aspect of any dental service for the handicapped. Introduction to the dentist should start at an early age, as soon as the teeth begin to appear. By arranging regular dental check-ups for the mentally handicapped person, a trusting relationship can build up and the dentist can be seen as a friend. In this way potential problems can be identified and dealt with early, and dental disease can be prevented.

Mentally handicapped adults living in long-stay hospitals have previously had their dental care provided by the hospital dental service. As these men and women move into the community, the more able may be treated within the General Dental Service. Many mentally handicapped people, however, because of psychological and behavioural problems or additional physical handicaps may feel they are unable to cope with treatment or have difficulties in gaining access to care. These individuals may be more appropriately cared for within the Community Dental Service where the expertise and time should be available to deal with the special needs of this group of patients.

References

BASCD (British Association for the Study of Community Dentistry) (1988) *The Home Use of Fluorides for Preschool Children: A Policy Statement*, BASCD, London

Shaw, L., Harris, B.M., Maclaurin, E.T., *et al*. (1983) Oral hygiene in handicapped children: a comparison of effectiveness in the unaided used of normal and electrical toothbrushes. *Dental Health*, **22(1)**, 4–5

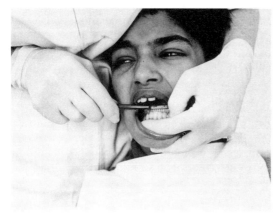

Figure 9.1

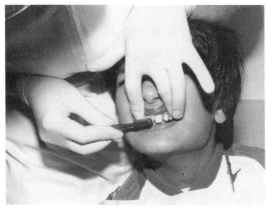

Figure 9.2

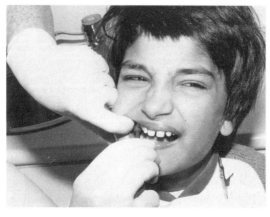

Figure 9.3

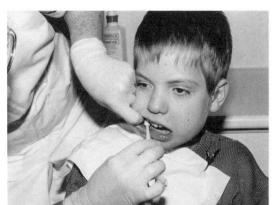

Figure 9.4

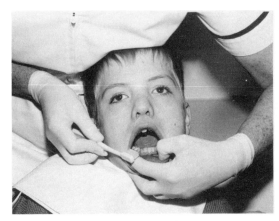

Figure 9.5

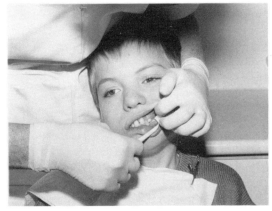

Figure 9.6

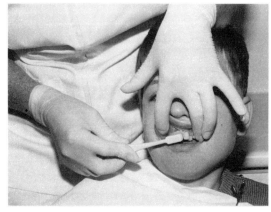

Figure 9.7

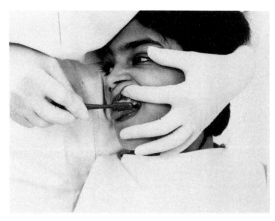

Figure 9.8

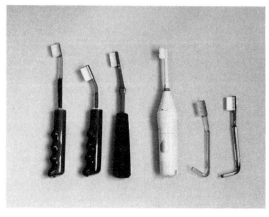

Figure 9.9

9.4 Physiotherapy

Eleanor Wilkinson

(For reasons of clarity, the physiotherapist is referred to as 'she' and the client as 'he'. Female clients are included throughout, as are the many male physiotherapists working in this field.)

Physiotherapy specifically for mentally handicapped people was first introduced about 25 years ago, for the benefit of hospital residents. The large mental handicap institutions housed people of all ages who had additional physical problems, which included cerebral palsy and other neurodevelopmental deficits. Some years before, physiotherapy for children suffering from cerebral palsy had been revolutionized by the work of Karel and Berta Bobath, who described abnormal postural reflexes in children, and developed a comprehensive rationale of treatment (Bobath and Bobath, 1987). This, and other paediatric techniques, were adapted and developed to cover a wider range of age and disability. Other well-tried treatment methods were enlisted, and new ones developed. Another branch of the profession began to grow, and now has a thriving clinical interest group, the ACPMH (Association of Chartered Physiotherapists in Mental Handicap.)

Today the populations of the mental handicap hospitals are much smaller, but the need for physiotherapy remains as great as ever. Skills that have been built up over the years are being practised in new situations. This challenge is being met by community mental handicap physiotherapists, who may be supported by specialist departments, or work as members of community mental handicap teams. Although ex-hospital residents use some generic health services successfully, experience has shown that specialist support is still needed, and this applies particularly to physiotherapy.

Physiotherapy for people with mental handicaps is indicated in many conditions or situations which impair potential for independence. The physiotherapist often knows the client or resident already, and identifies difficulties with which she can help. There may be self-referral, or a doctor, nurse, parent, teacher, or other concerned person can refer. In all cases, the physiotherapist should make contact with the client's general practitioner or consultant (if this does not already exist), and study any relevant medical history. She will also make an assessment; this includes a careful evaluation of the client's strengths and needs, and forms the basis for a treatment plan which sets attainable goals.

Conditions and situations encountered by the physiotherapist

The physiotherapist's involvement is usually due, directly or indirectly, to the client's neurological deficit. When there are severe physical handicaps, continuing physiotherapy management is indicated, and periods of low-level input, or simple monitoring, are punctuated with more intense interventions. One advantage of this continuous, informal contact is that many problems can be identified and dealt with before becoming intractable. Fractures, soft-tissue injuries, arthritis, chest infections, and orthopaedic surgery will also involve physiotherapy. Admissions to other hospitals are usually short, with early discharge home or to respite care, when the physiotherapist will continue or initiate a treatment programme.

Clients can be described according to their type of handicap, or by age group.

People who have cerebral palsy

The aims of physiotherapy are four-fold:

1. Inhibition of pathological reflex activity (which causes spasticity, muscle imbalance, unwanted movements and a variety of other difficulties) by good handling and positioning methods. If inhibition is not practised from a very early stage, the client remains wholly or partly immobile, prevented by abnormal postures from attaining functional movement. Permanent stiffness and deformity often result, varying in severity from a tight heel tendon, leading to poor walking balance and painful pressure on the ball of the foot, to complete body rigidity and asymmetry. At worst, this prevents the client from attaining any useful position from which to bear weight, use his hands, or achieve social contact and communication.
2. To initiate and reinforce the mature movements and postural control which are essential for independence at any level. These abilities are intrinsic in all basic mobility and self-care skills, as well as in recreational, sporting, and artistic activities. Once achieved, purposeful movement improves self-image, confidence, and physical fitness.
3. To enrich sensorimotor experience, which is always deficient when there is poverty of movement.
4. To share skills with parents, carers, and all who have day-to-day contact with the client, and to involve him with his own self-management.

Functional movement depends on the attainment of good stability, and on interpreting information about body position and spatial relationships.

People with simple motor delay or other neuromotor handicaps

Other clients do not present with obvious abnormal reflex activity, but show generalized delay in attaining milestones such as sitting, crawling, and walking. Muscle tone is (often grossly) low, posture is poor, and there is a tendency to overweight and low exercise tolerance. There might be recurrent or chronic respiratory infections, congenital heart defects, or sensory handicaps. The commonest condition characterized by simple motor delay is Down's syndrome. Others show delayed and patchy motor development, late onset or progressive neuromotor dysfunction. The aims of treatment will be adapted to suit the client's individual needs.

The young adult

The multiply handicapped child will usually have had contact with a physiotherapist at his school. Until recently, this contact probably stopped at the age of 18 or 19, unless the young person became a hospital resident. Hospital admission at this stage is now unusual, and physiotherapists are working in many adult training centres, hostels, and client's homes. Here they are treating not only young school-leavers, but other adults who may have had no contact with therapists since their school days. Progress can continue into the third, fourth and even fifth decade. However, development needs encouragement, and hard-won abilities must be used if they are not to be lost.

It is possible for a client to attain a new skill after months, or even years of apparent lack of progress. It is doubly important for severely cerebral-palsied young adults to continue their physiotherapy management and to expand their movement experience after leaving school (Golding and Goldsmith, 1987).

The older adult

Problems of the elderly tend to be more prevalent among mentally handicapped people than in the general population, and onset is often very much earlier. Arthritis, parkinsonism, soft-tissue injuries and fractures (linked to poor balance, epilepsy, and osteoporosis), venous insufficiency, and varicose ulcers are only a few of the conditions the physiotherapist is called upon to treat. The overall aim of treatment is to help the client to achieve or prolong independence and mobility. This will prevent, or greatly reduce, the incidence of chest infections, pressure sores, contractures, and many other conditions. If prevention is not possible, many of these problems will respond to specific physiotherapy techniques (Cash, 1973, 1974).

The roles of the physiotherapist

The paediatric physiotherapist

The child with special needs and his family can be supported by a paediatric physiotherapist, or by a mental handicap physiotherapist with paediatric training, who is able to continue and broaden her contact with the client after he leaves school. In the first case, the child's treatment should eventually be handed over to a therapist working with adults who have mental handicaps, care being taken to ensure continuity. In either case, her approach will be modified by the client's learning difficulties. The therapist's choice of treatment method will be influenced by her experience and training; there are many well-tried and well-documented techniques (Levitt, 1977; Finnie, 1974; Bobath and Bobath, 1987).

The hydrotherapist

One of the most useful facilities a physiotherapist can have is a purpose-built hydrotherapy pool. The severely handicapped client can float free and relaxed without the relentless restriction of gravity. Often far more movement (active and passive) can be obtained in the warm water than is possible elsewhere, and primary water skills can be practised before progressing to a group situation in a larger pool.

The member of a multidisciplinary team

There is usually a team of people involved, professionally or otherwise, with every person who has a mental handicap. Beside the client himself, there may be parents, teacher, nurse, occupational and speech therapists, doctor, social worker, and psychologist. As part of this team, the physiotherapist teaches parents and care staff how to handle and position the severely handicapped, and how to help all clients to attain their maximum independence. She is also the link between client and specialists such as orthopaedic consultant, orthotist, wheelchair technician, and bioengineer. The physiotherapist may be a full member of a community mental handicap team, involved as an adviser, or take referrals from the core team – depending on the type of team operating in the area.

The recreational therapist

The physiotherapist's goals are often achieved by using the motivation and enjoyment generated in recreational therapy.

Swimming
This is a skill that can add an extra dimension to the life of someone who is severely handicapped. For him the teaching method of choice is the Halliwick Method, as developed by the Association of Swimming Therapy (Association of Swimming Therapy, 1981). A group of swimmers learns, through carefully planned activities and games, to be safe and at home in the water without buoyancy aids. All the activities are designed to teach predetermined skills, using trained instructors in a one-to-one ratio with the swimmers. The group leader is likely to be a physiotherapist with Halliwick training. For this type of swimming group, it is desirable to have the use of a pool which has been heated to a comfortable temperature.

Other, more traditional methods of teaching are possible with more able groups, when the number of helpers and the water temperature are not so critical.

Riding
Physiotherapists find that riding is a most useful therapy for many of their clients. Riding is a symmetrical activity, which utilizes balance and whole-body coordination in a very enjoyable way. The rider learns to control his progression, sometimes for the first time, and to relate to and communicate with the pony. The Riding for the Disabled Association is the parent organization of 670 local groups all over the United Kingdom. Trained voluntary helpers are the mainstay of every group. The Chartered Society of Physiotherapy has a Riding for the Disabled Specific Interest Section.

'Keep-fit' and group exercise
Exercise groups are tailored to suit the clients. A group might be designed for profoundly or multiply handicapped people of any age, elderly ambulant or semi-ambulant clients, hyperactive or clumsy children, or physically able but behaviourally disturbed young adults. Some groups are led by a physiotherapist alone; some

involve several disciplines. The venue could be an adult training centre, hospital ward, physiotherapy department, or school. Good weather will often entice a group out of doors. Sometimes activities are planned along early developmental lines, in which case the class will probably take place on floor mats. Another format is the circle of people seated on chairs or stools. More able clients can run relay and obstacle races, or play indoor hockey and other team games. Most sports and pastimes can be adapted for wheelchair users. Useful equipment includes balls of all sizes, hoops, small rings, beanbags, light batons and the multicoloured exercise canopy. Appropriate music can be an essential element, but indiscriminate use of music is to be avoided. The aims of group activities range from reinforcing appropriate behaviour, to teaching therapeutic handling methods to a group of staff. Other aims may be the improvement of cardiovascular fitness, spatial awareness, balance and coordination, body awareness, or range and strength of movement.

The aids and equipment adviser

Aids and equipment which are purpose-made enable clients with physical handicaps to have better and more independent lifestyles than if they are limited to 'normal' household furniture.

Positioning equipment
To prevent the onset of positional deformities, and to provide comfort and security, children and adults with severe neuromotor handicaps must have a variety of supported positions throughout the day and night. They therefore need equipment such as standing frames, side-lying boards, and specialized seating. There is now a bewildering variety of this type of equipment on the market, and experience is necessary to negotiate the maze of catalogues, exhibitions and sales literature. The best plan is to try before buying – either by asking for the item to be sent on a sale or return basis, or (preferably) by visiting another centre where it can be tried out by the client. If money can be made available for an equipment library, some of these expensive items can be lent to families and adult training centres where they can be tried out for a longer period. Suitable easy seating can provide an occasional alternative to the wheelchair, and Kirton Designs Ltd. have a good range of specialized chairs, or will make a chair to individual requirements. Other invaluable equipment items are various types of standing frames supplied by Rifton, Joncare, James Leckey, and Nottingham Aids. Kirton Designs also make simple foam wedges and cylinders, and the Multiwedge for adults who need more control to lie prone comfortably. The physiotherapist can make equipment using fire-retardant high-density foam cut with an electric carving knife, assembled with thixotropic glue and upholstered in Ambla. A friendly joiner can be asked to make one-off wooden pieces to the clients' measurements.

Orthotics
It can be convenient to organize a regular clinic, when a number of clients need to be seen by the orthotist. The physiotherapist will bring her knowledge of the client to the assessment and fitting process. Suitable shop-bought or stock shoes and boots can be adapted in most cases to give the client a stable walking base, but surgical footwear may be necessary . Nowadays there is a choice for special footwear, which is available in a variety of styles. Items like spinal jackets, ankle-

foot orthoses, surgical footwear, and protective helmets are individually measured, cast, or moulded by the orthotist.

Walking and mobility aids
If a client has balance problems, his walking base may have to be enlarged by using an aid ranging in size from a simple walking stick to a Rollator, Mobilator or Forearm Support Walker. For others who only walk as a therapeutic (as opposed to a functional) activity, there are the Arjo Pilot and the Meyland Walker.

Wheelchairs
Assessment of client's needs and choice of wheelchair involves the therapist and wheelchair technician, and possibly an orthotist if a moulded seating shell is necessary. The priority is a good functional sitting position, enabling the client to propel himself if possible. If this is not realistic, an electrically propelled chair could be feasible. Every wheelchair must be suitable for the daily living situation, and questions must be asked about portability and car transport, width of doorways and manoeuvrability, and whether the chair is for continual or occasional use. Some clients who cannot propel with their arms can get around by using their feet to move the chair along the floor.

The physiotherapist working with people who have mental handicaps learns to use a flexible and innovative approach to each new challenge. She must be patient, persistent, and eternally optimistic. It is indeed a privilege when clients and their families regard her as a friend as well as their therapist.

References

Association of Swimming Therapy (1981) *Swimming for the Disabled*. E.P. Publishing, London
Bobath, B. and Bobath, K. (1987) *Motor Development in the Different Types of Cerebral Palsy*. Heinemann Physiotherapy, London
Cash, J.E. (1973) *A Textbook of Medical Conditions for Physiotherapists*, Faber & Faber, London
Cash, J.E. (1974) *Physiotherapy in some Surgical Conditions*, Faber & Faber, London
Finnie, N.R. (1974) *Handling the Young Cerebral Palsied Child at Home*, William Heinemann Medical Books, London
Golding, R. and Goldsmith, L. (1987) *The Caring Person's Guide to Handling the Severely Multiply Handicapped*, MacMillan Education, Basingstoke
Levitt, S. (1977) *Treatment of Cerebral Palsy and Motor Delay*. Blackwell Scientific Publications, Oxford

Addresses of organizations and equipment Suppliers

Riding for the Disabled Association,
Avenue 'R',
National Agricultural Centre,
Kenilworth,
Warwickshire CV8 2LY

The Chartered Society of Physiotherapy,
14 Bedford Row,
London WC1R 4ED

Association of Swimming Therapy,
Secretary: Ted Cowen,
4 Oak Street,
Shrewsbury SY3 7RH

Kirton Products (Specialised Easy Seating),
6, Rookwood Way,
Hollands Road Industrial Estate,
Haverhill,
Suffolk CB9 8BP

Rifton (Positioning Equipment),
Robertsbridge,
East Sussex TN32 5DR

Joncare (Positioning Equipment),
7 Ashville Trading Estate,
Nuffield Way,
Abingdon,
Oxon OX14 1RL

James Leckey Design (Positioning Equipment),
Design House,
Kilwee Industrial Estate,
Dunmurry,
N. Ireland BT17 0HD

Nottingham Rehab (Positioning Equipment),
17, Ludlow Hill Road,
West Bridgeford,
Nottingham NG2 6HD

Remploy Ltd., Medical Products Division (Mobility Aids),
415 Edgware Road, Cricklewood, London NW2 6LR

Arjo Hospital Equipment Ltd. (Arjo Pilot Walking Aid),
SPD Building, Acre Road,
Reading,
Berks. RG2 0SU

Meyland Walking Aid. Made in Denmark.
Supplied by:
Aremco,
Grove House,
Lenham,
Kent ME17 2PX

9.5 Art therapy

Simon Willoughby-Booth

When faced with an artwork, perhaps an incomprehensible mass of lines on a sheet of paper or a roughly shaped piece of clay, how can one begin to make sense of this experience? In what way does what one sees relate to its maker, to his or her needs and emotions and to the process which must have happened to create it? There is no easy means to enable us to see through the medium of the artwork to the creator on the other side; but with a sensibility for the nature of the creative process and for the relationship between therapist and client, it is possible to begin to understand the inherent meaning of the work and its dynamic in a therapeutic context. An artwork is a reification of the thoughts and feelings of its creator, and through it, these mental activities have a concrete existence distinct from the person who makes it. The artwork becomes an agent for the transmission of some aspect of the reality inhabited by its maker to the person who perceives it, and that act of perception represents an attempt to empathize with that other reality. Art therapy utilizes this empathic link as a means of helping the person living with disability, illness or disturbance, to deal with its effects.

Art therapy is an enabling process: enabling people with learning difficulties to utilize their own creativity in making artwork; enabling them to establish a sense of their own identity within the therapeutic relationship; enabling the expression and recognition of their needs; enabling client and therapist to address and begin to meet these needs; enabling and promoting durable change and personal growth. Some of the fundamental human needs that may be addressed during art therapy are the acquisition of self-esteem; the control of one's personal space and environment; the formation of meaningful relationships and the development of effective interactions. This is not intended as a definitive list but any one of the above might be of profound importance to a person with learning difficulties, who is often ill equipped to recognize and successfully meet such needs, and unable to articulate or acknowledge them concretely.

The role of the therapist is to facilitate the client's engagement in artwork and, through the medium of the art experience, to build a rapport with the client in response to his or her needs and expressed wishes. By adopting and developing appropriate strategies of intervention (or non-intervention), the therapist enables the client to advance towards a more autonomous situation; over which she or he has control and within which she or he functions effectively. By building a relationship centred on the process of making artwork, which is a non-threatening and enjoyable experience, the therapist is able to observe and interact with the client and build up an understanding of that person as a unique individual. In order to clarify some of the above points and to relate them to real, human situations;

the following descriptions of three people's involvement in art therapy will make clearer the actual process.

Claire

Claire was in her mid-teens at the time of her initial contact with the Art Therapy Department, which was during group sessions conducted to assess the needs of five young people from a special school. During sessions, Claire appeared to be isolated, to have very limited relationships with her peers and school staff, to have some degree of visual impairment and to be non-verbal. She preferred ritualized activities and was uninterested in using art materials spontaneously and appropriately.

To give a new format to the paintings done by the group, a large sheet of paper was put up on a screen, instead of on the table. Claire passed the screen and paused to examine the tray of paints beside it. With prompting and encouragement, she made some marks on the paper with a big brush and to support and validate what she was doing, some marks were made on the paper alongside her own. In subsequent sessions she was encouraged to paint and continued attempts to relate to her were made, by painting alongside and sharing the big sheet of paper. When the group sessions ended, it was decided to continue one-to-one work with her because of her growing response to painting. Primary aims at this time were to establish rapport, to make her aware of the shared activity, and to try to develop interaction through the act of painting.

During initial one-to-one sessions, Claire was encouraged to explore the range of marks she could make with crayons and paint. By working together on a shared sheet of paper, it was felt that she might become aware of, and later respond to, the marks made beside her own. A comfortable way of working was established, starting each session with a vigorous crayon drawing and then working into this drawing with paints. The balance of control in the drawings shifted progressively to Claire as her awareness and responses developed. The first clear indication of progress was her increasing attention to the colours in the painting, as she watched which ones were used and then chose the same colours herself. This became the basis for a simple game; taking turns to choose a colour and matching it with the same colour.

A similar awareness was shown, of the marks made in paint and crayon. At first, Claire's technique was to load her brush with paint and then to dab it rapidly and repeatedly onto the area in front of her. Gradually she began to extend her repertoire of marks, using bolder, sweeping movements in lines and curves. As the sessions progressed, she was offered increasing control over the direction of the work and given opportunities to make choices about materials and ways of working.

Four years after the first group sessions, Claire left school and her art therapy sessions had to be brought to a close. The final session was a manifestation of the changes that had taken place in Claire herself and in the relationship to her therapist. When she entered the art therapy room, she checked that paper was prepared; and when asked what she wanted to do she fetched a box of crayons, made sure that there was a clear space around her and began to draw energetically. For about 5 minutes she worked all over the paper, filling it with curving lines and sweeping elliptical marks, drawing as fast as she was able. She then paused to scrutinize the whole drawing. Searching through the box of crayons, she chose a different colour and proffered it to the therapist. When she got no response, she seized the therapist's hand and pressed the crayon into it. Keeping a firm hold on the hand, she led him to the paper and pointed to an empty space. When he persisted in refusing to respond, his hand was put on the paper, whilst Claire made drawing gestures and made him start to fill the gap. Before the space was completely filled in, Claire redirected the work to another part of the drawing and this process was repeated rapidly wherever there were blank areas. She had clearly determined that some areas needed further work and that this was a task for the therapist. It appears that she felt a need for a safe, containing boundary around the large forms she herself had drawn. Compliance, albeit with a show of reluctance, showed that her work and decisions were valued and respected. She was very able and confident in her control of the session and she had obviously enjoyed it. It is uncertain whether or not she really appreciated that this was her last session and it is regrettable, in view of the progress made in art therapy, that her involvement had to be curtailed before it had ceased to be fruitful. The making of artwork, in the context of a supportive and facilitating relationship, is central to the process and effective outcome of therapy. For Claire, art therapy provided a bridge to help in her transition from an intensely self-oriented life to a more appropriate relationship with her environment.

James

In a group, the art process becomes the focus of the group members' activities and interactions and a foundation for shared learning and development. Art therapy groupwork is a particularly effective approach as it removes the intense concentration on one-to-one interactions and creates multiple options for action and reaction, in a situation which, as the group develops a culture and cohesiveness, is safe and supportive. James is in his mid-forties and has attended art therapy for many years, spending as much time there as he possibly can each day. He is involved in an art therapy group which meets once a week for 2 hours.

The five members of the group function non-verbally and all the members have marked difficulties in communication and interaction. The two therapists who work with them use a mixture of verbal and gestural communication to direct and respond to the group's proceedings. The aim of the group is to provide a structured framework of art and other activities such as movement or music, which provide a forum for non-verbal interactions which will enable group learning processes to take place. Issues with which the group have had to deal include dependency, dominance, negotiating for time and space and how to maintain individuality within a group culture. Evidence for the existence of these, very typical, group therapy processes has been derived from observation of the group's behaviour, interaction and approach to its work, as well as from the actual artwork.

After the group had been meeting for some two and a half years, it was clear that James' engagement in the group was hindered by his difficulty in asserting himself and maintaining his own space in group paintings. Although he always began painting at the same time as the others, his territory was very quickly surrounded and then obliterated. This situation would, in most people, provoke anger and frustration and it was clear that James, whilst remaining apparently passive, was seeking a way forward. Several strategies were tried, to reinforce his obvious desire to contribute to the painting and to support him in asserting his own needs. When these were unsuccessful, it was decided to abandon the large collective works (12 ft × 5 ft), that the group were working on, and to see what would happen if each person had a big sheet of paper to himself.

At the start of the next session, James chose a palette of greens and white and immediately began work on one of the sheets of paper. He worked with great concentration for about 30 minutes and completed three paintings. It appeared that he knew exactly what he wanted to do and was exploring the effects he could create in a very 'painterly' manner, trying different ways of laying on the paint and mixing colours together. The impression given was that he had an already evolved method of painting but required the right situation within which he would be safe to try it out. This confidence was maintained and when, after several weeks, the group again tackled a shared painting, he was able to define and maintain his space within it. This simple and unobtrusive intervention led to an alteration in the dynamic of the group which helped James to extend his role in the group's work.

Michael

Art may be used in many different ways, according to the needs of the person involved. Michael is a very talented painter, despite his mental and physical handicaps, who uses the art therapy room as a studio, which reinforces his identity as an artist. He is an articulate man who can describe the importance of his work and his need to paint. Art therapy offers a supportive environment and in his work he can give reality and meaning to his feelings and express thoughts that might be rejected in other settings, such as his many paintings of nude women; and where he can take risks and work through emotions which are potentially threatening and overwhelming.

When his father became terminally ill, Michael discussed many of his feelings about this in art therapy, describing the course of the illness and how it affected him, with great calm. He informed the staff of the department when his father was re-admitted to a hospice and he realized that death was imminent. He had continued to work on his paintings throughout this period and in the fortnight before his father died, his work suddenly changed. Without any preliminaries or explanation, he painted two pictures; both are portrait heads, which are totally unlike all his other work. Both are powerfully expressive works in strong colours which vibrate and are clearly charged with his feelings. He has never chosen to talk about them but they must be seen as part of his preparation for the separation and loss, and a means of externalizing and coming to terms with feelings which were potentially too dangerous to be talked about with anyone else. The paintings played an essential, if tacitly unmentioned, part in Michael's successful working through of the process of grieving.

Conclusion

The ultimate aim of art therapy is to create, for the person with learning difficulties, opportunities for positive, lasting change and growth. The art therapist's understanding of the processes of making artwork and the many levels of thought, feeling and behaviour which may affect this process, provides a means of influencing and facilitating the client's ability to take advantage of this situation. As has been described above, change and growth in art therapy are the correlates of the individual's needs and it involves giving the client autonomy to achieve such change for him or herself, within the security of the therapeutic relationship.

No one should be referred to an art therapist merely because she or he likes drawing or needs to be occupied as the individual must have the capacity to progress through positive involvement in art experiences. The art therapist's assessment of the potential client will take account of responses to art media, to the art therapy environment and to the therapist, and will include an appraisal of the needs of the individual; made in conjunction with that person wherever feasible or with carers or other appropriate people. Through this process, goals for therapy can be established. The outcomes of a period of therapy can be measured in a number of ways: changes in behaviour, interaction, communication and engagement may be observed and the client may be able to verbalize his or her own views. The artwork produced in sessions will change and develop and provide tangible evidence of what is taking place. The whole functioning of an art therapy service may be evaluated by using models of service evaluation derived from the principles of normalization; to establish whether a high quality service has been created and maintained, which positively values service users and makes a significant contribution to their quality of life.

Art therapy is accessible to almost everyone, though it may not always be the most suitable approach. Some people are quite unmoved by art experiences or it may not be appropriate for their level of development and art therapy is not a panacea. Although a person may have difficulties in learning, communication, behaviour or other areas of their lives and despite physical or other handicaps, artwork and the creative process are exciting and effective therapeutic instruments, which promotes the growth of the individual towards a fuller and more effective life.

9.6 Music therapy

Jeanette Montague

Introduction

Every human being, irrespective of race, creed, age or intelligence, is a natural and gifted musician. Elements of music are melody, rhythm and harmony. They can exist separately or together to produce music. Each of us is made up of a series of complex rhythmic functions – pulse beat, heart rate, cell activity, brainwaves, metabolic rate. We each have a rate of functioning which is comfortable to us. When circumstances dictate that we have to function above our normal rate, we become stressed and pressured. When our environment dictates a slower rate of functioning we feel under-stimulated, bored and frustrated. Each one of us needs optimum conditions at work and in leisure, for our own rhythmic balance and needs to be met. Similarly, human beings speak, sing, chant, vocalize, sigh, groan, cough, cry. They interact with their environment not only through the rhythmic channels but also through melodic expressions. The newborn baby's cry has pitch, intonation, melody. The tribal chanting of ritualistic fragments are pitched and melodic. The vocal sounds of the child with profound learning difficulties are pitched and melodic. The voiced sigh of the old person tired of life is a melodic representation of her mood and feelings.

When elements of music happen together, we have harmony. Our environment is a musical masterpiece to which we all contribute. Every individual member matters to the end product. Where one member drops out, the place cannot be filled in the same way. This chapter focuses on the section of the orchestra we call 'people with a mental handicap'. It explores the contribution made by this section and shows that a player is a player no matter where they sit.

Setting the scene

Preparation for music therapy sessions is important. If an individual's contribution is to be valued, nurtured and developed, the therapist must provide optimum conditions, conducive to work of high quality. Consideration is given to such things as:

1. *Time of sessions* – is the client more responsive at certain times?
2. *Escort facilities* – Will shortage of staff mean that sessions have to be cancelled frequently?
3. *Transport* – Can non-ambulant clients be brought to sessions regularly?
4. *Accommodation* – Is the therapy room suitable for the client?

5. *Seating* – Is it appropriate?
6. *Distraction* – Is the level of stimulus appropriate; is the room quiet and free from unnecessary noise (e.g. works, machinery outside window)?

The stage is constructed around the individual and the scene is being set for him to take his chosen place with dignity.

Materials and resources

The therapy room contains some equipment. It has been selected with care, to provide each client with a range of experience, and a choice of media through which to work. The basic tools are a piano, drum and cymbal, selection of percussion instruments and audio-visual materials. Added to that, depending on clients' needs, will be specific items such as gong, swarmandal, vibraphone, harp, tabla, sarod, tumbadora. All are of excellent quality so that one feels uplifted, relieved, valued and respected when using them. A client with little mobility and stereotypic finger movements can play the harp, swarmandal or psaltery. The client with involuntary leg movement can make loud, low sounds on the bass drum, with his foot. The client who holds on tightly to objects will grasp the solid bar chimes, making them sound. The deaf and partially sighted client with limited sensory experience will explore the large gong with its ridges and bumps, harmonics and strong vibrations and glinting rays of light as the sun strikes its copper/bronze surface.

Referral and assessment

Appropriate referrals are made on behalf of clients who have communication and/ or behavioural difficulties. Also for those who have little self-confidence or awareness, or those with sensory problems. Martha, aged 18 years, has been referred by a medical officer. She is described on the referral form as 'the most mentally handicapped person ever seen on the ward', 'responds to nothing' and 'does not communicate or make eye contact'. A music therapy assessment session is arranged. Martha arrives in her wheelchair. She is tall and heavy. Her head hangs down and her hands lie motionless on her legs. There are 3 minutes of silence at the beginning of the session, then the index finger of her right hand twitches. The bodhran, a large lightweight skin-covered drum, is placed under her right hand so that when the same finger twitches again it makes a tiny sound on the drum. The therapist responds with an equally small sound on the same drum.

Some time later Martha coughs and concealed in the cough is a transient pitched sound. The therapist, who is also a highly trained musician, focuses in on the same pitch and responds vocally to it. There are now two channels of interaction open; index finger involuntary movement and vocal sound. The composition is underway. It is a quiet piece, almost like a primordial vision, elements awakening after a long rest. Later Martha's hands are cupped together by chance. There is a small gap between them. Two of the solid bar chimes are fed through the gap. The slightest movement of Martha's hands, legs or body, causes the two bars to sound against each other. When the sound is fairly loud, she lifts her head back and produces a strong single vocal sound.

The therapist improvises a plainsong-type melody to the syllables of Martha's name. It is strong and based on one sound, just like Martha's. The interactions develop as the two participants get to know each other on equal terms. Martha moves her foot. The bass drum is placed in front of it. Her strong shoes make a loud sound on the drum. She does it again and again. When the bar chimes are sounded on her right side she turns slightly towards them. When they are sounded on the left she does not move. There is sustained eye contact twice. Martha, like all of us, has a story to tell, needs to express, strengths to shake. The assessment shows that she is very much an individual, with her own distinct vocabulary. She responds to sounds, close physical contact and sensory opportunity. She is able to sustain eye contact, hears sounds at least from one side. Most of all she communicates with her environment and those around her. Most of us when we listen to music hear the tune, the catchy rhythm or the dramatic loud sequences. We can, however, turn to look further and listen more intently to appreciate that without the inaudible pizzicato or the seemingly insignificant repetitive arpeggios hidden in the depths of the harmonies, the tune would be less of a tune and the rhythm much less catchy. The assessment of suitability for music therapy looks not at the ability to sing or play instruments but at the whole person. It identifies strengths and needs in a general way and can aid diagnosis.

Aims and objectives

Aims in music therapy sessions do not differ from aims established for general improvement of quality of life. The means of achieving specific aims will differ in that the tools are music instruments and the technique is musical improvisation. The aims of music therapy may be identified as follows:

Communication	*Awareness*
Language comprehension	Awareness of self and of self in relation
Object discrimination	to others
Expression of feelings	Body awareness
Develop vocalizations	Name recognition
Eye contact	Relationship building
Develop verbal/non-verbal communication	
Socialization	
Motor skills	*General*
Increased control over involuntary movement	Utilize residual hearing
	Utilize residual sight
Gross and fine motor skills	Increase concentration/attention span
Meaningful use of hands	Decrease self-mutilation
Reaching and grasping	Reduce panic/anxiety
Relaxation	Increase motivation
Weight bearing	Express character/personality
Walking	

The music therapy process

Music therapists trained in different ways, use a variety of approaches in their work. The approach described here is client centred, non-directive and interactive. Following assessment of the client, the therapist has an overall view of the various strengths and needs. It has also been possible to learn something of the vocabulary – verbal and/or non-verbal – of the client. Armed with this knowledge, the therapist can then embark on the process of forming a relationship, building trust and security and getting to know the client better through the music they jointly produce. Within this relationship it is possible to experience feelings *with* the client, and also to acknowledge and hold the feelings, value them and interpret them. The response of the therapist in the music played may be 'I hear what you are saying' or 'I understand you feel very angry about this' or 'it is difficult for you to say what you want to say'. There are ways in improvization to communicate these responses through music. Clients communicating through music tell us about themselves in the content of their improvizations. For someone with low self-esteem, lack of confidence and reduced motivation, it may take several sessions before they feel comfortable enough to make a vocal sound. When that sound is eventually produced it is important that the therapist:

1. Acknowledges it by responding in some way.
2. Reinforces it by reacting in a musical way which enhances the sound.
3. Values it – by treating it as a valid and respected musical sound and communication.
4. Develops it – by treating it in specific musical ways, to open the idea out, expand on it and yet retain the familiar elements of the first utterance of the client.

Clients grow and develop in their music making, so that the therapist sees change, the musical interactions undergo transformation and the client experiences a freeing and release of pent up feelings and unexpressed communication. The process continues until there is a natural ending or until aims have been achieved. The process is monitored and recorded by video or audio means and written reports.

Case illustrations

Rachel is 24 years old. She is spastic quadruplegic, epileptic, non-ambulant. She is blind and perhaps deaf. She has no speech and language and is described as having no means of communication whatsoever. In session one, Rachel was introduced to the therapist and told where and when her music therapy sessions were to be. She was made physically comfortable and the session proper began. After a long period of silence Rachel's hand (which was lying limp on her leg) was gently placed on the swarmandal. The instrument was held at an angle so that Rachel's fingers on their own rested on the strings. The therapist withdrew all support so that Rachel, unaided, rested her hand on the instrument. Gravity eventually ensured that her hand came back to rest on her leg. As it slid down, her fingers and long nails plucked the strings of the instrument, causing it to sound. She had produced a series of notes, a rhythmic pattern, a musical fragment. The therapist replied. The process began again. Rachel's hand was gently and repeatedly placed on the instrument and allowed to, in its own time, return to rest on her leg. In the process, each time, she produced different music. Different, because each time her hand rested on different strings, and it moved down the strings at a different rate. Together then, client and therapist took turns to play music, communicating and interacting.

Over the next two sessions this same process continued. By session four, Rachel's wrist was seen to move slightly upwards in the direction of the instrument. This developed into a definite upward movement of her wrist and her index finger was poised ready to rest on a string. The instrument was carefully placed where her hand was about to land so that she always succeeded. Once on the strings, in her own time, the hand came down, her fingers making music on the strings as it went. By the end of session six, Rachel was able to recognize the therapist's voice, show excitement and anticipation when the swarmandal was heard, engage in turn taking activity, be an equal partner in a communication, use her hand, arm and fingers in a meaningful way. She had started to produce contented vocal sounds and moved her eyes when pleased and when she heard a response to her own sounds.

Joseph is 28 years old, with mild learning difficulties, emotional insecurity, word finding difficulty and inappropriate expression of anger. He often chose the harp to play in his music therapy sessions and would engage the therapist in 'intellectual' conversation about the intricacies of harp tuning. It took 7 months before the real issues and difficulties in his life were expressed. In session 25 Joseph had, as usual, chosen to play the harp. Therapist and client together improvised on the low thick strings. The piece lasted 15 minutes. At the end there was a long silence after which the question was asked 'what did that music sound like?' Joseph responded 'it is like the toilets in my ward. There is never any toilet roll. If there is toilet roll, there is no lock for the door. I hate going to the toilet in the ward. I try to keep it in.' The harp was turned round and another improvization played. This time Joseph took the high sounding strings. It lasted for 12 minutes. When asked to describe this music, Joseph said 'it is Cornton and Burnhill hostel. Having a cup of tea with friends – going to a concert – making your own tea – getting some peace and quiet'.

Together we explored the idea that Joseph had, through the two improvizations, said very fluently how he felt about his situation. On the one hand, subjected to inadequate toilets in a ward, where he tried to 'keep it in', and on the other, hopes of a life in the community and what that would mean. When asked verbally to express feelings about these two areas, Joseph would simply hang his head and exhibit his word finding difficulty at its worst. Given a non-threatening medium in which to work he was able to express fluently and openly how he felt about important aspects of his life.

Conclusion

Music therapists, in touch with their own music and creativity, aim to find and facilitate the creative process and music inherent in every client they work with. All of us are part of the whole, and each sound or movement produced by the client is part of the whole musical scenario. Utterances, however random or seemingly insignificant, are valued and respected. The environment must be conducive to therapy, and the materials carefully selected and skilfully used. Appropriate referrals will talk of communication and behavioural problems and not of musical ability. Aims and objectives link with every other discipline in the interdisciplinary team. The process respects the client as an individual and gives him the baton. A player is a player no matter where they sit. Any player can take the baton if and when they choose.

9.7 Occupational therapy

Linda Renton

Occupational therapy has much specialist knowledge to offer in the field of mental handicap. The core of occupational therapy is the therapeutic link between activity and dysfunction. The occupational therapist promotes functional independence through the analysis and application of relevant activity.

> 'The profession of occupational therapy has grown steadily over the last 50 years and continues to grow at a rate of 6% a year. Occupational therapy is the treatment of physical and psychiatric conditions through specific activities in order to help people reach their maximum level of function and independence in all aspects of daily life. Its approach is a holistic one, and aims to rehabilitate where possible, to maintain where total rehabilitation is not possible, to assist to readjustment where conditions are deteriorating, and at all times to consider quality of life.'
>
> (Craft, Bicknell and Hollins, 1985)

The process of occupational therapy

The occupational therapy process is highlighted in Figure 9.10 and shows the stages from initial client contact to discharge. It also identifies the basic assessment types and the three stages of treatment.

Assessment

'Any assessment, from informal evaluation to specific testing and diagnosis, aims to gather objective data which will help in the making of appropriate decisions.' (Peck and Hong, 1988). These decisions are usually client related and involve needs, future goals and training concerns.

There are six main reasons for assessment. These are: for screening purposes, to identify current level of functioning, as a diagnostic tool, to determine potential for training, to establish a baseline for training and to record and monitor progress and change. The occupational therapist may be involved in any of the above areas, and assessment is always carried out before a treatment plan is formulated. There are many different kinds of assessment utilized by occupational therapists and it is dependent upon the therapist's specific area of work as to which assessments are appropriate. Assessments utilized by occupational therapists can relate to: general

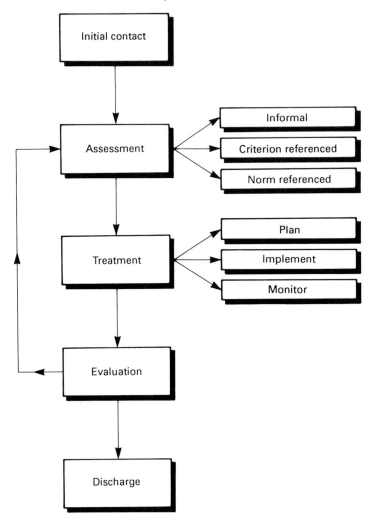

Figure 9.10 The treatment process in occupational therapy

ability, physical ability, hand function, perception, communication, play and interaction, self-care, social independence, independent living and work and leisure.

There are three levels of assessment, and the occupational therapist may well utilize all three. These levels include informal assessment, criterion-referenced assessment and norm-referenced assessment. Criterion-referenced assessment involves information gathering regarding clients abilities with no comparison of results to the performance of a sample group and norm-referenced assessment involves comparison of collated data with a sample group. These comparisons are researched and validated. Assessment can therefore be described as the means through which objective data can be gathered.

Living skills

The occupational therapist is concerned with activities of daily living or living skills. These are the activities which are carried out in the course of a normal daily routine. One can immediately appreciate the problems associated with attempting to categorize, assess then treat problem areas in the daily functioning of clients. One method of identifying and categorizing daily living skills is described by Peck and Hong (1988). This method involves breaking down living skills into three main levels: basic, intermediate and advanced living skills.

Basic living skills are those that are necessary to 'use' the body, make needs known and to learn. Skill in these areas allows the client to participate in and interact with their environment and social group and provides the basic building blocks for the development of personal care and self-help skills.

Intermediate living skills are those that apply to basic control, function, and communication skills. This involves perceptual/conceptual understanding, play, recreation and self-help skills. Clients who have independent mastery of intermediate living skills are able to care independently for themselves, apply their communication and interaction skills in a socially accepted manner but still require high levels of support.

Advanced living skills are those that make it possible to live independently in the community. This is one of the most complex of all training levels and includes budgeting, cooking and use of community facilities.

This categorization of living skills enables the occupational therapist to identify, assess and treat specific areas of dysfunction.

Treatment

As Figure 9.10 shows, treatment can only take place after appropriate assessment has been carried out. The client's abilities, needs, potential or diagnosis are identified, through assessment, and the occupational therapist can then 'develop programmes aimed at maximising ability and minimising disability' (Anstice and Bowden, 1985).

The treatment programme is made up of a programme of activities for the individual, aimed at treating the identified areas of dysfunction through activity. Although areas of dysfunction are usually highlighted, it is important to promote the positive areas of functioning.

An occupational therapist's treatment plan includes the following information:

1. Basic client data; name, date of birth, address, unit number.
2. Presenting problems.
3. Positive attributes (personal, social, cognitive practical).
4. Current treatments (medication, intervention from other disciplines).
5. Treatment aims.
6. Treatment objectives and strategies.
7. Future considerations.

The treatment plan is regularly monitored and reviewed, and clearly recorded.

To show how an occupational therapist might carry out treatment, an example from each of the basic, intermediate and advanced living skills will be highlighted below.

Hand function – basic living skill

Many clients with mental handicap also may have associated physical problems. Difficulties in hand function are not uncommon. Peck and Hong (1988) described hand function as not only depending on the motor control of the trunk, shoulder girdle, arms and hands, but also on visual, perceptual and cognitive development. Hand function is made up of reach, grasp and release and a general developmental delay may frequently present as a problem after assessment of a client. Occupational therapy may include the following aims:

1. To encourage hand–eye coordination.
2. To develop observation, tracking and scanning skills.
3. To develop reach, grasp and release.

Activities to meet these three broad aims could include bilateral work, e.g. clapping, tearing paper (collage work) and drawing (involving one hand stabilizing the paper and one drawing). Computer work/activities could also be utilized including the use of adapted hard- and software, e.g. specific programmes, microvitec touch sensitive screen, joystick and adapted switches.

Dressing – intermediate living skill

Dressing and undressing are frequently highlighted, after assessment, as areas requiring development for clients. To achieve independence in dressing some basic prerequisite skills are required. Klein (1983) outlined suggestions for teaching approaches and techniques to dressing. Dressing and undressing involves functional sequencing (movement patterns), serial order sequencing (ability to choose, match and coordinate clothes), and appropriate clothes for age, activity or weather conditions).

A specific problem area, frequently highlighted after assessment, may be that of lack of independence with lower limb garments. The aims of occupational therapy may include:

1. To break down the specific skill into component parts and then teach it to the client using the appropriate method, e.g. chaining, prompting, etc.
2. To offer a variety of activities to further develop the skill, e.g. physical ability, balance and hand function.

Activities to meet these aims could include the obvious activity of dressing. The occupational therapist could see the client regularly for dressing practice and could teach the basic steps to facilitate dressing independence. Although the beginning and end of the day may well be the most appropriate times for this, clients may frequently attend hydrotherapy, swimming or other activities, and this would be an ideal time to carry out treatment. Activities to develop general physical ability could include: parachute work, gymnastic ball games, floor games and computer games, using appropriate adapted switches, e.g. floor-pads, foot-switch. Hand function has been discussed above.

Budgeting – advanced living skill

There are many complex advanced living skills. Community living skills are practical skills required for community living. Budgeting is one such skill, made up of: coin recognition, simple arithmetic, money handling, shopping, planning and in some cases banking, menu planning and home accounts. Many clients require help in the area of budgeting as they have often lived in an institution for many years with little opportunity to develop independent budgeting skills.

The aims of occupational therapy, in this case, may be:

1. To develop skills in money handling, coin recognition and arithmetic.
2. To offer opportunities to carry out budgeting skills, in appropriate settings, e.g. post office, café and local shops.

Activities to meet these aims could include money dominoes, board games and 'counting' games, e.g. darts, sports and computer. There are also computer programs available which work specifically on budgeting skills, e.g. coin recognition, use of concept keyboard and games involving purchasing items. Other activities could also include the opportunity to practise skills in 'real' settings, e.g. regular visits, with reducing guidance to shops, cafés, banks etc.

Hopefully, by highlighting some general examples, from each level of living skills, an insight has been given into occupational therapy with clients who have a mental handicap. However, it should be remembered that the examples given are general in nature, and that frequently occupational therapy programmes are very specific.

Multi-disciplinary team work

Occupational therapists are committed to a multi-disciplinary approach to treatment, and a continual development of relationships with all members of the team is seen as vital in relation to the treatment of individual clients:

> 'An accurate understanding of the true extent of another Therapist's expertise, and an acknowledgement of area of overlapping interest and skills should lead to more appropriate referrals and expectations.' (Hollins, 1985)

A new model for multi-disciplinary teamwork in the community is emerging, that of the community mental handicap team, and occupational therapy can contribute to these emerging teams in two main ways. The first is as a professional team member to be involved as and when appropriate to contribute to the treatment of clients using the skills and techniques of occupational therapy. The second is as a core member of the community mental handicap team. The generic training of occupational therapists equip them with many skills relevant to the role of core team members, and occupational therapists have already established themselves as both core and team members.

Blundy and Prevezer (1986) conclude their article on community mental handicap teams by stating that 'role overlap in community mental handicap teams can be used positively to increase the understanding of other professionals enhancing and consolidating the working relationships between team members'.

Further contribution of occupational therapy

Occupational therapists are not always only involved in direct client contact. To utilize their skills most effectively they may frequently find themselves in the position of advisor, teacher or consultant. This can be highlighted if an example is given of a number of clients who are to be 'resettled' from hospital to a jointly funded (Health Board and voluntary agency) residential accommodation. Occupational therapy could offer training to the newly employed staff group on topics such as: role of occupational therapy; purposeful use of activity, assessment, programme plans, group work and activity analysis. The occupational therapist could also offer advice regarding the purchasing of equipment, e.g. recreational activities, creative equipment, aids to daily living equipment and adaptations that may be required. The occupational therapist could also offer ongoing support and involvement in developing programmes of activity for clients relating to enhancing their levels of independence and also in the monitoring and evaluation procedures.

Occupational therapists can also be involved in creating systems change within an organization or service. The increasing role of occupational therapists in policy decision making provides opportunities to guide service developments in line with underlying clinical philosophies, and the occupational therapists clinical knowledge contributes to the policy decision making procedure. The recent reorganization of the National Health Service has created opportunities for occupational therapists to influence policy making. Unit management teams, who manage and plan for mentally handicapped people, usually include an occupational therapist who is therefore in a position to contribute to the planning and development of services to mentally handicapped people.

In conclusion, occupational therapy has much specialist knowledge to contribute in the field of mental handicap and can be described as promoting functional independence through the assessment and treatment of dysfunction using specifically selected activity.

References

Anstice, B. and Bowden, R. (1985) The role of occupational therapy in mental handicap. In *Mental Handicap* (eds Craft, M., Bicknell, J. and Hollins, S.) Bailliere Tindall, London

Blundy, C. and Prevezer, K. (1986) The occupational therapist as a member of the community mental handicap team. *British Journal of Occupational Therapy*, **1986**, 107–110

Craft, M., Bicknell, J. and Hollins, S. (1985) *Mental Handicap*, Bailliere Tindall, London

Hollins, S. (1985) The dynamics of teamwork. In *Mental Handicap* (eds Craft, M., Bicknell, J. and Hollins, S.) Bailliere Tindall, London

Klein, M.D. (1983) *Predressing Skills*, Communication Skill Builders, Arizona

Peck, C. and Hong, S. (1988) *Living Skills for Mentally Handicapped People*, Croom Helm, London

Further reading – occupational therapy

Armstrong, J. and Rennie, J. (1986) We can use computers too. *British Journal of Occupational Therapy*, **49**, 297

Anderson, C. (1983) *Feeding. A Guide to the Assessment and Intervention with Mentally Handicapped Children*, Jordanhill College, Glasgow

Bracegirdle, H. (1987) Occupational therapy with mentally handicapped people. *British Journal of Occupational Therapy*, **50**, 334

Brands, D. and Phillips, H. (1980) *Gamesters Handbook,* , Hutchison & Co, London

British Journal of Occupational Therapy (1986). Mental handicap edition, **49**

Dearling, A. and Armstrong, H. (1985) *The youth games book*. Intermediate Treatment Resource Centre, Glasgow

Erdhart, R. (1982) *Developmental Hand Dysfunction*, Ramsco, MD

Fawdry, J. and Jackson, B. (1986) *Creative Ideas*, Winslow Press, Winslow

Harvey, F. (1986) Review of the assessment of people with a mental handicap. *British Journal of Occupational Therapy*, **49**, 119

Hogg, J. and Raynes, N. (1987) *Assessment in Mental Handicap*, Croom Helm, Kent

Kierman, C. and Jones, M. (1989) *Behaviour Assessment Battery*, NFER Nelson, Berks

Warner, J. (1981) *Helping The Handicapped Child With Early Feeding*, Winslow Press, Winslow

Wood, M. (1983) *Music for Mentally Handicapped People*, Souvenir Press, London

10

Specialist health services

10.1 Community nursing

Pauline Kemp

Introduction

The traditional role of the nurse providing custodial care in the large institutions began to change and evolve in the early 1970s. This was largely the result of the Government White Paper – *Better Services for the Mentally Handicapped* – which was published in 1971. The emphasis then shifted from hospital care to community care, nurses began to see that they had a role outwith the institution and gradually began to emerge from behind the hospital walls. Initially they were involved in the aftercare of discharged residents who were moving back to the community, but gradually the service expanded to deal with people who had never and would never live in a hospital.

Further impetus for the development of community services came with the Jay Report published in 1979 (OHSS, 1979) which dealt specifically with mental handicap nursing and care. The main proposals included recommendations for joint training based on existing social work qualifications, and whilst this has not generally been implemented, it has led to a more holistic and socially aware training for nurses in mental handicap.

Community nurses now play a major role in the care in the community of people with a mental handicap. This role may be as part of a community mental handicap team organized on multi-disciplinary lines or as part of a discrete community nursing team. However, nurses choose to function in the community; their worth as an integral part of a comprehensive strategy for people with a mental handicap is well recognized.

The principles embodied in the United Nations Declaration of Rights of Mentally Handicapped People (1971) and Wolfensberger Principles of Normalisation (Wolfensberger, 1972) form the foundations on which community care is based. Although an emphasis on care in the community has theoretically been present since the Mental Health Act of 1959, it was not until the seventies and the United Nations declaration that a real determination to change attitudes and policies emerged.

Development of Community Nursing Service

As stated above, community nurses emerged in the early 1970s providing aftercare for discharged residents of hospitals. Often the services started with only one nurse and was dependent on his or her adaptability in meeting the very different needs of people with a mental handicap living in a community setting after many years in an institution. Not only the client, but the nurse too had to change the way they viewed a given set of circumstances. The development of the service relied to a large extent on the innovation and skills of this new breed of mental handicap nurse, with the emphasis being placed on keeping people out of hospital if at all possible and ensuring a normal life in the community.

Particular to the role of the community nurse was the rehabilitation and habilitation of people with a mental handicap including the provision of a meaningful daytime occupation. Whilst this latter point may, by some people, be seen as theoretically the province of Social Services, in many areas such services were very limited and often the only professional involved in community care for the mentally handicapped was the community nurse.

Given the poor provision by local authorities, many Community Nurses found themselves setting up and running group homes and hostels and finding alternatives for their clients as they were discharged from hospital. Some of these alternatives have included for example supported landladies or landlords obtained by advertising. Provision of daytime occupation for the first clients discharged from hospital involved going to Job Centres, liaising with the Disabled Resettlement Officer and sometimes finding 'live-in' jobs in places such as boarding schools and nursing homes. Underlying all this was the need to provide support to maintain these people in their new community settings.

The client group that community nurses found themselves dealing with in the early years was very different from the current client group. Then, the people who were moving out of hospital had much greater potential for rehabilitation to independent living. Some of the clients were able to live on their own, some got married, many would never have been referred to a hospital had today's criteria with regard to admission been in operation. Indeed, many would no longer be classified as mentally handicapped. However, the increasing emphasis on community care by successive governments has led to developments by local authorities, housing associations and voluntary organizations which provide non-institutional care for people with a greater degree of handicap. Inevitably then, the client group that community nurses deal with has become more handicapped, requiring different types of support and an expansion of skills. In the face of this changing pattern of community care, nurses have had to be and have shown themselves to be highly adaptable.

Community nursing today

The present-day community nursing service still involves the aftercare of people discharged from hospital, but has now expanded in many areas to provide a domiciliary service for all people with a mental handicap wherever they are. This is now the largest component of a comprehensive community nursing service. It also provides specialist nursing input to special schools, liaison with statutory and voluntary agencies, and a demand led impetus for new, often innovative community developments.

Joint project with voluntary associations have provided opportunities for staff to work in residential community settings which are jointly managed by the community nursing service and the voluntary association. As before, the emphasis is still on rehabilitation and habilitation and a lifestyle based on The Principles of Normalisation (Wolfensberger, 1972).

Function of domiciliary service

As noted above, the domiciliary service is now the largest component in community nursing. The remit for such a service includes the prevention of inappropriate admissions to hospital, the support of families and others who are caring for a person with mental handicap at home in a hostel or other community residence, often on a crisis intervention basis, assessing and monitoring the health-care needs of their client, and ensuring the provision of other appropriate services. These functions are best carried out within a multidisciplinary framework such as a community mental handicap team (see Chapter 1).

The role of the community nurse

In 1985 the Royal College of Nursing published a document titled the *Role and Function of the Domiciliary Community Nurse for People with a Mental Handicap*. This document was intended to define the role of the community nurse as it was apparent that uncertainty and differing practices were leading to a fragmentation of the service. In it, however, the document recognizes the need for flexibility when describing the community nurse's role and it is therefore not intended to be a dogmatic prescription of the job. They saw the role as involving most, but not all of the following:

1. *Advising on:*
   (a) Prevention and minimization of the effects of handicap.
   (b) Developmental training.
   (c) Behavioural problems.
   (d) Social training and interpersonal relationships.
   (e) DSS benefits.
   (f) Other local and national resources.
   (g) Further education.
   (h) Health education (including sex education).

2. *Monitoring and evaluation of:*
   (a) Planned intervention.
   (b) Development of services.
   (c) Behaviour programmes.
   (d) Social training.
   (e) Administration of specific medications and their side-effects.
   (f) Health-related needs.

3. *Promote:*
   (a) Self-help groups.
   (b) Parents workshops.
   (c) Teaching forums to promote self-help skills.

4. *Liaise with:*
    (a) Voluntary organizations.
    (b) Statutory organizations.
    (c) Primary care teams.
    (d) Community mental handicap teams.
    (e) Private sector.
    (f) Other involved professionals.
5. *Offer counselling and advice to:*
    (a) Individuals.
    (b) Families/carers.
    (c) School/work/recreation.
6. *Report:*
    (a) Deficiencies in service.
    (b) Identified future needs.

Whilst this is a summary by the RCN of the role and function of a community nurse in mental handicap, many of the components may be carried out by keyworkers from other professional groups in conjunction with a community nurse from within a community mental handicap team. The nurse's membership of a community mental handicap team is seen as essential in reducing isolation. Inevitably there will be an element of 'role blurring' within a multi-disciplinary team, e.g. between community nurses and social workers. This should not be seen as detrimental to positive teamwork, rather it should facilitate an efficient and needs related service for clients.

The following description of a community nursing service will serve to further amplify the role of the community nurse within the parameters detailed in the RCN document.

Planning and implementation of a community service

Planning a community service today requires a commitment from health boards and social services to a properly funded and comprehensive community care strategy. It is essential that relevant demographic data and the implementation dates of future services are adequately assessed so that realistic staffing and an appropriate service can be achieved. The intention should be to enhance existing services. However, community services have to evolve and often start with less than ideal conditions.

The National Development Group have recommended that community nursing services should provide one community nurse trained in mental handicap for a population of 25 000. This is clearly an ideal, but should be the aim of every developing service.

The evolution of the service is determined largely by identification of client needs; essentially it is demand led. In an ideal world, the demand should be identified and planned for, before it arises. In reality this is not practicable. However, liaison with existing services and potential consumers should provide a reasonable assessment: of the role and need for a planned community nursing service; how it will interact with existing services; what the expectations of the service are; how people can be referred to the service; and what the potential expansion of the service is, thus ensuring better communication and teamwork.

Example of a developing community nursing service

In an area such as Edinburgh City and West Lothian with a population of 562 000 approximately, which is served by one large hospital for people with a mental handicap, the community nursing service has been developing since 1972. At that time there was one community nurse, there are now 43 staff in the community service of which 13 (including the nurse manager) provide a domiciliary service. These trained staff are supported by four nursing assistants. The current nurse to population ratio is therefore 1:43 000. The active case-load is restricted to 25 and so inevitably there is a waiting-list of clients. This ensures two things – excellence of service to clients and also evidence to support its continued expansion. Community nurses cannot provide a good service if they are trying to deal with a case-load in excess of 25, the time and commitment preclude this.

The service has its own operational policy which provides clear statement of its philosophy and function – the promotion of as normal a life as possible for all people with a mental handicap, the prevention of unnecessary hospital admissions and the provision and servicing of a comprehensive community care strategy.

Staff deployment

Initially community nurses were based in the local hospital. Further development of community services has enabled the community nursing service to be based nearer its client group with the domiciliary nurses working in areas which are conterminous with local social work divisions. Instead of working from the hospital, most now have bases in health centres, social work resources or in voluntary organizations and work in conjunction with other professionals under the umbrella of the community mental handicap team. This improves communication and teamwork for the professionals, but more importantly provides a more accessible centre for clients and their families in an environment that is more acceptable than a large institution often at a distance from population centres.

Breadth of activity

As stated above, the domiciliary nurses function as part of a community mental handicap team. Within the team the nurse will use a systematic approach of assessment to identify and meet the needs of individuals. This can be exemplified by the following case study.

James is an 18-year-old young man with a moderate mental handicap and a history of childhood epilepsy. He has been taking phenobarbitone for many years, but has not been assessed since leaving the paediatric service. He lives at home with his parents and two younger non-handicapped siblings. Referral to the community nurse via community mental handicap team was instigated by the families GP because of behaviour problems.

Initial assessment by the nurse revealed that James was having temper tantrums and outbursts of destructive behaviour in response to his parents' attempts to place limits on him. His siblings had a considerably greater degree of freedom than James despite being junior to him. They also had continued in the education system where as James had left school at 16 and had no adult training centre or further education placement. In the evenings they had local clubs and other leisure activities to attend, James had nothing except the occasional outing with parents – these were often terminated early as a result of James' disruptive behaviour.

Following the initial assessment, the nurse reported back to the community mental handicap team and arranged:

1. Re-assessment of James' physical and mental state, including assessment of his need for continued anti-convulsant medication.
2. Social work involvement with James and the family, liaising with them over referral for an appropriate day placement.

The nurse provided continuing input to James and the family to enable James to participate in more age-appropriate activities and to support his parents in learning to treat James as an adolescent growing up and not as a child. Putting James in touch with local clubs and his parents in touch with parent support groups has proved successful in alleviating James' boredom and his consequent anger and frustration. He now has an appropriate day placement at a local adult training centre and is gradually being weaned off phenobarbitone as there is now no indication for anticonvulsants. His behaviour has improved, but he is by no means an angel. Nevertheless, his parents feel more secure and supported in caring for James and are learning to treat him as a maturing adolescent.

In this case the nurse has been involved in provision of advice, monitoring and evaluation, liaison and counselling as detailed in the 1983 RCN document referred to earlier in the chapter.

Other community staff placements

As noted above only 17 of the 43 staff are involved in the community domiciliary service, the remaining 27 are deployed as follows:

Nine staff seconded to joint projects between the health board and two voluntary agencies providing residential care for 29 people with a mental handicap. The projects are jointly managed by the community nursing service manager and the voluntary agency who also supply staff. Seconded staff retain Whitley Council conditions of service and are managerially accountable to the CNSM.

A network of support services is built into each project with the aim of using generic services as far as possible and specialist services only when required.

The experiences of these staff who have been seconded from the hospital have confirmed the view that the ventures provide a means whereby staff can expand their horizons in regard to providing care for people with a mental handicap. Staff are able to work with smaller groups of residents, learn new skills from other professionals and vice versa, be involved in innovative and exciting patterns of care and see the personal growth of themselves and the residents they care for in a less restrictive more normal environment. The experience of teamwork and a commitment to the philosophy of the voluntary organization are important aspects of the secondment which, hopefully, will have benefits if these staff choose to return to the hospital to work, or move onto other places.

Thirteen staff are in a community based hostel, run by the health board, which provides rehabilitation or long-term care for up to 20 residents with two beds for respite care which are under the control of the domiciliary service.

Two staff are deployed in education, working in a school for people with profound learning difficulties, a large number of whom also have health care needs associated with their handicap. In addition, they provide a domiciliary service for certain pupils with severe problems to provide continuity between the school and the home. Within the school, they are involved in training staff in management of epilepsy, setting up programmes in toilet training, feeding, behaviour management, etc. for the pupils and in working with the team of visiting professionals such as physiotherapist, speech therapist, occupational therapist and psychologist.

Training

Those whose numeracy is good will realize that the total number of staff so far accounted is 41. The remaining two staff are seconded for a period of 1 year to the Diploma in Community Mental Health Care Course at a local college for further education. Such training is important for those nurses who are part of the domiciliary service to enable them to function as independent practitioners. However, the courses should be seen as an adjunct to continuing in-service education and not as a substitute. All nurses who transfer into the community service should be regarded as being in a learning environment for at least the first 6 months and should then, within the first 2 years be seconded to a relevant post-registration course. It is important that staff gain experience in the community service before attending a post-basic course to maximize the learning and also to ensure that they are committed to working in the community as such work does not attract special duty payments, etc. that are associated with hospital work.

Future developments

Nurses in the community service have already come a long way from providing an aftercare service for people discharged from hospital. Increasingly, they are expanding their involvement into resources run by agencies other than health boards. The continuing rundown of large hospitals which provide residential care means that people with severe and profound mental handicap are now cared for in the community and their consequent health care needs require increasing involvement in education, day services, respite and residential care by community nurses with specific training in mental handicap nursing. Parents and others, who have cared for the majority of people with a mental handicap in the community are now much more aware of service availability, and the emphasis has shifted from service provision to service need. It is no longer acceptable to say 'that is all we can offer', now it is a question of 'what do you need?' and of providing the service to meet the need. It is recognized that no one statutory or voluntary agency can meet all an individual's needs, and community nurses in mental handicap will be working as part of a multi-agency, multi-disciplinary service, through secondment, joint funded posts or from within the domiciliary service.

Hopefully, this chapter has given the reader an insight into the extent of a community nurse's role within mental handicap nursing and care, and the importance of working within a multi-disciplinary team to ensure the provision of a comprehensive service. However, it is important to remember that 'a good community nurse should know when his or her job finishes and someone else's begins' and that 'quality is more important than quantity'.

References

Department of Health and Social Security (1971) *Better Services for the Mentally Handicapped*, DHSS, London

Department of Health and Social Security (1979) *Report of the Committee of Enquiry into Mental Handicap Nursing and Care* (the Jay Report), (Cmnd 7468–1, HMSO, London)

United Nations (1971) *Declaration on the Rights of the Mentally Retarded*, UN, New York

Wolfensberger, W. (1971) *The Principles of Normalisation in Human Services*, National Institute on Retardation, Toronto

Royal College of Nursing (1985) *The Role and Function of the Domiciliary Community Nurse for People with a Mental Handicap*, RCN, London

10.2 Psychiatry

Bill Fraser

The recognition of emotional disorder in people with handicap is difficult and psychiatrists with special interest in the developmentally disabled are necessary to help GPs in early detection and treatment. Treatment can mostly be carried out by the GP, the community mental handicap nurse and occasionally recourse to temporary admission to hospital. In the immediate future there will continue to be a need for psychiatry provision within specialist mental handicap hospitals but increasingly general psychiatric hospitals are admitting people with mental handicaps. Psychiatrists working in the field of mental handicap are especially exposed in the multi-disciplinary environment in which they operate to scrutiny of the special skills which they can offer. Psychiatrists must continuously define and refine their skills and shed inappropriate work that can be done by others.

A person with a severe mental handicap may, like a person of normal intelligence, become anxious, depressed. In fact, the stresses which he or she faces are likely to be greater than that of people with normal intelligence and his or her psychological vulnerability also greater. Because the diagnosis of clear-cut mental illnesses is often complex, there are difficulties in establishing the true rates of prevalence of mental illnesses amongst people with mental handicaps. Relatively little is known about the natural history of mental disorders in people with mental handicaps. In a longitudinal study of children in Aberdeen followed up until they were 21 years old, Koller *et al.* (1983) found 59% who had displayed some form of behaviour disorder so that they came to the attention of the authorities during their childhood or adolescence. Corbett (1979) in his study of children in Camberwell found 6% of children with severe mental retardatioan showed adjustment reaction; 4% conduct disorder; 4% neurotic disorder; 2% isolated habit disorder; 10% severe stereotypies and pica; 4% hyperkinetic behaviour disturbance with 17% childhood psychosis. Among adults he found a prevalence of 46% for significant psychiatric disorder.

It is important to nip transient emotional disturbances such as adjustment reactions in the bud, as the disorders may become progressive in a vicious circle of ignorant management, negative social attitudes, experience of failure by the person with a handicap and his caregivers and enhanced negative feelings by everybody concerned.

Most mental illnesses do not show themselves until the adolescent stage has been reached, compared with mental handicap which occurs with the beginning of life or soon after. Any of the forms of mental illness which may occur in the fully developed mind may also occur in people with mental handicaps; however, the lower the IQ, the more difficult it is to recognize mental illness as the diagnosis is

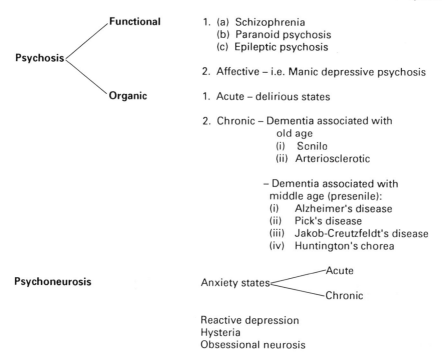

Figure 10.1 Common types of mental illness

largely dependent on verbal communication: thus the diagnosis of mental illness in people with mental handicaps is made more often in those whose intelligence is towards the upper end of the handicap range.

Mental illness is principally divided into psychosis and psychoneurosis. A person suffering from a psychotic illness loses contact with reality, whereas in neurotic illness, contact with reality is maintained.

Psychoses are divided into functional and organic psychoses. Functional psychoses are those in which function is disturbed but there is yet no demonstrable physical cause to explain the symptoms. Organic psychoses are those in which there is a demonstrable physical cause, i.e. tumour, infection, change in blood vessels, etc.

The more common types of mental illness may be classified as shown in Figure 10.1.

Functional psychosis

Schizophrenia

This illness is characterized by symptoms that interfere with the patient's thinking, emotions, drive and motor activity and may result in a gradual deterioration of personality. The incidence in the general population is 0.85%; it is higher in the relatives of schizophrenics. In most cases, the illness begins between the ages of

15 and 25: the predisposing personality is often introverted or 'schizoid'. Typically, the schizophrenic is of asthenic build. Recently there is some evidence to suggest that several genetic lesions predispose an individual to the condition. The prognosis is better in atypical forms of the illness, i.e. where it has an acute onset, a precipitating factor, where the personality is extrovert and the build pyknic, where the patient is realistically disturbed by his symptoms and where there is no marked family history.

Schizophrenic illnesses have been traditionally classified into four types and all four may show the characteristics of each other. Although these four types – hetrophrenic, catatonic, simple and paranoid – merge into each other and have little theoretical basis, the terms are still part of psychiatric usage. Schizophrenic means 'split mind' and in the schizophrenic there is dissociation between thinking and feeling. The major features of the illness are:

1. *Disturbance of thinking* – There is loosening of associations and disconnection of thoughts ranging in severity from vagueness in thinking to a stage where the patient's utterances cannot be understood at all.
2. *Disturbance of emotions* – The patient's expression of emotions is not in step with his conversation; he may sit with a rather fixed smile on his face even if being asked about a recent bereavement of a close relative.
3. *Disturbance of drive or volition* – The patient is lacking in the will to do anything constructive and may spend time in bed or sitting staring into space often without realizing that he is so inactive.
4. *Disturbance of motor activity* – This may range from stupor to wild excitement and overactivity. Patients may allow their bodies and limbs to be placed in unusual positions which are maintained indefinitely.
5. *Primary delusions* – A delusion is a false belief with no basis in reality. A delusion that appears out of the blue in fully developed form in the setting of clear consciousness and that is immediately accepted as valid by the patient is a primary delusion and is characteristic of schizophrenia: for example, a patient who has gone to a party may suddenly feel that everyone is hostile to him and wants to kill him.
6. *Hallucinations* – A hallucination is a perception that has no basis in reality. Hallucinations may also occur in other mental illnesses. Auditory hallucinations are the most common in schizophrenia; the patient may hear voices commenting on his every action. Visual hallucinations as well as hallucinations of touch, taste and smell may occur.

It is common to distinguish between positive and negative symptoms in schizophrenia; positive symptoms representing an active disturbance of the brain, negative symptoms reflecting a loss of normal brain functions. The terms *type 1* and *type 2* symptoms of schizophrenia have been used to characterize respectively *positive symptoms* (delusions, hallucinations and thought disorder) which are well controlled by psychotropic medication; and *negative signs* (affective flattening, apathy and povery of speech) which are largely unaffected by medication. There is some evidence from computerized tomography that 'negative sign' schizophrenics have larger lateral ventricles. One question to be asked is whether chronic schizophrenia follows positive and negative presentations in the acute illness in an equally predictable sequence. There is some evidence that type 2 schizophrenics are more likely to go on to a chronic stage, and also that some people who are of normal intelligence develop a chronic (defect state) schizophrenia indistinguishable from mild mental handicap. The term 'thought disorder' is woolly and imprecise. It does seem that much of the strange speech of schizophrenics is not due to some theoretical 'thought disorder' but involves deterioration in grammar, fluency and ability to form a text, and resembles mild dysphasia.

Treatment
Schizophrenic symptoms can be modified by the phenothiazine and butyrophenone groups of drugs. In the acutely disturbed patient chlorpromazine (the best known of the phenothiazine group) or haloperidol (the prototype of the butyrophenone group), would be used; where the patient is withdrawn and uncommunicative, a less sedative phenothiazine such as trifluoperazine would be used. In both very overactive and very withdrawn patients where the condition is acute ECT may be used. Relapse can to some extent be prevented by injections of long-acting phenothiazines, given at 2-, 3-, or 4-weekly intervals. A community psychiatric nursing service plays a vital part in rehabilitatioan by ensuring that patients, discharged from hospital, receive maintenance therapy and in advising relatives on further management.

Paranoid psychosis
This can be recognized in people with mild mental handicaps; it is usually a phenomenon of middle and old age, and there is a high incidence of impairment of vision and hearing in patients who develop paranoid delusions in later life, just as there is in normally intelligent adults who develop paranoid illnesses at a late age.

Epileptic psychosis
There is a higher incidence of schizophreniform psychosis occurring in association with epilepsy than could be expected by chance, the psychotic experiences growing out of the personality change and semi-confusional epileptic phenomena.

Diagnosis

The differentiation of schizophrenia from depression in people who are non-verbal is extremely difficult. There is no defined constellation of non-verbal symptoms of schizophrenia.

There is evidence that psychotic disorders in people with mental handicaps run a more benign course than in the non-handicapped population.

Schizophrenic and paranoid psychosis would be difficult to diagnose in patients with an IQ much below the upper end of the moderate range of mental retardation. A schizophrenic or paranoid psychosis may produce an apparent drop in the level of intellectual functioning as assessed on intelligence testing, but the premorbid level of intelligence is a more accurate indication of the patient's intellectual potential.

Several authorities have more or less agreed on a prevalence rate of 3.4% amongst residents of mental handicap hospitals. This excludes patients with stereotypies, mannerisms and major impairment of social interaction, i.e. persistent developmental disorders of the autistic or atypical autistic disorder categories. The schizophrenia prevalence rate for people with mental handicaps living in the community is not known but it is higher than for the general population.

Manic depressive psychosis

This illness is characterized by mood swings from elation to depression; it is predominantly an illness of middle life, though the first attack may be earlier. Between attacks, the patient returns to his normal personality. It may present as mania or depression or a mixture of both. The patient may have one or two attacks only in a lifetime, or repeated illnesses. Chronic depression and chronic mania can occur, and more rarely there may be continuous alteration from mania to depression. The predisposing personality is typically extrovert and subject to mild mood swings. Twelve per cent of the children of an affected parent are affected. There is strong evidence of three genetic linkages, one with the gene concerned with the manufacture of tyrosine, hydroxylase or brain amine. Women are affected more than men. Prognosis is best where the attack is typical (opposite to schizophrenia), worse where there are manic episodes, and worst of all if there are episodes of mania and depression.

Depression
The onset may be sudden or insidious. Typically, the patient feels at his worst in the mornings and mood improves towards evening. The highest incidence of suicide is in the early morning. The depressed patient feels hopeless, unworthy, guilty and possibly hypochondriacal. If delusions are present they are depressive in content; the patient believes that he has cancer or that he is infecting everyone around him. Hallucinations are rare but, if they occur, take the form of voices making insulting remarks or of horrible scenes being enacted, i.e. they are depressive in content. The depressed patient is slowed in all his functions, and may become stuporous; appetite is poor, sleep is disturbed and there is early morning wakening with inability to return to sleep.

Rarely the depressive may be violent towards others, i.e. may kill other members of the family, rather than leave them in an evil world.

Treatment   In a severely depressed patient, ECT is the treatment of choice. Where the illness is less severe, one of the tetracyclic or tricyclic anti-depressant drugs would be used. Cognitive therapy can be a useful adjunct (see below).

Mania
Mania is rarer than depression. The patient is hyperactive. Prior to treatment, death from exhaustion was not uncommon. Ideas flash through the patient's mind, he is grandiose and may feel he has great powers. Mood is one of infectious gaiety but at times the patient may be very irritable and require great tact and patience on the part of the nursing staff.

Treatment   Mania can be treated successfully with haloperidol, droperidol, with phenothiazines in addition if necessary. ECT is sometimes useful. Where the patient is having frequent mood swings, lithium is used as a maintenance therapy.

Diagnosis

Affective disorders can be recognized in people with mental handicaps, mood change tending to be poorly sustained and in the manic lacking in the quality of infectious gaiety typical of the normally intelligent manic. Associated delusions tend to be naïve. Affective disorders can occur in adults with severe mental handicap, but diagnosis can be difficult the more severe is the handicap of the patient and may need to be based on a prolonged study of behaviour, weight and sleep patterns by observers who know the patient well, supplemented by a knowledge of mental illness patterns in the family.

Manic depressive illness is marginally easier than schizophrenia to diagnose in people with mental handicaps. Features associated with mania include increased motor output, vocalization, aggression and sleeplessness; and of depression decreased motor activity (or, paradoxically, wandering), poor appetite, sleeplessness or excessive sleep. Taking longitudinal accounts of the behaviour, weight, sleep patterns based on reports by caregivers and using Spectral Analysis can help to establish complex periodicity on a periodogram where the naked eye cannot immediately see a definite pattern of swinging moods or behaviour (Tyrer and Shakour, 1990).

In a long-stay mental handicap hospital Wright (1982) diagnosed 2.8% amongst the total group as having an active affective illness.

Organic psychosis

The effects of organic cerebral disease are more marked in people with mental handicaps than in the normal population. The normal mental changes which occur in old age and those associated with senile dementia appear much earlier and progress more rapidly in people with mental handicaps.

Organic mental illnesses are caused by anatomical or physiological disturbance in the brain or result from physical illness elsewhere in the body. The nature of the symptoms depends on the rate of development of the disease process. The most important system that distinguishes the organic psychosis from the functional is *clouding of consciousness*. This is a state of disturbed awareness which may vary from mild disorientation in time and place to coma.

Organic mental states may be acute or chronic.

Acute organic psychosis or delirious states

These may occur in association with physical illness such as pneumonia; the delirious patient is restless, has a poor attention span, his thinking is concerned with imaginary experiences and there may be hallucinations; he is disorientated in time and place. Sleep is disturbed.

Delirium may be drug induced; barbiturates taken in excess may give rise to confusion, ataxic gait, constipation, foul breath, acneiform skin eruptions and coma. It has to be remembered that delirium in people with mental handicaps may be caused by the toxic effects of anticonvulsants and dose levels should be kept under review; in this context it should be remembered that people with mental handicaps are more susceptible to the toxic effects of not only barbiturates and other anticonvulsants but also antidepressants and tranquillizers. Patients who have been on tranquillizers for some time should be advised to discontinue them gradually over a period of weeks rather than stop them suddenly, which may lead to unpleasant withdrawal effects and sometimes delirium. Similarly, alcohol withdrawal may be a cause of delirium.

Delirium may be caused by chemicals, e.g. those containing lead: where lead poisoning is acute, there is delirium, aphasia, convulsions and coma if untreated;

in chronic lead poisoning there is failure of concentration and memory, headache, deafness, transient speech defect and visual disturbance.

Chronic organic psychosis

The irreversible decline of mental functions produced by organic brain disease is termed dementia. The process begins with failure of recent memory, attention and slow, vague thinking. Mood is labile and shallow, judgement is impaired. There is progressive intellectual failure until at the end stage, at which the patient leads a vegetative existence requiring everything to be done for him. The dementias are divided into the senile and pre-senile groups as follows.

Dementia associated with old age

Senile dementia   Senile dementia occurs after the age of 70, is more common in females and there is an increased incidence in the families of those afflicted. The onset is insidious and there is steady and rapid deterioration of all aspects of intellectual functioning. Delusions and hallucinations may occur.

Arteriosclerotic dementia   There is degeneration of the cerebral blood vessels with secondary degeneration of brain tissue. There is patchy failure of brain function. Personality is preserved to a later stage than in senile dementia. There may be associated hypertension, cerebrovascular accidents, neurological signs and epileptiform fits.

The diagnosis of arteriosclerotic dementia in people with mental handicaps is difficult and would depend on a knowledge of premorbid level of functioning.

Dementia associated with middle age – pre-senile dementia

Alzheimer's disease   This condition begins in middle life with impairment of memory and loss of efficiency, accompanied by emotional disturbances and change in muscle tone. There is generalized atrophy of the cerebral cortex with the temporoparietal region being particularly affected, causing difficulty in speaking and senseless repetition of last words or parts of words of a sentence. There is loss of sense of position in space. The patient's gait becomes stiff and awkward. There may be convulsions, and in the terminal stage the patient leads a vegetative existence. More females than males are affected. People with Down's syndrome who survive into middle age are prone to develop a dementia whose neuropathology is identical with that of Alzheimer's. A gene responsible for the degenerative amyloid plaques and tangles found in Alzheimer brains has been located on chromosome 21, but there is still dispute as to its importance.

The appearance of brain dysfunction in people with Down's in middle life is complicated by the increased likelihood of pseudo-dementia due to hypothyroidism. Sub-clinical hypothyroidism is more likely in people with Down's. By the age of 50 only 40% of people with Down's can confidently be said to be euthyroid. Regular screening of thyroid stimulating hormone, thyroid antibodies, thyroglobulin and microsomal antibodies are necessary.

The cognitive deterioration and changes in personality and harbingers of dementia are often subtle and hard to detect. Withdrawal from conversation, loss of interest in workshop activity, increased rigidity and irritability, occasionally inappropriate mischievousness, deterioration in gait – shuffling and loss of coordinated walking patterns – was found by Lott in a detailed study of individuals with early onset dementia. However, whether this could be attributed only to dementia or possibly to the effects of atlanto-axial subluxation which is quite likely to present as a gait problem and (as more sensationally reported) as paralysis due to sudden exercise causing abrupt flexion and extension of the neck. Urinary and faecal incontinence are late manifestations of the illness. At this time patients will show moderate or severe cortical atrophy on CAT scans. Such a clinical picture if fluctuating may be due to depression and a therapeutic trial of an antidepressant is worth trying

Pick's disease   In this condition the atrophic change affects the three outer layers of the cortex and, in particular, the frontal and temporal areas. Personality change occurs first, and the first indication may be uninhibited behaviour; speech defects occur, the patient omitting words or using them in a peculiar fashion. There may be increased sensitivity to pain. Epilepsy and disturbances of gait are less common than in Alzheimer's. The terminal stage is identical in both.

Jakob–Creutzfeldt's disease   This is a rare disease of middle life which begins with memory impairment and widespread neurological disturbance, causing tremors and spasticity of the limbs and disturbance of gait.

Huntington's chorea   This disease is transmitted by a single autosomal dominant gene and about half the offspring of an affected person can, therefore, be expected to develop it. In the majority of cases, the illness begins between 25 and 35, but it may be as early as 3 or as late as 70. It may thus be a cause of mental handicap where there is early onset.

Neurological symptoms may be preceded by mood change; the involuntary movements usually commence in the face, hands and shoulders, but an abnormality of gait may be the first sign. Memory may be surprisingly well retained even when the disease is well established. Depression is common, and there is a high incidence of suicide. The average duration of the illness is 10–15 years, with death taking place before the age of 60, but in some cases the disease is more slowly progressive.

Psychoneurosis

Anxiety states

All individuals experience anxiety at some time in their lives, e.g. prior to an interview or examination. In response to stress in the normal individual, there is an increase in the concentration of adrenaline in the blood, an increase in blood sugar, a rise in blood pressure and pulse rate, skin becomes pale and sweats, mouth becomes dry; respiration becomes deeper and more frequent; there is generalized trembling. There may be frequency of micturition, diarrhoea, nausea and vomiting. In prolonged anxiety states, there may be increased muscle tone, tension, restlessness, sleep and appetite disturbance, causing deterioration in general health. In psychoneurosis anxiety appears inappropriate to the situation or excessive in degree.

Acute anxiety states
An acute anxiety state may appear in people with mental handicaps as a response to stress in the same way as in the normally intelligent individual.

Chronic anxiety states
Chronic anxiety states may occur in people with mental handicaps in the higher ranges of retardation. There is generally an inherited predisposition, or history of insecurity in early life caused by loss of a parent by death or divorce. Stressful situations of many kinds, instead of producing a constructive response, may induce a state of continuing conflict in those individuals predisposed to the development of neurotic illness.

Treatment
Relaxation therapies are effective with people with mental handicaps if simply phrased. Relaxation therapies and manipulation of the environment can be combined so that, where possible, stressful situations are avoided. Yoga is documented as beneficial for anxious people with mental handicaps.

Neurotic or reactive depression

Reactive depression is a reaction to some external cause, e.g. death of a close friend, but is more intense than one would expect. It is distinguished from endogenous depression by the fact that there is a definite precipitating factor, a tendency for mood to worsen towards evening, inability to get off to sleep and frequent waking throughout the night.

In practice, there is overlap between endogenous and reactive depression, many patients having features of both.

Treatment
Mild tranquillizers may be helpful as there are often associated anxiety symptoms. The patient has to be helped to come to terms with whatever has been the precipitating factor.

In general psychiatry and the psychiatry of general practice in recent years, cognitive therapy has become important as an adjunct to antidepressants and in its own right as a way of treating depression. Beck *et al.* (1979) pointed out that many unpleasant emotions arise not from actual events but from how events are interpreted. Treatment includes a re-focusing of attention on to coping and pleasurable experiences, encouraging the patient to encounter pleasurable activities, and training in assertion and encouraging the person to think of alternatives to the irrational inferences that he or she makes (see Chapter 3).

Hysteria

Hysterical symptoms have a motivation which is unrecognized by the patient and there is often gain from the symptom. Hysterical symptoms may occur in any personality type in a setting of mounting emotional strain, e.g. marital strife may have caused strain for some time, when an argument, no more serious in itself than previous arguments, may precipitate dissociative symptoms, i.e. complete loss of memory or regression to the age before the marriage took place.

In conversion hysteria, the patient solves a conflict by producing a symptom such as paralysis of a limb, or blindness or symptoms of any other physical illness. People of lower intelligence are more likely to develop dissociative symptoms than those of superior intelligence.

Obsessional neurosis and phobic anxiety

An obsession exists when a person cannot exclude thoughts from consciousness, distinguishes them as unreasonable and attempts to resist them but cannot do so. Obsessions with sex and violence, death, dirt and germs are typical. Rumination is the term applied to repetitive obsessional thinking; compulsions are acts which the patient feels compelled to carry out. Phobic states where the anxiety is concentrated on a specific object, e.g. insects or dogs, are widespread among people with mental handicaps. Establishing the prevalence in moderate and severe mental handicap of neurotic disorder is well nigh impossible, but in Day's 1983 study of admissions over a 5-year period, 28% were diagnosed as neurotic, of which only 4% were moderately and none severely retarded. With the resettlement of people with mental handicaps in the community, it might be anticipated that more neuroses will occur with exposure to the stress of ordinary life.

Childhood psychoses: pervasive developmental disorders

Obsessional neurosis and withdrawn psychotic states must be distinguished from the rituals and social impairment of childhood psychosis.

Wing and Gold's (1979) classification of childhood psychosis is based on a degree of social impairment found on clinical examination. They identify three groups:

1. *Infantile psychosis* – The commonest group.
2. *Disintegrative psychosis* – A rare group where abnormalities usually begin after the age of 3 years.
3. Childhood schizophrenic where the child – usually a schoolchild – starts to develop signs of adult schizophrenia, e.g. delusions and hallucinations.

Positive prognostic features in children with infantile psychosis include the presence of useful speech before the age of 5 years.

The confusion of the terms 'autism' and 'childhood psychosis' has led to the introduction of the diagnostic category 'pervasive developmental disorders' to describe those children in whom multiple distortions of development have occurred. In DSM III distinction is made between pervasive developmental disorder and specific developmental disorders (e.g. the developmental language disorders). Sub-divisions of pervasive developmental disorder (PDD) include infantile autism (IA) where gross abnormalities of speech language and relationships occur in the first 30 months of life; atypical autism which does not meet all the criteria of autism but occurs in the first 30 months, and childhood onset of pervasive developmental disorder (COPDD) which may meet the criteria but occurs later (Tables 10.1 and 10.2) (see also Russell, 1984). Recently the American Psychiatric Association published a revised 3rd Edition of DSM (DSM III R, 1987) which notes that the age of onset differentiating Infantile Autism from other PDDs

Table 10.1 DSM-III diagnostic criteria for infantile autism

A.	Onset before 30 months of age.
B.	Pervasive lack of responsiveness to other people (autism).
C.	Gross deficits in language development.
D.	If speech is present, peculiar speech patterns such as immediate and delayed echolalia, metaphorical language, pronominal reversal.
E.	Bizarre responses to various aspects of the environment, e.g. resistance to change, peculiar interest in or attachments to animate or inanimate objects.
F.	Absence of delusions, hallucinations, loosening of associations, and incoherence as in schizophrenia.

Reproduced by permission of the *Journal of Mental Deficiency Research.*

Table 10.2 DSM-III diagnostic criteria for childhood onset and atypical pervasive developmental disorder

A. Gross and sustained impairment in social relationships, e.g. lack of appropriate affective responsivity, inappropriate clinging, asociality, lack of empathy.
B. At least three of the following:
   (1) sudden excessive anxiety manifested by such symptoms as free-floating anxiety, catastrophic reactions to everyday occurrences, inability to be consoled when upset, unexplained panic attacks.
   (2) constricted or inappropriate affect, including lack of appropriate fear reactions, unexplained rage reactions, and extreme mood lability.
   (3) resistance to change in the environment (e.g. upset if dinner time is changed), or insistence on doing things in the same manner every time (e.g., putting on clothes always in the same order).
   (4) oddities of motor movements, such as peculiar posturing, peculiar hand or finger movements, or walking on tiptoe.
   (5) abnormalities of speech, such as question-like melody, monotonous voice.
   (6) hyper- or hypo-sensitivity to sensory stimuli, e.g., hyperacusis.
   (7) self-mutilation, e.g. biting or hitting self, head banging.
C. Onset of the full syndrome after 30 months of age and before 12 years of age.
   Absence of delusions, hallucinations, incoherence, or marked loosening of associations.

Atypical pervasive developmental disorder in these studies defined patients who had symptoms before 30 months of age but did not meet criteria for autism. Since symptom onset before 30 months of age excludes a diagnosis of childhood onset the atypical category was utilized.

Reproduced with the permission of *The Journal of Mental Deficiency Research.*

is not valid; and we now have 'Autistic disorder' embracing IA and COPDD and a category for atypical cases – pervasive developmental disorder not otherwise specified (PDDNOS).

The hunt for a *basic cognitive deficit* in infantile autism has led to the discovery that autistic children have serious impairments in pretend play and in the ability to take account of other peoples' mental states. They do not develop a normal ability to see and feel and think things from another's perspective; to get into the other person's mind. Their mental development is uneven with frequently even precocity in tool using. Autistic people accordingly may treat and manipulate adults as objects without realizing what they are doing. This makes them relatively proficient in figuring out how things work, and defective in sharing knowledge with others and acquiring knowledge from others.

How do we distinguish behaviour disturbance from psychiatric disorder?

The psychiatrist is initially faced with a problem of *behaviour disturbance*. Behaviours are labelled as disturbed and reacted to as disturbed because:

1. The disturbed person behaves in an idiosyncratic or inappropriate manner. In other words, we have trouble understanding his behaviour.
2. The person's actions conflict with the smooth function and norms of the relevant social groups.

Behaviour disturbances create management problems. Further, the norms of contact vary between social groups and individual perception of behaviour disturbance is to a certain extent subjective. Another important point about disturbed behaviours is that their consequences are important. The disturbances negatively affect the long-term character of interactions with disturbed persons. Also, disturbed behaviour should be seen as dynamic rather than simply as instances of static categories. We know that behaviour disturbances in people with mental handicaps have complex origins: in the environment; in maladaptive learned behaviour; in fears, rational or irrational; in attempts by puzzled, immature individuals, ill-equipped for the roles expected of them and confused by their inability to communicate their intentions, to understand the intentions of others, to negotiate a role; in reactions to physical pain or discomfort and in superadded mental illness.

It has repeatedly been observed that psychiatric problems are common in people with mental handicaps but there is a lack of suitable objective assessment tools because the manner in which such individuals manifest psychiatric symptoms usually differs from non-retarded individuals; their expressive abilities are limited. The art of the psychiatrist in an interview with normal adults is picking up verbal leads. This evidence is not available in people with mental handicaps in the form of verbal content. In interviewing people with mental handicaps, the art is in picking up non-verbal leads and 'leaks'.

Scales, tests and checklists

What tests are available for emotional illness? What do they test and what are their most appropriate uses? The usefulness of an assessment instrument depends on the ease in use and speed of its administration; appropriateness(in terms of age, sex and level of disability); the numbers of domains and related items covered and evidence of the reliability and validity.

The problem of validity is particularly important because all behaviours are disturbed relative to norms which can and do vary. It is important to use tests that do not just basically count frequencies of behaviours which the authors feel intuitively to be deviant or which the rate perceives to be deviant, or which incorporate psychiatric jargon of syndromes, but are fundamentally ratings of behaviours salient to caretakers, nurses and parents.

The best known and most versatile scale is probably the *adaptive behaviour scale* but it is time consuming and does not weigh relative severity of behaviour problems. Each scale has its own advantage – and behaviours which it taps – the *aberrant behaviour checklist* (Aman *et al.*, 1985), for example, is designed to probe transient and subtle treatment *changes*. (Most scales are designed to portray *stable* behaviour traits.) Other useful scales include *Balthazar's scale*, the *behaviour disturbance scale* by Leudar and Fraser and the *psychosocial behaviour scale* (Espie *et al.*, 1988) which is a particularly good scale at clarifying hysterical behaviour. The psychiatric diagnostic scales which can be used with the mentally handicapped include *standard psychiatric interview* (Ballinger *et al.*, 1975) the *self-report depression questionnaire* (SRDQ, Reynolds, 1990), and *Psychopathology instrument for mental retarded adults* (PIMRA (Senatore *et al.*, 1985) which is based on the Diagnostic and Standard Manual for Mental Illness (DSM III). Reid and Ballinger (1987) have developed an assessment scale for personality disorders in the mentally handicapped.

Current frameworks of classification are multiaxial. Psychiatric diagnosis is one axis; medical diagnosis is another axis. Psychiatric diagnoses do not correlate well with behavioural disturbances. Behaviour disturbances and psychiatric disorders do not 'map on'. Behaviour disturbances may be due to any or all of the psychiatric disorders and the disorders may present as any or all of the behaviour disturbances commonly seen and identified in checklists, i.e. aggressive conduct, mood disturbances, withdrawal, antisocial conduct, idiosyncratic mannerisms and self-injurious behaviours (Fraser *et al.*, 1986).

The ethics of medication

The lobby against *ever* using psychotropic medication based some of its case on data from one research laboratory which was deliberately falsified to fit in with an anti-illness perspective of challenging behaviour (the Breuning case). This view is partly understandable. 'Blunderbuss' drugs had been used in the past, often in large dosage without definite objectives other than expediency. People with mental handicaps who are emotionally ill have an equal right to receiving precise medication, especially now that major tranquillizers and the new antidepressants are more refined, speedier in response and precise so that proper baseline/ABA designs are feasible and drug effectiveness monitored. Even when 'illness' cannot be detected, there is sometimes a clear indication for the use of major tranquillizers for calming individuals and reducing stereotypies – but only in combination with a behavioural management programme, e.g. anger control, assertiveness training, cognitive therapy, etc. The move away from polypharmacy in the use of anticonvulsants and the use of computer programs displaying behavioural and epileptic profiles makes the choice of the best program and the correct medication easier.

References

Aman, M., Singh, N., Stevant, A. and Field, C. (1985) The aberrant behaviour checklist. *American Journal of Deficiency*, 485–491

Ballinger, B., Armstrong, J., Presley, A.S. and Reid, A.H. (1975) Use of standardized psychiatric interview in mentally handicapped patients. *British Journal of Psychiatry*, **127**, 540–544

Beck, A.T., Rush, A.J., Shaw, B.F. and Emery, G. (1979) *Cognitive Therapy of Depression*, Guildford Press, New York

Corbett, J. (1979) In *Psychiatric Illness and Mental Handicap* (eds James, F. and Snaith, R.), Gaskell Press, London

Day, K. (1983) A hospital based psychiatric unit for mentally handicapped adults. *Mental Handicap*, **11**, 137–140

Espie, C., Montgomery, J. and Gillies, J. (1988) The development of a psychosocial scale for the assessment of mentally handicapped people. *Journal of Mental Deficiency*, **32**, 395–404

Fraser, W.I., Leudar, I., Gray, J. and Campbell, I. (1986) Psychiatric and behaviour disturbance in mental handicap. *Journal of Mental Deficiency Research*, **30**, 49–59

Koller, H., Richardson, S.A., Katz, M. and McLaren, J. (1983) Behaviour disturbance since childhood in a 5 year birth cohort of all mentally retarded young adults in a city. *American Journal of Mental Deficiency*, **87**, 386–391

Lott, I.T. (1982) Down's syndrome ageing and Alzheimer disease: A clinical review. *Annals of the New York Academy of Science*, **396**, 15–27

Reid, A.H. and Ballinger, B.R. (1987) Personality disorder in mental handicap. *Psychological Medicine*, **17**, 983–989

Reynolds, W. (1990) Depression in persons with mental retardation, In *Advances in Developmental Disorders. A. Research Manual* (eds Barrett, M.R.P. and Matson, J.L.). JAI Press, Greenwich, CT

Russell, O. (1984) *Mental Handicap*, Churchill Livingstone, London

Senatore, V., Matson, J.L. and Kazdin, A.E. (1985) An inventory to assess psychopathology of mentally retarded adults. *American Journal of Mental Deficiency*, **89**, 459–466

Tyrer, S. and Shakour, Y. (1990) The effect of lithium in the P of aggressive episodes. In *Key Issues in Mental Retardation Research* (ed. Fraser, W.I.). Routledge, London, pp. 121–129

Wing, L. and Gould, J. (1979) Severe impairments of social interaction and assorted abnormalities in children: epidemiology and classification. *Journal of Autism and Developmental Disorders*, **9**, 11–29

Wright, E.C. (1982) The presentation of mental illness in mildly mentally retarded adults. *British Journal of Psychiatry*, **141**, 496–502

11

Social services

Victor Chlebowski

Introduction

This chapter on social services for people with learning difficulties (as people with mental handicaps have became more recently known) will show how the supports to this client group have developed. This process has developed largely as a result of changes in thinking and legislation. The chapter is divided into three sections:

1. Social Services support to individuals and their families (fieldwork or client services).
2. Alternative patterns of care and supported placements (residential and day care or service provision).
3. Benefits and welfare rights (finances and resources).

This introduction takes as its theme, the view that social services are politically reactive and the development of service provision is affected accordingly. At national level, central government dictates the policies which will be implemented by the local authorities and hence the priorities social services will accord to particular client groups. At a local level, social workers in England and Wales are employees of County or Borough Councils, and in Scotland, of the Regional Councils. This means they have both the national perspective to contend with, and also the dominant group of local politicians.

Historical perspective

Until the mid 1800s people with learning difficulties mainly lived at home, if they survived birth and childhood at all, owing to the social and health deficiencies. It could be argued that this was truly a time of care in the community. Family life changed, however, with the industrial upheavals of the 1850s and the associated social consequences.

People 'not suited' to work in the factories of that time were removed to institutions. In those days such institutions were a cross between asylums and 'specialized education centres' for people with learning difficulties (but also people with a mental illness or a physical handicap), of every age.

The calibre of institutions varied enormously, but the educative role soon became overtaken by the need for long-term/permanent 'hospital' care and ushered in the age of care out of the community. Legislation and the current thinking shaped attitudes and priorities still apparent in some people today.

The 1913 Mental Deficiency (Scotland) Act excluded the 'mental defective' from the welfare and social agencies (including education) that the non-handicapped citizen would attend. It effectively 'legalized' care, out of the community. This Act, and its English and Welsh counterpart, set up a principle which to an extent still exists within legislation today, i.e. the 'duty to perform and provide', but without enforcing local authorities to act. In 1913 local authorities were merely recommended to undertake certain action which they were not enforced to take. In this case, the setting up of Mental Deficiency Committees.

Today social services have in certain areas of England and most recently in Wales, taken initiatives to promote care but based on central monetary involvement. Earlier, in the 1920s and 1930s, it was the voluntary organizations' influence on legislation together with government committees, that had brought about many clients resident within their homes, coming within the care of the local authorities. However, as in 1913, this care remained the result of recommendation rather than requirement.

In the late 1940s and the early 1950s, improvements in provision heralded the care in the community philosophy now in vogue. Specifically, these improvements highlighted supervision, guardianship, training and occupation for those living in the community. Within the educational field, children requiring 'special education' were identified, effectively reversing the picture created prior to the First World War.

Both the England and Wales and the Scotland Mental Health Acts of 1959 and 1960 respectively allowed patients within hospitals informal status, and local authorities began creating their own special social work fieldwork, residential and day care developments.

Despite such progress, studies (e.g. in 1966 Jean Moncrieff's Political and Economic Planning Study on Mental Subnormality in London), in the home, showed many of the main concerns that are still apparent today. These included: the shortage of money spent on the increasingly ageing group of carers; poor quality of social work help received; and that the support offered to families (the main carers for people with learning difficulties) was 'slight in contact, and sporadic in application'.

In the 1970s, government white papers and surveys, e.g. the Health and Welfare Development of Community Care 1972 (Blue Book) Recommendations on Services for People with a Mental Handicap, showed the direction that was to be taken, e.g. recommending 1.2 places in hospitals per 1000 population. Such recommendations without the provision of government monies consistently failed to indicate how these targets were to be achieved.

The Seebohm Report in 1968; the 1971 White Paper, *Better Services for the Mentally Handicapped*; the Peter's Report in 1979; the Barclay Report in 1982; and the Short Report 1985, were all influential in the thinking about care in the community, but once more failed to stipulate how local authorities were to meet their recommendations. Local authority social services have therefore made their own priorities and developed their own provision accordingly.

Social services support to individuals and their families (fieldwork/ client services)

It can be argued that social services fieldwork support has developed according to the priority each individual local authority has given to it. Linked to this are local government policies and attitudes of the time, often heavily influenced by central government financial backing. Increasingly, parental pressures on elected members and service providers, as well as a growing movement of self-advocacy amongst people with learning difficulties themselves, has dictated the progress of this service.

Supports to clients can be for clarity and ease of understanding divided into the fieldwork and residential day care models. Fieldwork can be further divided into that provided by area or patch social work teams within a given locality and by social workers based within health settings such as hospitals, health centres or out-patients clinics.

There are further categories of client support such as transport, occupational therapy, registered carers, welfare benefit advice, leisure and/or occupation provision that do not fit neatly into any straight demarcation between fieldwork and residential and day care.

Area or patch teams within a given locality

Generally speaking, Regions in Scotland and the Boroughs and Counties in England and Wales are divided into Divisions or Districts, and within these are located area or patch teams. It is not uncommon for these Area Teams to have a specialist worker or group of workers whose remit it is to provide help, information and support to individuals or families who have an interest in, or need for assistance with, issues relating to people with learning difficulties.

A recent piece of legislation, the Disabled Persons (Services, Consultation and Representation) Act 1986, is an attempt to improve the effectiveness and coordination of services to all people with disabilities, not just people with learning difficulties. Succinctly, it gives all people with disabilities the right to:

1. Appoint representatives to act on their behalf.
2. Make formal representations about services provided for them.
3. Be consulted about the development of services through organizations of disabled people.

Not all parts of the Act have been implemented in England and Wales nor in Scotland (the Act does not apply to Northern Ireland). However, it is likely that the Act will have a significant bearing on social services and social work departments. The Act calls upon social work to provide services according to the needs of individuals, based on appropriate assessments and representations.

Assessment, whether this is undertaken by a social worker or other professional colleagues, such as a Community Occupational Therapist is an important tool around which supports for individuals and their families can be provided.

The following supports could be offered by the social worker, depending on the range of the relevant local authoritys' provisions available:

1. *Point of contact* – As the area team will have a fairly high profile within any given community, the allocation of the client group within overall priorities, may provide a link person. This can introduce individuals and their families to a whole range of potential contacts or services, depending upon the need, age of the person and service requested.
2. *Information about benefits and resources* – The social worker is in a position to provide information about resources and facilities in addition to being a contact or link point.

3. *Counselling and facilitating* – A number of models exist which may be of benefit to any individual seeking support, relief or assistance:
   (a) Individual or family casework.
   (b) One-to-one counselling with the 'client'.
   (c) Group work.
   (d) Individual support focusing on a specific problem or issue (e.g. written support to assist a housing transfer application.
   (e) Facilitating a process that ensures the client partakes in the stages to be undertaken (e.g. in-budgetting or a self-help domestic programme).
4. *Advocacy* – Much prejudice and ignorance still remains for many people with learning difficulties and their families. An educative function is very often required within the context of addressing attitudes held by certain individuals. Involvement in local community groups, such as social clubs and drop-in centres, is one aspect of the advocacy or educative function, in which social workers can support individuals and their families.
5. *Planning* – In planning support services, 'users' of such services are increasingly becoming involved themselves and promoting their needs and aspirations. Nevertheless, planning whether it be for a specific counselling service, the development of a daytime/occupational resource, or at joint planning levels with multi-agency participation, social workers will be involved and can provide advice and direct support.

The adoption and long-term or permanent fostering of children with learning difficulties is now a common enough event to warrant specialist Family Finding Teams being created, assisted by relevant legislation. Amongst the other specific statutory and specialist duties undertaken by social work agencies are the occupational therapy (e.g. practical aids and adaptations) and the home care (e.g. home help) roles.

However, specific mention should be made of the work undertaken by the Approved Social Worker in England and Wales and the Mental Health Officer in Scotland. Their functions are enacted within two specific pieces of legislation within The Mental Health Act, 1983 in England and Wales and the Mental Health (Scotland) Act, 1984. These appropriately trained social workers have experience in dealing with matters referred to in the respective Acts both relating to people with a learning difficulty as well as those who may also have a mental illness. The social worker's tasks cover practical advice, consultation giving and consent within the meaning of the Acts, as well as the undertaking of specific roles to do with guardianship and detention as defined within the relevant sections of the aforementioned legislation.

Many of these roles and duties are also relevant within social work in health care settings.

Social work teams within health care settings

Service varies in different parts of the country. However, it is not unusual to find social workers attached to specific hospitals for people with learning difficulties. The main remit of these hospitals tends now to be 'rehabilitation' or 'resettlement' of residents back into the community (although treatment, assessment and respite functions still continue within many hospitals). The focus of social work teams within these settings is therefore geared to this task, and to ensuring that the individual or groups of individuals are appropriately supported and maintained in their new setting.

Social workers in these settings are working not only with the resident, but also health service staff (medical, nursing, therapies, etc.), relatives and/or friends of the client. Additionally there are the different support services available within social work agencies as well as those in voluntary organizations, education authorities, housing associations, etc., all of whom will be offering services to all people with learning difficulties, in hospital, or living in the community.

An important aspect of hospital social work is the provision of social work assessments designed to inform the work of the clinical team. In acknowledging many of the principles of normalization and self-advocacy, and in accepting the rights of individual clients, many social work departments have embraced an open access policy. This has ensured that social workers may write down assessment or other information about the client and (subject to certain limitations, as laid out in the Access to Personal Files Act 1987, and its accompanying Regulations implemented in April 1989) that person has the right to see that written information.

Another part of social work within a hospital setting, is the provision of advice and support to residents and families about the changing role of the hospital and the consequences of hospital retraction and the developments geared towards care in the community. The social worker along with the charge nurse can be seen as having a crucial role in communicating, e.g. the reasoning behind inter-ward moves for residents because of ward closure, or the cessation of a particular function such as respite care provision, within the hospital setting.

The picture of hospital care within the UK has dramatically altered over the past two decades. The social worker has played a significant role in finding alternative accommodation but equally importantly, day and leisure care facilities for this client group. Equally the social worker has been involved in ensuring that only appropriate admissions to hospital are made, where the need is clearly for medical and/or nursing care. This ensures that families and clients are able to use community based resources if their needs can be so met, as an alternative to the hospital provision.

One of the sections of the Disabled Persons Act 1986 referred to earlier, but which has yet to be implemented is that which relates to 'Persons Discharged from hospitals'. In general, Section 7 of this Act states that the 'hospital managers' must notify the health and local authorities of the area where the person intends to live, and that the individual is being discharged. These authorities in turn must assess the person's need for the services they provide, with the implication that provision for these individual needs should be made.

This Act probably goes the furthest yet in trying to ensure that care in the community becomes a reality for all that wish it. However it still leaves local authority social services departments exposed to central government cash restrictions on their spending, which may in turn constrain service development within certain client groups.

Social work has expanded into other NHS settings such as out-patient clinics and health centres. Referrals to social workers involving families in counselling work, advice and practical assistance etc. may be made by a range of professionals. Social workers location in, or attachment to, such settings has increased over the past two decades, further extending the multi-disciplinary and agency remit allied to health care settings. This facet helps ensure that social work intervention is possible and available at whichever point the client comes into the NHS setting.

Social support services

Social work has a further contribution to make in terms of support services, for example their transport provision, ranging from big fleets of large buses to often discreet, non-stigmatizing, neutrally coloured smaller vehicles. Sometimes these are contracted out. Usually they have escorts and are often adapted for specific needs, e.g. equipped with a tail-lift.

The provision of Domiciliary Carers and Home Helps for individuals and their families within their own homes has been another helpful contribution to service support.

Finally the promotion of the 'social welfare' catch-phrase, embodied in most of the recent social work legislation, introduces other services and options for support. Cash assistance to individuals, e.g. for holidays, welfare advice, financial support to local community ventures, e.g. drop-in clubs, lunch clubs etc., are other services often provided.

Alternative patterns of care and supported placements – residential and day care/service provision

The Griffiths Report *Community Care: Agenda for Action* (1988) recommended the establishment of a Minister of State responsible for community care. A key role for the social services departments would be to employ case managers who in turn would assess the needs of individuals and put together packages of care including fieldwork and residential and day care.

Lady Wagner's *Positive Choice* Report, also published in 1988, reviews the role of residential care and also the whole range of statutory, voluntary and private residential establishments. Its remit was to report on their effectiveness in responding to the changing social needs of this decade. Wagner sees residential care as part of a continuum within care in the community. 'People who move into residential establishments, should do so by positive choice, and living there should be a positive experience', providing a better quality of life.

It is important to distinguish between the need for accommodation and for services. The former should be offered only as an alternative to a service which could be made available within the home. The basic principles to be followed should embody the rights of a citizen to enjoy much of what is desired within the concept of normalization. This means setting goals for people with learning difficulties, and achieving these by ordinary means, that are valued by the local community. Within community care arrangements there should be a range of alternatives and a choice of resources from which individuals and their families could select according to their needs.

Alternative patterns of care should first concentrate on support provided within the home or home-like equivalent. Examples of this are 'Domiciliary Carers' (individuals who have been assessed and matched as appropriate) who go into a person's own home to offer support. This may take the form of practical care such as lifting, dressing, toileting, etc.; or occupational assistance such as helping a person to use a computer, or visiting day services outside the house, etc.

A progression from this is a Befriending Scheme geared to a specific social relationship with an individual in their own home or to assist in offering an opportunity to go to outside social activities, such as swimming, the cinema, evening classes, etc.

Another source of support is centred on a matched family offering care in the form of a Share the Care provision according to an agreed contract for respite.

The above examples could be pursued in any combination of supports within the home, providing respite or relief for the main carers. These supports should be based on a declared need, precise planning, clear assessment and monitoring, appropriate training of service providers and effective operational support.

A second line of residential care is traditional support in buildings, e.g. staffed houses or hostels. With the advent of the Griffiths recommendations and DSS (Department of Social Security) board and lodging payments, 'registered accommodation' within the terms of social work legislation, is becoming more prevalent. This may be established by a private individual or by a voluntary organization (both conforming to stipulated regulations). The advent of the National Health Service and Community Care Act 1990 will further expand this provision by allowing the purchasing of buildings on a social work, contracted or agent-provided basis.

These resources are often autonomous. They may function as separate establishments; or may form a core and cluster provision; or may be informally linked with other similar establishments.

Local authority resources tend to offer a range of residential services often within the same building. These may include assessment; short-term care; training and preparation services; respite care; longer term/permanent care; and emergency placements.

Over the years, the provision of centres, whether they are called occupational centres, social education centres, adult training centres or resource centres, has been made by the social services for day care. In recent times there have been real indications that not only educational, but vocational and social developments in daytime services should take place. Government-sponsored schemes (most recently Employment Training) have engendered specific responses from agencies such as Mencap, SSMH and the Shaw Trust, when in the past they were under the aegis of the Manpower Services Commission. In particular 'Sheltered Placement Schemes' have afforded opportunities to individuals capable of producing at least 33% of a non-handicapped person's output. The 'New Training Programmes' have also focused on people with learning difficulties emphasizing that 40% of the individual's time will be spent on direct training, when linked to short-term employment opportunities.

Such vocational initiatives have also been matched by developments within local authority resource centres. The rationale of many resource centres involves the radical addressing of the philosophy behind the provision of centres moving towards localized services focused on a resource building but adopting an 'inside out' approach, i.e. using facilities already used by the local population, but with the help of extra staff support. The clients concerned are also playing an increasing part in decisions about their programmes of activities. Many centres have fostered the development of consumer committees. The range of activities available for day-care attenders has also increased. A small sample of these could include woodwork, craftwork, glass making, cement making, swimming, horse-riding, printing, gardening, drama, computer use, athletics and film making.

Such facilities are open to the whole range of abilities associated with people with learning difficulties. The special needs of those with a profound or severe handicap are beginning to be met by the use of enhanced staff levels and by the skills and experience of a range of specialist staff who may provide physiotherapy, occupational therapy, movement or music therapy, etc. within these settings.

The older person with learning difficulties may also be involved in a drop-in centre or lunch-club type of facility, or the use of a social club, or other ordinary community facility.

Benefits and welfare rights

This is a vast and complex subject. There are a host of specialist publications that address this subject matter, e.g. the *Disability Rights Handbook*, updated each April by the Disability Alliance, and the *Rights Guide to Non-Means Tested Benefits* and the *National Welfare Benefits Handbook*, published separately by Child Poverty Action Group. Within each region there are a range of Welfare Rights Advisors attached to local authority social services and social work departments, as well as voluntary organizations, the Citizens' Advice Bureaux and Department of Social Security Offices. Benefits, the amounts paid and the criteria applied change frequently, often on an annual basis. These factors must be borne in mind within this section, as the information provided is only correct at the time of writing and is subject to change.

There are a number of other issues to be considered when addressing basic benefits: benefits can be non-means tested (i.e. dependent on specific individual criteria, not the individual's own finances); contributory (i.e. dependent on National Insurance contributions); and/or non-contributory (i.e. available if certain criteria are met but not dependent on National Insurance contributions). Some benefits may also have tax implications.

Some of the specific benefits which may assist people with learning difficulties and their families may include:

1. *Income support* – Intended to meet regular weekly needs.
2. *Social fund* – Intended to meet exceptional expenses.
3. *Mobility allowance* – Intended to assist those with mobility problems.
4. *Attendance allowance* – Intended to assist those requiring exceptional care or supervision.
5. *Severe disablement allowance* – Intended for those without National Insurance contributions to qualify for sickness and invalidity benefits.
6. *Invalid care allowance* – Intended for those who cannot work because they are caring for someone.
7. *Community charge rebate* – Possible 80% assistance to pay community charge rates.

Income support

This is a means-tested benefit to assist people who do not have enough money to live on. If a person's income works out less than the amount that Social Security calculates they need to live on, then the difference between the two amounts is the income support entitlement. Income support qualification is generally dependent on the following conditions. The person must live in the UK; be aged

18 or older, or 16–17 and pass other tests; must not be working 24 hours or more a week (the same applies to their partner); must not be in full-time non-advanced education; must be available to work; and must have less than £6000 in capital (this sum includes any held by their partner if applicable).

The applicable amount of income support is made up of a personal allowance (a basic scale rate, reviewed each year) for a single person or a couple. There is a dependent's allowance rate for each dependent child. There is also a client group premium which is an allowance payable on the satisfaction of certain criteria, e.g. a disability premium taking into account people with learning difficulties.

Income support is a 'passport' to other types of help such as housing benefit and also the community charge rebate. People living in Residential Care Homes, Nursing Homes, Hostels and Board and Lodgings will receive an 'accommodation charge' to cover the amount paid, including meals where these are provided, on the qualification of a set criteria within this benefit.

The social fund

This is a system divided into two where payments are made either due to the applicant's legal entitlement, with no set budget (e.g. maternity payments, funeral expenses, cold weather payments); or based on discretion subject to constraints whereby interest-free loans or alternatively grants are made (e.g. for removals, fares, bedding etc.).

This latter system consists of the following sources of benefit:

1. Budgeting loans.
2. Crisis loans.
3. Community care grants.

Budgeting loans are payments used to assist people on income support to pay for something they cannot afford. Usually they are given to help pay for a large one-off expense and so spread the expense over a longer period of time. Savings over £500 will reduce the loan pound for pound, but the minimum load is £30 with a maximum of £1000.

Crisis loans are intended to assist a person's need to meet an emergency or the consequences of disaster. Though no minimum loan exists, it too has a maximum of £1000.

Both these loans are required to be paid back.

Community care grants are for people in receipt of income support or eligible for it, who are facing special difficulty arising from their special circumstances and in particular to support the general policy of care in the community. If a person has savings of over £500, a community care grant will be reduced by the amount of the extra savings. There are suggested maximum grants, e.g. £500 for a single person setting up his or her own home, or £400 for minor structural repairs and maintenance costs. It is worthwhile noting that the grant tends to be awarded to more able individuals. Difficulties may be encountered when a less able person leaves a long-term hospital (for example) and requires staffing support, and is looking for assistance with buying a bed. The grant is intended amongst other things to be awarded to assist an individual to stay in the community rather than be in care, or another example is to pay for fares in order for an individual to be visited where that person is ill or is in need of a relative's or close friend's company.

Mobility allowance

This is a weekly non-taxed payment for people who have walking difficulties. This must be caused by a physical condition. However, if an individual's mental handicap is accepted as having a physical cause, then the qualification criteria may also be met. This is where the person is either unable to walk; virtually unable to walk; or the exertion required to walk would, in itself, constitute a danger to life, or would be likely to lead to a serious deterioration in health. Distances walked at one time and the quality of walking, could also be considered as reasons to apply. Applicants should be at least 5 years old (applications three months prior to the fifth birthday will be considered) and not have reached the age of 66 (providing medical conditions have been satisfied before the age of 65). Once qualified, the allowance, if conditions continue to be satisfied, will continue until the 80th birthday. People who are registered blind and also those who are registered profoundly deaf are also now being treated by the DSS as eligible.

There are associated benefits attached to receipt of this allowance, for example the Orange Disabled Badge Scheme and exemption from vehicle excise duty. There are legal and practical problems surrounding mobility allowance claims for people with learning difficulties and others with severe mobility problems. However, with assistance (e.g. from a Welfare Rights or Citizens' Advice Worker) it is still possible for some of these individuals, including those who are autistic, or deaf/blind, to qualify.

Attendance allowance

This is a weekly, non-taxed benefit for people who need attention or supervision, either frequently or continually during the day in respect to bodily functions or to avoid substantial dangers to themselves. Similarly, this could apply to prolonged or repeated attention at night. Anyone aged 6 months or more can qualify (there is no upper age limit) providing the qualifications are met. The allowance is paid at two rates, lower and higher. If the day conditions and the night conditions are met, the higher rate of the allowance will be paid.

Attendance allowance is a passport to other benefits, such as the disability premium or Invalid Care Allowance.

Severe disablement allowance

This is a weekly, non-taxed cash benefit for people who have been incapable of work for at least 28 weeks but who do not have enough National Insurance contributions to qualify for sickness or invalidity benefits. The applicants have to be over 16, but under 60 years if a woman, and 65 years if a man.

The benefit which has four possible routes for qualification, depends upon whether:

1. The person had a former non-contributory invalidity pension or housewives non-contributory invalidity pension.
2. The person first became incapable of work on or before his or her 20th birthday.
3. The person who though not eligible through (1) or (2), is however, incapable of work and is assessed as being at least 75% disabled (always rounded up to 80%).

4. If not eligible under (1), (2) or (3), the person must show a loss of physical or mental facility, such that the extent of the resulting disablement amounts to not less than 80%.

Invalid care allowance

This is a taxable, weekly benefit for people of working age who cannot work because they are caring for a severely disabled person. A person must spend at least 35 hours each week caring for a person who in their turn must be in receipt of attendance allowance or constant attendance allowance.

It should be noted that income support beneficiaries will have this reduced by the amount of the invalid care allowance. However, it does have some advantages such as counting towards Class I National Insurance contributions.

Community charge rebate

(Note: this is not a DSS benefit, but a welfare right). A person registered to pay the community charge will get a bill each year covering 1 April in one year to 31 March the next. If the individual cannot afford to pay the full amount they may be able to get a rebate.

Those on income support will automatically get a rebate and will be told how much they have to pay. (Everyone will have to pay at least 20% of the community charge and all of the water charge.) Those owner-occupiers who got a rate rebate in Scotland up to 31 March 1989, will also be assessed automatically. Those who have already applied for a community charge rebate, if eligible, will be told how much they have to pay. Local Community Charge Rebate Offices will advise of eligibility.

Some people will be exempt from the charge. To be exempt, the person must be entitled to either invalidity pension; attendance allowance; constant attendance allowance; severe disablement allowance; disablement benefit with unemployability supplement; war disablement pension with unemployability allowance; or be over pensionable age.

Carers of persons with a severe learning difficulty, who are not getting any of the above benefits, should seek advice, since the person may be entitled to claim one of them.

It is now the case that anyone who receives a qualifying benefit because they have a mental impairment (i.e. attendance allowance or constant attendance allowance or entitlement to exemption on the grounds of severe mental impairment which is to ensure that nobody loses their original exemption) should qualify for exemption by right. Doctors now have only to certify that impairment is mental rather than physical. In view of this it may be prudent to apply for exemption if it is possible that the person with learning difficulties may qualify. This exemption should be sought from The Local Community Charges Registration Officer. Different rules apply to people staying in places like Hospitals, Hostels and Nursing Homes and therefore advice should be sought for them from this officer.

Other benefits

Other benefits have become established as a result of voluntary organizations' campaigns. For example, a national organization known as Disablement Income Group (whose main objective is to campaign for a national disability income including a disablement cost allowance) were instrumental in 1971 in having the Attendance Allowance and Invalidity Benefit introduced as social security benefits to severely disabled people. They have most recently (June 1988) become involved with the *Independent Living Fund* for 'very severely disabled people who can only live at home if they have a lot of paid help'. The fund is an independent discretionary trust. Its aim is to prevent such people from having to enter residential care if they cannot afford the support. Furthermore, it may enable people in residential care who are capable of living independently to do so. The fund's life will have a limited timescale and is now further limited to people between the ages of 16 and 74 and who are in receipt of full Attendance Allowance. Further information should be sought from the Independent Living Fund, PO Box 183, Nottingham NG8 3RD.

The Family Fund, administered by the Joseph Rowntree Memorial Trust, is another government financed resource. This particular fund is for severely handicapped children under the age of 16. It tends to provide set lump-sum grants for specific items which arise as a consequence of caring for such a child with special needs, e.g. washing machines, payment of driving lessons, specialized equipment.

Further information should be sought by writing to the Family Fund, PO Box 50, York, YO1 1UY.

It is not commonly known or understood that trusts in general exist in abundance and financial assistance could be forthcoming from a whole host of philanthropic and established sources, if certain criteria are met. It is advisable to start any quest for such resources in the local library, which should have a *Directory of Charities* available for perusal.

More specifically there is a scheme which provides a lump-sum payment for handicap caused by vaccine damage. The leaflet HB3 which describes this is *Payment for People Severely Damaged by a Vaccine*. A payment of £20000 is available for people who suffered permanent and very severe damage as a result of vaccination under a routine public-policy vaccination programme. The £20000 award is available only to people who make (or made) their first claim for help under the scheme on or after 18 June 1985. A claim made earlier restricts payment to £10000. The date of the vaccination makes no difference.

In addition *Urban Aid* and *European Economic Community Social Funds* (innovatory programmes) may also be available; details of these are available through local Regional, County or Borough Councils.

Supplementations from Social Services Departments for attendance at places of occupation or residence may be made available to assist individuals with learning difficulties and their families. Social services departments may also consider assisting with costs of holidays and councils may offer schemes where bus travel is free.

No comprehensive list or guide has been attempted or is claimed to have been produced within this section. Further advice on these benefits and resources should be obtained by contacting one of the following: local social services departments, Citizens' Advice Bureaux, or any Department of Social Security Office.

References

Access to Personal Files Act 1987, HMSO, London
Barclay, P.M. (1982) *Social Workers: their role and tasks*, HMSO, London

Charities Digest 1990 (96th edn) An Alphabetical Digest of Charities, Family Welfare Association, London

DHSS and Welsh Office (1971) *Better Services for the Mentally Handicapped*, HMSO, London

Directory of Grant Making Trusts 1989 (11th Compilation) Charities Aid Foundation, Kent

Disability Rights Handbook (15th edn April 1990–April 1991) Disability Alliance Educational and Research Association, London

Disabled Persons (Services, Consultation and Representation) Act 1986, HMSO, London

Griffiths, Sir Roy (1988) *Community Care Agenda for Action 1988*, A report to the Secretary of State for Social Services by Sir Roy Griffiths, HMSO, London

Lakhani, Beth and Read, J. (1990) *National Welfare Benefits Handbook* (20th edn 1990/1991) Child Poverty Action Group, London

Mental Deficiency (Scotland) Act 1913, HMSO, London

Mental Health Act 1983, HMSO, London

Mental Health (Scotland) Act 1960, HMSO, London

Mental Health (Scotland) Act 1984, HMSO, London

Moncreiff, Jean (1966) *Mental Subnormality in London. A Survey of Community Care. Political & Economic Planning.* Report, London

National Health Service & Community Care Act 1990, HMSO, London

Petos, D.A. (1979) *A Better Life. Report on Services for the Mentally Handicapped in Scotland,* Scottish Home and Health Department and Education Department, HMSO, Edinburgh

Rowland, M. (1990) *Rights Guide to Non Means Tested Benefits* (13th edn 1990–1991) Child Poverty Action Group, London

Scottish Home and Health Department and Scottish Education Department (1972) *Services for the Mentally Handicapped*, Blue Book, Edinburgh

Seebohm Report (1968) Report of the Committee on Local Authority and Allied Personal Social Services, HMSO, London

Short, Renee (1985) Second Report from Social Services Committee Session 1984–85, *Community Care with Special Reference to Adult Mentally Ill and Mentally Handicapped People*, House of Commons, HMSO, London

Social Work (Scotland) Act 1968, HMSO, London

Wagner, Lady Gillian (1988) *Residential Care: A Positive Choice*, HMSO, London

Useful addresses

Disablement Income Group, Millimead Business Centre, Millmead Road, London LN7 9QU

Disablement Income Group (Scotland) ECAS House, 28–30 Howden Street, Edinburgh EH8 9HW

European Economic Commission Social Fund, The Commission of the European Committees, Directorate General Employment, Social Affairs and Education, European Social Fund, Rue de la Loi 200, 1049 Brussels

Manpower Services Commission, Moorfoot, Sheffield S1 4PQ

MENCAP, 123 Golden Lane, London EC1Y 0RT

Scottish Society for the Mentally Handicapped, 13 Elmbank Street, Glasgow G2 4AQ

Shaw Trust, Caithness House, Western Way, Melksham, Wiltshire SN12 8DZ

Urban Aid Programmes (England and Wales), Department of the Environment, 2 Marsham Street, London SW1P 3EB

Urban Aid Programmes (Scotland), Industry Department for Scotland, Urban Renewal Unit, New St. Andrews House, Edinburgh EH1 3TA

12

Community mental handicap teams

Sally Cheseldine

Why community mental handicap teams?

Most people with mental handicaps live with their own families or independently in the community. These numbers are increasing with the progressive closure of large mental handicap hospitals, and it only seems logical that to provide support for these people, there should be a parallel development in community services.

However, in the early 1970s it became evident that although people with mental handicaps have a right to the same 'generic services' (i.e. primary health and social care) as anyone else, they were not receiving the help they needed. These general community-based services, as opposed to *specialist* services for people with mental handicaps, meant that professionals received a broad-based training and might only come across one or two people with mental handicaps in their area. Without the necessary training and experience they would lack the expertise to provide the appropriate help.

In response to a growing awareness of these problems, the National Development Group for the Mentally Handicapped in its pamphlet, *Mentally Handicapped Children: a Plan for Action* (1977), recommended the setting up of Specialist Community Mental Handicap Teams (CMHTs), consisting of both NHS and local authority staff.

The overall purpose of a CMHT would be to provide a support service for people with mental handicaps and their carers, from cradle to grave within their local community. Three specific functions were identified:

1. To act as the first point of contact and to provide advice and help.
2. To coordinate access to services.
3. To establish close working relationships with relevant local voluntary organizations.

It was envisaged that one CMHT would operate in each local area with a population between 60000 and 100000, and would consist of two 'core' members: a community mental handicap nurse and a social worker. These two full-time workers would be backed up by a range of other specialists, such as a clinical psychologist, speech therapist, consultant psychiatrist and an occupational therapist.

It is worth noting that the concept of the CMHT as proposed by the National Development Group differed from the proposals of the Court Report which recommended the setting up a *District* Handicap Team (DHT). A DHT would deal with all children with any type of handicap, and would ensure that they stayed in mainstream services for children with needs being met by people experienced in child care. The CMHT model is the one that has been adopted in most areas but service providers are now aware of the need to consider the child as a *child* first, and not assume that any problems are simply due to a mental handicap.

A major concept proposed by the National Development Group was that of a named person, or 'keyworker', for every person with a mental handicap, who would act as the point of contact for all services, and ensure that a coordinated plan was implemented. This person might be a social worker or a community nurse, or could come from one of the other agencies in contact with the family.

The CMHT would also act as a resource centre for information on facilities and services in the area, available to parents, people with mental handicaps and the service providers. This might include information on social security benefits, grants, where to go for help with housing or employment, and local voluntary organizations who might be able to provide help.

What happens in practice?

There is no definitive statement as to what a CMHT should do, or who should be in it, and it is arguably a more helpful approach not to look for one. This allows for change and flexibility so that a service can be needs-led and cater for individuals, rather than expecting people with mental handicaps to be a homogeneous group who 'fit' into whatever service the statutory bodies choose to provide.

Individual teams differ from district to district, depending on the size of the geographical area covered; whether there is a mental handicap hospital within the district; whether health, social services and education have the same boundaries within an area; whether there is one building to house all the members of the CMHT; and whether there is a policy for joint planning and funding between health and social services.

Some teams provide a service to adults only, others deal with all ages. Some specifically exclude people with mild learning difficulties, some only operate this policy with children up to school-leaving age.

Inevitably this can lead to confusion: whose 'responsibility' is a child with a mild learning difficulty attending a school for children with severe learning difficulties? What about the child with Down's syndrome attending mainstream school?

Plank (1982) found many different team structures and practices, and wide variations between teams in a number of features, such as membership, base, referral policy, parent participation and assignment of keyworkers. Cotmore, Sinclair and Wistow (1985) also reported variation in membership and activities, but identified a similarity in overall role – identifying needs, and then developing support systems and resources to meet these needs.

CMHTs are involved in both short-term and long-term planning for the individual and the service as a whole, and try to move away from a model of crisis intervention. This involves maximum cooperation between different agencies so that efforts are neither duplicated nor assumed to be carried out by another part of the service.

Membership of the CMHT

The core membership of a CMHT typically consists of a social worker, a community mental handicap nurse and a clinical psychologist. In larger CMHTs there may be more than one 'core team' to cover different age groups or different geographical 'patches', and several other people may be involved depending on the needs of the person with the mental handicap. These may include a consultant psychiatrist, occupational therapists, rehabilitation officers, home support workers, nursing auxiliaries, social work assistants, pre-school teachers, liaison health visitors and volunteer coordinators. In addition to this large group of paid professionals who link into the CMHT, many voluntary groups provide important sources of help and support, e.g. Mencap (SSMH in Scotland), Council for Voluntary Services and citizens' advocacy groups. Many areas are also now starting to invite the service users, i.e. people with mental handicaps, and their families or advocates, to advise on service provision. This is a sensible way of developing needs-led services and ensuring a powerful voice in the call for better services.

The role of individual members of the CMHT

The role of the keyworker, irrespective of their professional discipline, is to provide a contact point for the mentally handicapped person and their family, to ensure they have access to relevant advice and services, and to coordinate input and long-term planning with other professionals and agencies. In some teams the keyworker stays with the person and his or her family from birth or diagnosis, onwards. In others, the keyworker may change as a child moves on to requiring services from the adult sector of the team. There may also be differences in the extent to which the keyworker is involved in day-to-day input with the individual. Inevitably there will also be changes in keyworker due to either the client or the professional moving areas or changing jobs. In all cases the Community Team must ensure that the individual, his or her family, and the other agencies involved know who is taking over as the contact person.

The role of specific professionals within the team will necessarily alter as a child grows and becomes an adult, and eventually old age takes over. There may well be overlap in the service offered by different disciplines, and who does what may be determined by current needs of the client groups, and the individual interests of the professionals. With the multi-disciplinary nature of CMHTs there can be input from more than one team member at any one time, and useful reinforcement of support and advice can be given in this way.

When a handicapped baby is born, or the diagnosis of a handicap first made, the initial contact the parents have with the CMHT is likely to be with the social worker, or other counsellor trained in supporting parents through these traumatic early days. This support may extend beyond the parents to grandparents and brothers and sisters, and whether a child is taken home to the family or rejected and offered for adoption, the family will need this support.

Once the baby arrives home, and during the pre-school years, there may be involvement from a specialist health visitor, or a liaison health visitor whose role is to support the local health visitor in providing advice on child development to the family. Soon the clinical psychologist may start to be involved, looking at the child's rate of development and identifying needs and developing intervention strategies for meeting these needs. These interventions may be focused around a system such as 'Portage', or be less structured, but generally recognize the need for, and the importance of, support for parents in home-teaching systems. The community nurse is likely to be very involved with this work.

Input to the family in the pre-school years may then include assessment of development and advice about facilitating this (psychologist and community nurse), advice about social service benefits (social worker), advice about special equipment and adaptations (social worker and occupational therapist), advice about specific physical disabilities (speech therapist, physiotherapist and community nurse), and family support and provision of respite care (social worker). These are only *some* aspects, and there should of course also be access to all ordinary health and social care facilities for children.

At nursery school age and with the approach of full-time school attendance, the CMHT should have strong links with the Education Department. This may take the form of enlisting or providing support for the child to attend a local playgroup or nursery and then a mainstream school, or in working closely with staff and parents while the child is attending a special school.

During the school years the team may take on a collective role of ensuring the young person has access to the same community amenities as other children. Home support workers or nursing assistants may enable the child to attend non-segregated play schemes during the holidays (i.e. local schemes that take all the children from an area, rather than merely 'integrated' schemes which are set up for handicapped children and invite equal numbers of non-handicapped children along); youth and community workers may help in providing access to local youth clubs, the Boy Scouts or the Girl Guides.

If there are problems or difficulties during the school years which cross the boundary between school and home, members of the team may be involved, and so the existence of a keyworker is no less important at this stage. While many fears and anxieties may lie dormant during the school years, they typically re-awaken as school leaving nears. Late adolescence is the period when young people are more likely to be referred to the CMHT, and, in the past, it has been the time when people with mental handicap were most likely to be admitted to mental handicap hospitals. The reasons for this may be manifold: the ordinary problems of adolescence are compounded with those of mental handicap; parents are that much older and may be unable to cope; services for adults may not be appropriate for young people leaving school, or may not be as well developed.

The overall role of the CMHT at this time is to help individuals and their families to prepare for the changes that adulthood brings, and to develop long-term plans to meet the needs of the person with mental handicaps, and ultimately prevent admission to a mental handicap hospital. This may be done through Individual Programme Planning which gives everyone who is involved the chance to put forward their suggestions or ideas, but particularly keeps the client as the most important person in the decision-making process.

As with the service to young children, there will be some overlap of roles, but input may include advice on benefits and housing options; help in deciding on and providing day care; assessing and teaching independent living skills; developing leisure interests; and dealing with problems and difficulties. Support to parents and families should not be neglected either – many families assume that it will always be their role to 'care' for their mentally handicapped member, and it is often at a crisis point, when the second parent dies, that the CMHT is suddenly called in to 'find somewhere' for the client, or to provide emergency cover to enable him or her to stay in their own home. Yet with sensitive counselling and planning a positive move from the family home can be arranged before a crisis is reached, so that the client moves to his or her own home, with the appropriate level of help, within the positive framework of family support. If the plan is that the person should stay in the family home, then the family should be encouraged to talk this over with those people who will actually be giving the support.

When the idea of community care was first being mooted, it was often suggested that an intensive level of support would be required at first, which could then be faded out as skills were acquired. While this may be the case for some people, for others it would be unrealistic. Even very able people who do not require living-in staff support, may require weekly visits for the rest of their lives, or indeed increasing levels of support as they grow older. As adults are being encouraged to live independently and make decisions for themselves, they are increasingly 'opting out' of local authority day care provision. Enabling access to work situations and appropriate social and leisure settings is becoming a major aspect of CMHT work. Alongside this is the need for specific skills to be taught, whether they be budgetting and shopping skills, social interaction skills or community awareness. Team members may find themselves doing one-to-one work, or may work through others, such as care assistants, nursing assistants or families.

As people with mental handicaps grow older they risk what has been called the 'double jeopardy' of old age *and* mental handicap. This is a relatively new phenomenon because in the past old age was so rarely achieved by this section of society. Yet in spite of the large proportion of society who will one day be old, services for elderly people with mental handicaps are only just starting to get off the ground. It has largely been CMHTs who have innovated the development of this side of the service, in response to an unmet need. The emphasis is very much on developing a positive approach to retirement, rather than a running down, and links are being established with age-appropriate local services such as Age Concern. There may also be special needs for this age group, for example, needing help to maintain existing friendships after leaving an ATC, particularly if people cannot travel independently; coping with the loss of friends and family who die; the effects of dementia on already shaky life skills. Once again, all members of the CMHT may be involved.

Whatever the age of the client, and whether the client is able to speak for him or herself or through another person, the priorities and general role of a CMHT will remain the same – to facilitate maximum independence and a valued lifestyle with whatever support is necessary for the individual with a mental handicap. This requires high levels of communication between different service providers and agencies and is more likely to be achieved at grass-roots level where there is a neutral community base to house the multidisciplinary team, and a management level where there is respect for the skills each discipline brings to the situation, and a policy of joint planning, funding and training.

Where to next?

The specific roles and functions of the CMHT will always be subject to some change – as new needs are identified, as more clients move from hospitals and hostels into the community and as policy makers allocate resources to the service.

Teams are already responding to needs, for example, setting up befriending schemes to link individual mentally handicapped people with individual volunteers in recreational activities, enabling self-advocacy and citizen advocacy schemes to get off the ground, setting up home-from-home respite schemes for children and adults, and looking at alternatives to day care and residential services provided by statutory bodies. The response to greater numbers of people with mental handicaps living in the community rather than in hospitals or hostels may be to employ more 'hands-on' workers who have day-to-day contact with the client group, but who are supervised and led by the CMHT for that area. Indeed this is one of the issues developed in the Griffiths Report (1988), where it was suggested that community services should be social work led, but that health, particularly community nurses and clinical psychologists, would have a major role in innovation and service development.

It is becoming increasingly evident that a 'core team' of one social worker, one community nurse and one clinical psychologist will not be enough to provide a service to a district with a population of 100 000. The emphasis on providing a community service to all people with a mental handicap means that hospitals will be used less, if at all, in the management of behaviour that presents a great challenge to the service. While care givers may not require an emergency support team, they may well require more staff for a temporary period and long-term support in the management of behaviour problems. It is unrealistic to expect the same community nurses and psychologists to provide this while at the same time maintaining a high quality, non-crisis orientated, service to their other clients.

A great deal of both public and professional education is required for community living to be successful, and much of this can be achieved by the CMHT. The public can be educated in quiet, unobtrusive ways by seeing clients being enabled to use community amenities on an individual basis. Other professionals, such as dentists, chiropodists and even staff in local general hospitals can be educated and supported in their treatment of people with mental handicaps, by CMHT staff helping clients to attend local facilities and emphasizing their need for appropriate treatment, i.e. seeing the relevant ailment, rather than the label 'mental handicap'.

To summarize, it was suggested earlier that there is no 'correct' model for a CMHT. By being aware of this and by regularly reviewing their input and response to needs, each CMHT should be able to ensure that it changes with the changing demands of the service consumers.

Case history 1

Mrs Oswald was already 16 weeks pregnant before she realized it – she was 42 and had assumed that her missed periods were due to menopausal changes. She knew of the risk of having a child with Down's syndrome at her age, but decided not to take up the offer of amniocentesis, saying that the baby would be welcomed to the family whatever its condition. Nevertheless she experienced great trauma when Katie was born and diagnosed as having Down's syndrome, in spite of being told the news sensitively with her husband by the consultant paediatrician.

The CMHT was notified of Katie's birth within 12 hours, and the team social worker arranged to visit at the same time as the paediatrician the next day. At this stage shock was the predominant reaction, with Mr and Mrs Oswald feeling confusion and disbelief and needing sympathy and emotional support. Gradually their reaction turned to one of sorrow and grief – at the loss of a healthy baby, followed by feelings of anger, guilt and failure. The social worker allowed the parents time to talk about these feelings, and discussed very factual aspects of the condition. He also suggested that Mr and Mrs Oswald might like to meet another parent of a Down's baby – a suggestion that was warmly received.

Katie was physically fit and at 10 days old she went home. The social worker continued to visit on a regular basis as the named 'keyworker' and when Katie was 3 weeks old he was joined by the liaison health visitor. She provided practical help in managing Katie, emphasizing the need to stimulate her and not just think of her as a 'good' baby who slept well. Mr and Mrs Oswald already had two children, boys aged 15 and 13, and so already had good, basic parenting skills.

The boys were delighted at having a sister, although they had to put up with a fair amount of teasing from the other boys at school about having a handicapped sister. The social worker was involved again and spent time with the boys both individually and with the wider family, helping them to develop ways of responding to such taunts.

As Katie grew she passed through developmental milestones rather later than usual. She sat up at 14 months and tried to stand at 18 months. Mrs Oswald wanted to help her as much as possible and knew from her local contact with Mencap and the Down's Syndrome Association that home teaching packages were available. The clinical psychologist had been involved in assessing Katie's developmental level and introduced Mrs Oswald to the Portage system of home teaching. The areas of physical development and communication were identified as priorities, and fortnightly visits were made to the family by the community nurse to help in identifying specific goals and devising ways of attaining them.

At 2½ years an individual programme plan meeting was held, attended by CMHT staff, the local health visitor, the pre-school teacher and Mr and Mrs Oswald. It was decided that Katie's needs were very much the same as any other child of that age, and a place in the local playgroup would go a long way towards meeting those needs. The social worker, community nurse and pre-school teacher would act as a link between the family, the CMHT and the playgroup, and very soon Katie settled down to five mornings a week there.

Case history 2

During her years at a special school for children with severe learning difficulties, Barbara had acquired many skills. She could handle money and buy basic provisions, and she could find her way from home to the local shops and library. There was little involvement from the CMHT other than a phone call from the keyworker to her parents every 3 months to check that all was well, and to ask if they needed any help. The keyworker also attended 'statement of educational needs' meetings when they were held at the school.

It was at one of these meetings, when Barbara was 15, that her parents expressed a general concern over her social isolation. She already attended the Gateway Youth Club once a week, with other students from her school, and was collected and brought home by the Mencap minibus. Barbara, however, had said she would like to attend the local church youth club which met every Thursday and Sunday, but she did not know anyone else who went there. Her parents were keen that she should join in this activity, as they were already members of that church.

The keyworker arranged a meeting with a youth and community worker from the local authority, a community nurse and the youth club leader, at which they identified what support would be needed to enable Barbara to attend. Barbara already knew her way to the church hall, although she had only ever been with her parents, and they considered it inappropriate for them to accompany her to a youth club, so she might need help to get there and back. Once at the club there were several activities which were new to Barbara, such as table-tennis and badminton – so she might need help to learn them. She might also need support in actually meeting the club members and making new friends.

Barbara was highly motivated to learn new skills and the community nurse involved her closely in planning the goals. The task of getting to and from the club was broken down into stages and she was helped by the youth and community worker to gradually do more and more on her own. The club leader asked for volunteers to teach the new activities to Barbara and this in turn helped her to meet new people. Over time the friendships extended beyond the club to other social activities.

As Barbara approached school-leaving age at 19 the CMHT was again involved in helping her and her parents to make the transition from children's to adult services. A series of meetings was held, attended by all the school-leavers and their parents. The social worker talked to the group about post-school options and arranged visits to day centres, hostels and the local Further Education Centre. The psychologist led discussions about what 'adulthood' had meant for the parents, and how it might be different for their sons and daughters. For Barbara and her parents this was the first time that the idea of a positive move away from home had been considered, and it raised a lot of emotions and fears that had lain dormant for many years.

Her parents now knew which members of the CMHT should be contacted from the adult side of the service; they asked for help from the community nurse and psychologist in assessing Barbara's skills, and from the social worker in helping them to look at positive ways for Barbara to spend her day, and in exploring housing options.

Case history 3

Tony's parents died within 3 months of each other – his father from cancer and his mother from a stroke. They had always assumed that Tony would go and live with his sister and her family when this happened, but when it came to the crunch her husband said that *his* family came first, and that 'social services are there to cater for people like him'. The CMHT had known the family for many years and had anticipated this possibility, and a bed was quickly found for Tony in a local hostel.

Tony was 30 years old and had never spent time away from his parents, apart from going daily to the Special Needs unit at the local adult training centre (ATC). He was doubly incontinent, could walk, could feed himself with a spoon, and communicated using a few basic Makaton signs, such as 'drink', 'eat', 'mother', 'father' and 'hello'. His evenings and weekends were spent sitting in front of the television, or going on family outings to the shops or to visit relatives.

When his father had died first, Tony's mother had not wanted him to know, saying that he wouldn't understand anyway. He did not attend the funeral. His behaviour, however, suggested that he was very aware of the change that had occurred. At home he kept getting up at night and climbing into his mother's bed; at the ATC he wandered aimlessly around the room stopping only to gaze out the window. He did not cry nor did he mention or sign 'father'.

When his mother died, again Tony's sister did not want him to attend the funeral. The social worker and psychologist talked to her about Tony's need to grieve and say 'goodbye' and a compromise was reached where Tony didn't travel in the family car but with his ATC instructor, whom he knew well.

At the hostel the psychologist worked with the staff to help them recognize some of the signs of loss and bereavement that Tony might show, because he had lost not only his parents, but also his home and a total way of life. The community nurse and the ATC instructor arranged times for Tony to go to the old house, so that he could maintain a link and also so that his skills could be assessed in the environment he knew best. On the basis of this it was calculated that he would need nearly 100 hours of staff support to live in the house, which the CMHT could not offer immediately.

Nevertheless the tenancy of the house was maintained in Tony's name and the Social Services department agreed to transfer the monies used to give him a hostel place to supporting him in his own home. The costs were eventually reduced by two of Tony's friends from the ATC joining him in the house.

One year later Tony was still showing some signs of bereavement – he would still occasionally get up in the night and go to what had been his parents' bedroom. However, his routine at the ATC had returned to normal, he carried photographs of his parents with him and often showed them to people, and he had started to do many more activities in the evenings and at weekends.

Case history 4

Henry was 62 years old when he wrote to the superintendent of the mental handicap hospital he had lived in for nearly 40 years asking to go home. He had been sent there by the courts when he was 23 years old because of a petty theft he had committed, and because it was known that he was 'of unsound mind', as the records described him, and it was felt that a prison sentence would not help him.

He was one of five children and attended the local school where he learned to read and write. When he left school at 14 he worked as an odd-job boy for a local shop, whose manageress ultimately accused him of theft. During his years at the mental handicap hospital he visited his home town at least twice a year, and so was aware of the changes that had taken place. His letter to the superintendent pointed out that if he *had* gone to prison, at least he would have served his sentence by now, and he felt that he had been 'incarcerated' (his word) for long enough and would like the chance to spend the rest of his life near his family.

The manager at the hospital contacted the CMHT to ask for help, and the psychologist and community nurse went to meet Henry. He expressed interest in a local residential hostel and it was suggested that he should have a few short stays there to get to know the staff. This would also help him to get to know the area better and hopefully give him ideas about where he would like to live in the longer term. It also enabled the CMHT to assess what level of support Henry would require to live in the community.

Over a period of 6 months Henry decided that he definitely did want to leave the hospital, but that he would prefer to live with people of his own age group.

The local social services department had an agreement with the Regional Health Authority on joint funding of community care projects, and received an annual 'dowry' for Henry from the RHA which would help to fund support staff. The CMHT's assessments had shown that while he would need help with activities of daily living, Henry did not need 24 hour support.

Having visited several flats and houses occupied by people of a similar age, also supported by the CMHT, Henry decided he would like to live in a warden-controlled accommodation, i.e. a one-bedroomed flat with kitchenette and toilet, in a block of 20 flats occupied by other older people (not known to the CMHT), with a resident warden. Two peripatetic home-makers were appointed who visited him daily and, supervised by CMHT staff, taught him basic independence skills and also helped him to get to know the neighbourhood and local services.

A volunteer of a similar age was found through a Befriending Scheme, and helped Henry to find out about local facilities for people of his own age, e.g. lunch clubs, swimming for the over-fifties, and concessionary theatre trips. His only disappointment has perhaps been his family, who were opposed to his return. This was an important issue for the CMHT to discuss, but it was felt that Henry was their client, and his wishes were most important.

References

Cotmore, R., Sinclair, R. and Wistow, A. (1985) Five faces of care. *Community Care*, **27 June**

Court Report (1976) *Fit for the Future – The Report of the Committee on Child Health Services*, Cmnd 6684, HMSO, London

Griffiths, R. (1988) *Community Care: Agenda for Action*, HMSO, London

National Development Group for the Mentally Handicapped (1977) *Mentally Handicapped Children: A Plan for Action*, Pamphlet No. 2, DHSS, London

Plank, M. (1982) *Teams for Mentally Handicapped People*, CMH, London

13

Psychological therapies in mental handicap

William R. Lindsay

This chapter will outline some of the psychological methods that have been adapted for use with people with a mental handicap and to look at the literature on their effectiveness. Treatments will include cognitive therapy approaches, approaches which have been employed in anxiety management and treatment approaches aimed at helping anger and aggression in people with a mental handicap.

Assessment of cognition and emotion

In the past when assessing the private world of people with a mental handicap we have usually asked carers and relatives. A reasonably extensive literature has developed on emotional problems of clients using standard interviews with significant others or symptom check-lists filled out by staff members. However, recent developments in assessment techniques have moved towards more reliable and systematic methods of asking clients themselves to judge the extent and nature of their cognitive and emotional difficulties.

Lindsay and Michie (1988) and Michie and Lindsay (1988) reported work on the Zung Self-Rating Anxiety Scale (Zung, 1971) and the Zung Self-Rating Depression Scale (Zung, 1965), two assessments used extensively with other populations. They found that standard presentations of the scales produced very low reliability scores and they redesigned the test with two major considerations in mind. Firstly the language and concepts were simplified and put into local language to ensure understanding. Secondly they truncated the graded multiple choice answers to a simple presence or absence of the symptom or feeling.

Kazdin, Matson and Senatore (1983) and Helsel and Matson (1988) have adapted the Zung Scales using an extensive explanatory preamble, some initial 'trial' questions and a multiple choice format. The graded multiple choice options were accompanied by a bar graph which was a pictorial representation of the answers (see later). All the above methods employed allowed subjects to respond reliably.

These studies demonstrate that if the therapist takes some care, then reliable and valid assessments of the private feelings and thoughts of people with a mental handicap can be gathered. However, it may be that the clinician will wish a more flexible instrument to judge problems and strengths and feelings or self-concept. Gowans and Hulbert (1983) considered the difficulties of using standard tests with people with a mental handicap. They felt that imposing a preconceived structure on self-concept might force the client to consider himself in a novel or indeed foreign and unaccustomed manner. Such an assessment may omit areas which the individual himself or herself might feel important. They suggested the repertory grid technique (Fransella and Bannister, 1977) might prove to be a useful method, more sensitive to individual differences and personal considerations. Oliver (1986) reported a case study of a girl with Down's syndrome whose IQ was in the 40's. Using simple, clear constructs he developed a personal assessment of the subject which gave fascinating insights into her self-concept. Although this is only a single case study it is a good demonstration of how such a personal and flexible assessment might be conducted.

Analogue and lickert scale assessments

One of the most common methods of assessment focused on personal considerations is an analogue or 'lickert' scale assessment. This is a graded assessment of a single dimension relevant to the person's problem. The scales have an infinite variety of uses depending on the individual problem being assessed. The person is asked to rate the problem from a little or none of the attribute; through moderate amounts of the attribute; to a great deal of the attribute. The scale could have a set number of answering points, usually 3–7, or can be completely flexible where the person simply makes a mark on a line indicating the extent they experience the attribute. Many emotions, feelings, and internal events can be assessed in this

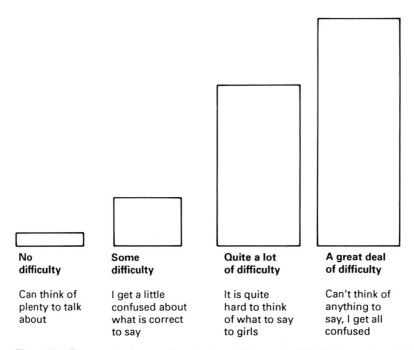

No difficulty	**Some difficulty**	**Quite a lot of difficulty**	**A great deal of difficulty**
Can think of plenty to talk about	I get a little confused about what is correct to say	It is quite hard to think of what to say to girls	Can't think of anything to say, I get all confused

Figure 13.1 Response to the questionnaire item: 'How much difficulty do you have thinking when you talk to girls? When you talk to girls can you think of what to say to them? Do you get all confused in your head when you talk to girls?'

way, including anxiety, depression, anger, confidence, difficulty in thinking, confusion, intrusive thoughts, one particular thought, etc. The person might rate duration of the internal event (from no time, through seldom, a little time, frequently, to constantly), or intensity of the internal event (from none, through some, quite a lot, a great deal, to as much as I can imagine experiencing).

With clients who have a mental handicap it is best to use a bar graph as a visual aid to help describe each answer point (as developed by Kazdin, Matson and Senatore, 1983), and supplementary questions to clarify the issue. Figure 13.1 is an illustration of a questionnaire item for difficulty in thinking.

In this way the person with the mental handicap is given a pictorial representation of the gradations in internal events. Some of the studies below will illustrate how these methods have been used.

Cognitive therapy

The expansion of interest in cognitive therapies did not reach clients with a mental handicap. This is true despite the fact that much of the basic therapeutic research was done with children and with some modification one could suppose that the techniques might be eminently suitable for people with a mental handicap.

Self-instructional training (SIT)

Meichenbaum (1977) hypothesized that voluntary motor behaviour in children was initiated and inhibited through verbal control. This control is developed through three stages. Firstly, adults and others control the child's behaviour through overt direction. Secondly, the child begins to control their own behaviour through speech and thirdly as the child's speech becomes internalized, so the control of behaviour becomes covert and internalized.

Meichenbaum and his colleagues then extended this work to compare the private speech of various categories of children (Meichenbaum, 1977; Meichenbaum and Goodman, 1971). Impulsive children tended to differ in the quality of their private speech and also used it in different ways. Their private speech was more imitative, more self-stimulatory and less self-regulating than more reflective children. Unlike reflective children it tended not to be sensitive to situational demands or changes.

Using these findings, Meichenbaum and Goodman (1971) attempted to treat hyperactivity by changing the internal dialogues – private speech – of the children.

During training the therapist modelled skills which the child then learned. In relation to a problem-solving task he defined the problem linguistically. He drew attention to the relevant features of the task and guided his responses to these relevant features. He reinforced himself for successful completion of stages in each task. All of these are skills which the child was encouraged to learn. As the training sessions progressed, so the tasks increased in difficulty and the covert dialogue increased in complexity. These methods produced significant improvements in the children on a range of cognitive ability tests when compared with placebo treatment and no treatment control groups.

The promise of this basic research has been fulfilled both in the outcomes of training programmes and in the extension of the methods to more and more complex aspects of cognition. Mayers and Craighead (1984) noted a wealth of positive research work which concentrates on the remediation of problems in cognitive processes in children.

Some of the basic elements of SIT seem suitable for adaptation to people with a learning difficulty. The basic elements of overt control to covert control, with the therapist helping the individual to form and then internalize the dialogue is a very practical way to proceed. The emphasis on self-reinforcement to supplant self-doubt or self-criticism seems again to be a simple directive which may be appealing to those of us who work with such clients.

Lindsay (1986) reported a series of cases in which the results of social skills training in people with a mental handicap appear to be related to changes in cognitions rather than to changes in behaviour. While these case studies were uncontrolled, they illustrated the possible effects of poor self-image, lack of self-confidence and antagonism to others in the development of adaptive social responses.

Meichenbaum (1974, 1977) has written that performance difficulties and social anxieties can be maintained by the negative self-statements which people say to themselves before and during a sequence of interaction or behaviour. For example, if one of our clients is going into a social interaction with a thought 'I can't think of anything to say', this thought will prevent him or her from developing positive coping strategies in that situation. The techniques do not assume that people are aware of their self-statements. Indeed some people with a mental handicap may not even have formed the thoughts linguistically. Nevertheless they are part of a person's approach to the situation and if the therapist asks about them they can be elicited. In addition, positive coping self-statements can be used during therapy whether or not the patient has experienced them beforehand.

This summarized extract is taken from a group which was learning how to ask someone out. The problems arose in the group when one man (John) flatly refused to do this section of the programme, although he had been quite keen on the group up to that point. The conversation in the group went as follows:

Therapist: 'Come on John you can have a go now, it's your turn to ask Sandra if she wants to go out somewhere.'
John: 'No! no! I don't do things like that.'
Therapist: 'Everyone has tried, it is your shot.'
John: 'You shouldn't ask girls out.'
Therapist: 'It is all right here John, you can do it here.'
John: 'No, it's bad, you can't ask girls out.'

Although this extract is short, already several self-statements have been elicited which would prevent John from ever asking anyone to go out with him. If he approaches this situation with self-statements such as 'I don't do things like that', 'you shouldn't ask girls out', and 'it's bad to ask girls out', then the power of these self-statements will prevent him from using any conversation abilities that he might have. It was then possible to examine these self-statements in more detail to investigate the basis for the feelings about asking girls out.

Therapist: 'Why should you not ask girls out?'
John   'Oh, because you're never allowed to do that.'
Therapist: Opens the discussion to the group.
Therapist: 'Is it all right to ask girls out with you?'

Others:	'Yes you can ask if they want to go out for a cup of coffee.'
	'Yes you can take them into town.'
	'Aye, it's all right to take a girl out if she wants to go.'
Therapist:	'Yes, it is important she should want to go. If she wants to go out for a coffee is it all right to go?'
Others:	'Yes, you could take her out.'
	'I would like to go out.'
Therapist:	'You would like to go out with someone would you Sandra?'
Sandra:	'Yes, it's good to go out.'
Therapist:	'John, everyone says it's all right to ask someone out and Sandra wants to go out. What do you think?'
John:	'It can't be all right, well it must be.'

By his non-verbal appearance John was clearly influenced by the others' attitudes. He was obviously beginning to wonder about the realistic basis for his self-statement. There followed 10 minutes of discussion on the propriety of asking a member of the opposite sex to go out with you. We also discussed appropriate places to go and which places would be easily afforded and which would be expensive. Towards the end of the discussion the therapist asked John whether or not he would be able to substitute a positive self-statement for a negative self-statement. Here the therapist attempted to challenge John's negative self-statements. He might have done so directly but instead opened the discussion to the group to gain opinions, which might challenge John's opinions.

Therapist:	'Can you say "it's good to ask a girl out?".'
John:	'Oh I don't know, I don't know.'
Therapist:	'Try this; say "it's good to ask a girl out".'
John:	'Oh I don't know, I don't know.'
Therapist:	'Well say; "you can ask a girl out".'
John:	'Can ask a girl out.'
Therapist:	'Good! well done! Now try it again, say "I can ask a girl out".'
John:	'Well, em, I can ask a girl out.'
Therapist:	'Now that's good! Say it again silently to yourself.'
John:	'I can ask a girl out.'
Therapist:	'Good! Now say it into yourself silently.'

John silently repeats the self-statement four times.

| Therapist: | 'Good John, now say it again to yourself and then ask Sandra if she wants to go out with you.' |

John repeats this again to himself and proceeds with the roleplay, asking Sandra if she would like to go out with him for a coffee.

As can be seen in this extract the therapist has formalized the negative self-statement of 'I shouldn't ask girls out'. The analysis of the rational basis for the statement has not been done at a sophisticated level. The therapist merely asked the other group members how they felt about asking girls out or being asked out. The other group members then challenged the basis of John's statement by indicating that they felt it was perfectly in order to ask girls out. One member in the group said she would like to go out. Therefore, if the others thought it was all right, we were able to put it to John that his self-statement was at odds with the general opinion.

The second section of the extract was aimed at having John substitute an encouraging self-statement for the ones that were preventing him from entering into the social exchange. It is always best to substitute the simplest appropriate alternative and in this case it was the converse of his negative self-statements. Although he was somewhat reluctant to try a more positive cognition he had been persuaded by the previous discussion in the group. The important point was to use the discussion which had persuaded him and summarize it into a positive self-statement which could be used in future and which would remind him of our analysis of his approach to the interaction. Therefore the simple self-statement 'I can ask girls out' was used in this case.

The therapist might also have challenged the basis of John's thoughts directly. In the following extract taken from Lindsay and Kasprowicz (1987) the therapist challenges the negative self-statements 'I can't do this', 'this is terrible' and 'I feel bad' in a girl who was asked to talk about a recent trip she had taken.

Therapist: 'What do you think will happen to you?' [if you talk to us about your recent trip]
Margaret: 'I don't know.'
Therapist: 'Will anything happen?'
Margaret: 'I don't know.'
Therapist: 'Will you fall down?'
Margaret: 'No.'
Therapist: 'Will somebody scare you away?'
Margaret: 'No.' (Laughs.)
Therapist: 'Will somebody hit you when you talk to them?'
Margaret: 'No.' (Still laughing.)
Therapist: 'Will you sit on a seat and it will break?'
Margaret: 'No, don't be silly.' (Laughing.)
Therapist: 'Well what will happen?' (Laughing.)
Margaret: 'I don't know.' (Laughing.)
Therapist: 'Will anything happen?'
Margaret: 'No.'
Therapist: 'So nothing is going to happen.'
Margaret: 'No.'
Therapist: 'So why do you feel terrible if nothing will happen?'
Margaret: 'I don't know.'

At this point the therapist was trying to challenge Margaret's self-statements of feeling terrible with two results.

Firstly the context of self-statements was framed. Meichenbaum (1974) wrote that 'it is unlikely that clients actually actively talk to themselves prior to treatment'. In this case it is doubtful that Margaret would have said to herself, 'I feel terrible, I can't do this, I feel bad' before she went into the interaction. It may be that individual self-statements become enmeshed into their emotions and do not reach the level of conscious thought. It could also be that there is no thought or self-statement – people just feel bad and so do not engage in what is making them feel bad. However, the fact that mediated self-statements are possible means that they can either be inserted into the chain of responses if they are absent or changed to more adaptive self-statements if they are present in the sequence of responding. By challenging an individual's elicited self-statements the therapist can increase their importance to a level where the individual may be able to use them in therapy. At any rate the context and usefulness of self-statements was established.

A second result was that, from her non-verbal response, Margaret showed that she understood some of the irrational nature of herself-statements. The therapist outlined some examples of 'terrible' events which could happen. By her increasing laughter in response to the suggestions it can be inferred that Margaret realized that those things were highly unlikely. Therefore the basis of the bad feelings was being challenged and undermined. The therapist then went on to elicit from Margaret positive coping self-statements which she could use, and finally she went on with the interaction.

In this study Lindsay and Kasprowicz (1987) found that four out of five people in the group increased their assessed 'confidence' after training.

It is important to keep the self-statements as simple and as natural as possible. Therefore, statements which the clients or their friends would use frequently might be the most powerful pieces of private speech to insert into a dialogue. Marshall (1989) used self-instructional training to increase the ability of adults with learning difficulties to complete an abstract task. The self-reinforcement which was inserted into the dialogue was the statement 'I'm doing brilliant'. Clear, direct self-statements such as this produced improvements in the performance after training and at 6 weeks follow-up.

Conclusions

There is a great deal of clinical research, knowledge and activity in the area of cognitive behaviour therapy. Unfortunately, at the moment, only a small amount of this clinical research has reached the area of people with a mental handicap. Much of the basic research linking changes in self-statements and cognitions to improvements in skill and behaviour shows that the procedures can be fairly straightforward and easily understood. This would suggest that the methods of cognitive behaviour therapy would be suitable as a procedure to be used with people with a mental handicap.

Treatments for anxiety and phobia

Before reviewing treatment methods for anxiety in people with a mental handicap, we must recognize that it may be difficult to define anxiety in individuals who have limited or no language or communication. For people with a mild mental handicap there is less of a problem since anxiety would be defined in terms much the same as those employed for the general population (DSM III, American Psychiatric Association, 1980). However, where language and cognition become more impoverished and individuals are unable to explain their feelings or are less able to understand the concept of anxiety, phobia, etc., then most judgements will depend to a greater degree on appearance and behaviour. Therefore, often anxiety will be assumed in individuals who present clinically with chronic restlessness and agitation, poor attention span, low concentration, verbal outbursts such as shouting and making noises or pronounced tremor. People would appear to become agitated and worried if asked to sit still or undertake a task for any length of time. If approached by others then the individuals will appear to become agitated by the social contact and either walk away, or appear extremely uncomfortable while the conversation is continuing. However, many will be unable to tell us about their feelings.

Novosel (1984) studied 53 adults admitted to a mental handicap hospital over a 6-month period and found that 57.5% scored in a range of 'pathological severity' for phobias. He discovered a wide range of objects and situations that were feared by patients.

As people are relocated from institutional settings to smaller community residences they may experience some of the pressures which living in town puts on us all. Therefore, two effects may surface. Firstly, problems which have been masked by the relatively restricted environment of a hospital, will become more acute as individuals live in a less controlled environment. Secondly as they are put under the pressures of community living they will develop the kinds of problems which we all experience and so will become as prone as the general public to difficulties with anxiety and phobia. All of these points stress the need for treatment approaches for individuals who have a mental handicap and also suffer from anxiety related difficulties.

Abbreviated progressive relaxation (APR)

The majority of clinical studies investigating the effects of relaxation techniques on people with a mental handicap have employed derivatives of progressive relaxation training. Bernstein and Borkovec (1973) operationalized procedures and dealt with 16 major muscle groups covering the whole body. The subject's attention was focused on the muscle group and the therapist then asked him to tense it for a period of 5–7 s. The muscle group was then relaxed while the subject's attention was maintained on the muscle group. This may then be repeated before the procedure moves on to the next major muscle group. The subject's attention is constantly focused upon the feelings of tension and relaxation in the muscles. The client is also encouraged to practise these exercises between sessions at home.

APR and people with a mental handicap

Case studies using the techniques of APR have been reported with some success. One study by Steen and Zuriff (1977) is worth specific mention since it dealt with an extremely self-injurious woman with a profound mental handicap who had been kept in full restraint for 3 years. APR methods were used only with her arms and the techniques were simplified so that the woman was given only the instructions 'tighten up' and 'relax'. Physical help was given to enable her to tense and relax her muscles and she was also reinforced for successful tension/release cycles. 150 relaxation training sessions were given in all and following treatment the amount of self-injurious biting and scratching fell to very low levels. At 1-year follow-up staff reported that self-injurious behaviour was still low and she was no longer held in restraint.

Lindsay and Baty (1986a) investigated responses to APR in four individuals suffering from chronic anxiety and agitation. Three of the four subjects responded to treatment as assessed by behavioural and physiological measures. Analysis of individual response patterns suggested that it took subjects around five or six sessions to begin to understand the demands of training and respond to treatment. This would mean that group treatments which had less than six sessions may not allow sufficient time for subjects to respond. Furthermore they felt that the paradoxical aspect of APR, in that people are required to tense their muscles in order to relax, was confusing for individuals with a moderate or severe mental handicap. The subject who did not respond positively treated the whole procedure as an active game, becoming more rather than less excited and agitated. If these effects were to prove more general than this case, then any therapeutic effects on individuals would be masked in a group comparison by others who did not respond to treatment.

In a further study Lindsay and Baty (1989) conducted APR in a group format, comparing it with another relaxation technique. They found that these effects were exacerbated in that when individuals became excited in a group they influenced other members of the group, thus causing a general rise in agitation rather than a relaxation effect. There were, however, significant reductions in rated anxiety after 12 sessions of APR, showing that the techniques could be effective in a group format.

General effectiveness of APR

McPhail and Chamov (1989) compared a group of six subjects who received 12 sessions of APR (four sessions per week over 3 weeks) with a control group who were in a story telling control condition. The subjects' disabilities were reported to range from profound mental handicap to mild mental handicap. They were chosen because they regularly showed disruptive behaviour in their work or activity groups and as well as being assessed for immediate relaxation effects, they were also rated on 17 categories of disruptive behaviour. Disruptive behaviour was assessed the day after training and at 12 weeks follow-up. The results showed a 'significant and substantial' reduction in disruptive behaviour in the subjects' receiving APR. There were no changes in the control condition. The authors felt that 'the effects of daily training ... were immediate and also cumulative'. However, at 12-week follow-up disruptive behaviour had returned to baseline levels.

Lindsay, Richardson and Michie (1989) also studied the generalized effects of APR. Measures were taken of agitated movement, agitated speech and general anxiety 1 hour after the completion of each of 12 treatment sessions and at 3-week follow-up. Subjects receiving APR showed a gradual reduction in measures indicating the generalized effects of relaxation training and although they did not reduce as quickly as other conditions APR eventually proved as effective as other techniques in terms of these generalized results.

Conclusions

There is now some evidence that a modified and simplified version of APR may be effective with people who have a mental handicap. It is certainly the case that the procedures are effective with individuals who have a mild mental handicap. Recent studies have shown that the techniques may also be effective with individuals who have a moderate or severe mental handicap.

One consequence of becoming a widely accepted technique is that inevitably the methods have become diluted by familiarity. I have often heard it said that so many people use APR in such a casual fashion that the treatment may fall into disrepute through lack of clinical effectiveness. Certainly in my own clinics individuals have said to me after I have suggested the use of relaxation techniques, that someone gave them 'a tape' in the past and it did not work. APR is a technique which should be woven into the person's lifestyle and tied to other procedures such as cue control and constructive tasks (see below). This is not a plea for elitism but for therapists conducting APR to be careful and thorough in their application of procedures.

Behavioural relaxation training

Because of difficulties in using APR with some subjects, Lindsay and Baty (1986b) explored the use of behaviour relaxation training (BRT). This is a technique developed by Schilling and Poppen (1983) when they found APR to be ineffective with learning disabled boys. BRT differs from APR in that it does not require subjects to tense their muscles, or perceive and understand the difference between tense muscles and relaxed muscles. Therefore it is a conceptually simpler, technique. The therapist models relaxed and unrelaxed behaviours in each of the major muscle groups (muscles groups are the same as in APR) and then asks the client to imitate the relaxed position. Verbal prompts and manual guidance are used as needed, and a great deal of prompting will be used in the initial stages of treatment. Schilling and Poppen found that BRT produced larger and more rapid changes in observed relaxation than control conditions. Lindsay and Baty (1986b) reported the effectiveness of BRT on four individuals with a severe mental handicap.

Lindsay and Baty (1989) found BRT to be effective when administered in a group format and to produce significantly greater reductions in observed anxiety than APR. In addition it did not have any of the previously mentioned drawbacks of APR, in that subjects did not misconstrue the demands of training and there was no misunderstanding that the purpose of group was an exciting game. Lindsay, Richardson and Michie (1989) found BRT to produce significant generalized reductions in agitation and anxiety more quickly than APR, although there was no difference between the conditions by the end of treatment.

Lindsay et al. (1989) compared BRT and APR in group and individual formats against a no-treatment control with subjects who had a moderate and severe mental handicap. Measures were taken before treatment, midway through the treatment course, after treatment and at a short 3-day follow-up. Subjects received 12 sessions of treatment at a rate of four per week. They were assessed using a behavioural rating scale and pulse rate. It was found that there were improvements on the behavioural rating scale for all conditions when compared with the control group but that the BRT conditions produced significantly greater reductions in rated anxiety than the APR conditions. There were no differences between the groups on pulse rate.

BRT seems to be a promising treatment approach with individuals who have a moderate and severe mental handicap. It does not appear to have the drawbacks inherent in APR. Because it is an essentially passive technique whereby people simply model relaxed responses, there is no paradoxical element where clients are expected to tense their muscles in order to relax. There appears to be no side-effect whereby clients might misconstrue the demands of training and become more rather than less excited.

Cue controlled relaxation

Cue controlled relaxation (CCR) is not really a technique by itself. It is an adjunct to any technique that is being used and although it has usually been used with APR, it is not included in the section on APR because it can be linked to any form of relaxation procedure. The essential aspect is that the relaxation effects are linked to a cue word so that eventually the subject will be able to relax to the cue word only, rather than a time-consuming relaxation procedure. This would have obvious advantages in terms of saving the therapist time and effort.

One of the best controlled case studies in the field was conducted on a young woman functioning in the borderline range of intelligence (IQ = 71) and who suffered from frequent psychomotor seizures (Wells *et al.*, 1978). Using a reversal design they established a functional relationship between CCR (linked to APR) and psychomotor seizures. The subject was instructed to vocalize the cue word covertly at the onset of each pre-seizure aura and this reduced the frequency of seizures. When she stopped using the cue word during an experimental reversal phase, the seizure frequency increased to baseline levels. The reinstatement of CCR procedures reduced seizures once again. Improvements were maintained at 3-month follow-up.

In most studies the word 'relax' was used as a cue word linked with the relaxation procedure. The word itself matters little, as this anecdote will illustrate. My colleague and I were treating a boy with a profound mental handicap who suffered from asthmatic attacks. When he had these asthmatic attacks he was treated with Ventolin and oxygen and the words 'Ventolin' and 'oxygen' would commonly be used as he was calming down from his asthmatic attack. Since these attacks were fairly frequent the words were used often. It became apparent that he began to use the words as a cue for calming down and ward staff would use the words 'Ventolin' and 'oxygen' in the absence of the treatment to calm him when he became excited. Indeed the important semantic nature of the cue word is that it may be understood by the client and that if others were to become involved in treatment (e.g. families, care staff, friends, etc.) then they feel comfortable using this cue.

Lindsay *et al.* (1988) used CCR linked to BRT with three men who had severe mental handicap and little language. They chose the words 'quiet and still' as cue words since they seemed more easily understood by the clients. They found that the men showed a quick, positive response to BRT and that the effects transferred to a cue word. This could then be used by ward staff and strangers to induce relaxation in the clients without using the BRT procedures.

Although relatively untested in people with a mental handicap, these case studies suggest that clients seem to respond to CCR. It is a helpful addition to treatment since it allows clients to relax quickly without having to proceed through a complete course of relaxation lasting up to an hour. Given that they may become calm relatively quickly it may allow the rest of the time to be spent in more adaptive and constructive pursuits (see below).

Biofeedback techniques

One of the earliest reports of the use of biofeedback with people who have a severe mental handicap was by Schroeder *et al.* (1977). They used EMG feedback and reinforcement to produce large reductions in self-injurious behaviour in two young men with severe mental handicap. There were also reductions in mean EMG amplitude. However, it is unsure whether or not the EMG feedback or the reinforcement techniques or both were producing the reductions in symptoms.

Calamari, Geist and Shahbazian (1987) found that a combined relaxation procedure was effective in relaxing subjects who had a range of intellectual deficits.

In this study the assessment and treatment measures were well described and improvements were seen in both physiological and behavioural measures. The combined relaxation treatment included auditory EMG biofeedback, APR, modelling and positive reinforcement procedures. Unfortunately the authors do not separate out treatment procedures and we cannot tell the relative effectiveness of each component. Therefore biofeedback procedures, although extremely poorly researched in the population, have been included in a well-designed study testing a package of treatment which was found to be effective in reducing anxiety in people with a mental handicap.

In vivo and exposure methods

One of the most common methods of anxiety reduction in relation to phobic symptoms is *in vivo* exposure. Marks (1981) has written that it is probably the treatment of choice for such problems, and recently Marks and O'Sullivan (1988) noted that effects maintain to long-lasting follow-up assessments and it is cost effective when compared with drug treatment.

The main feature of these treatments is that the client is exposed to real fearful situations under therapeutic conditions. Often these conditions will be graded so that the client does not meet an exceptionally fearful setting early on in the programme. Rather they would be introduced to a moderately threatening situation so that they could learn to become more comfortable with this before they progress to more anxiety provoking aspects.

There are several therapeutic elements contained in the procedure of exposure treatments. Most obviously the client is being confronted by situations of which they are phobic and so are being given opportunities, under therapeutic control, to control their anxiety and deal with it. Secondly the situations are graded so that the client does not habituate any improvements to one aspect. Rather, the threatening aspects of the phobic setting become greater as the client copes with each stage in the hierarchy. Thirdly, the client is learning from a very early stage in treatment how to cope with their own feelings of anxiety.

Luiselli (1978) treated fear of travelling in the school bus in a 7-year-old autistic boy. He involved the boy's mother in graded exposure to using the bus. He began simply with having him sit on the bus and worked up towards having him go to and from school by himself. Improvements had maintained at 1-year follow-up.

Lindsay *et al.* (1988) used *in vivo* exposure to treat fear of dogs in two women with a mild and moderate mental handicap. They reviewed some of the elements in exposure treatments, although the relative importance of these methods remains to be tested. The treatment components were as follows:

1. *Increased contact with the feared situation* – Increased contact is basic to treatment and from the very beginning clients are introduced to the feared situation under therapeutic conditions.
2. *Changing stimuli* – Attempts are made to ensure that subjects do not simply become familiar with one aspect or situation. Therefore the situation should be changed as regularly as possible. In this study seven different dogs were used, reducing the possibility of habituation to any one dog.
3. *Eliciting anxiety* – In an exposure treatment one of the main objects is to elicit anxiety in subjects so that they can immediately begin to develop strategies for

coping with the feared situation. While subjects are given help to develop various ways of coping with the phobic stimulus through approaching the situation and gaining some control over the situation, opportunities are presented throughout treatment for them to develop their own coping strategies. This is done by encouraging individuals to become more comfortable with aspects they find anxiety provoking. For example, one subject disliked small brown dogs, while another was more frightened of movement. Therefore they were introduced to those aspects of the stimulus and given a great deal of encouragement and praise for coping with their anxiety.

4. *Graded exposure* – The therapy sessions begin with a scenario which is moderately anxiety provoking, for example, in the case of dog phobia the dogs might be brought into the room but for the first 20 minutes are kept at the other side of the room away from the subjects. As they become more comfortable with this first situation the dog might be led closer to the subjects. In this way subjects are encouraged to learn how to cope with their anxiety in relation to the close proximity of the feared stimulus. As the session progressed and the dogs became increasingly close to the subjects, their anxiety would rise and fall as they perceived increased threat which would then subside. Towards the end of the first few sessions the therapist removed the dog to its original position at the other side of the room. Subjects' anxiety reduced markedly so that they now felt quite comfortable in a situation which 90 minutes previously they had found extremely anxiety provoking. The session ended with a relatively low level of anxiety.

5. *Modelling* – During each session the therapist would model non-anxious responses to the clients in relation to the feared situation. He or she would be in contact with the dog, giving it orders, walking it, moving it and in other ways showing control over the dog.

6. *Control over the feared situation* – This is an important part of anxiety management and becomes a more common technique as treatment progresses with each subject. It is linked to the behavioural test in the paper by Lindsay *et al.* (1989) in that all of the items on the behavioural test require a degree of control on the part of the subject over the dog. Subjects were encouraged with increasing frequency to give the dog orders, take the dog's lead, make it perform simple behaviours such as walking and sitting. In this way subjects developed feelings of control over the feared situation and also increased their interactions with the dogs.

7. *Generalization* – Generalization sessions were conducted after three sessions in the treatment room. During these sessions subjects went out to situations where they would be more likely to meet the threatening stimulus, in this case, strange dogs. They were then introduced to a new dog and encouraged to cope with this new situation using all the methods outlined above.

8. *Relaxation* – Where subjects are particularly anxious about sessions beginning or are reluctant to come to treatment sessions (especially at the beginning of the programme) relaxation exercises are used. [These have been outlined above.]

We are now in a position to recommend the use of graded exposure for the treatment of phobic anxiety in people with a mental handicap. Group and individual studies ranging over several different presenting problems have reported successful outcomes in at least the short term. However, we have established only that treatment may work and there remains a pressing need to investigate the important aspects of treatment and the durability of improvements in the client group. There remains a lack of comparative research looking at the effectiveness of the range of alternatives to *in vivo* exposure and the relative importance of each component of a complex treatment programme. We are also ignorant of which personal aspects change towards the phobic situation – the cognitive aspects, the behavioural aspects and the physiological aspects. There is some reason to feel that the nature of phobia in the client group may be different from other populations. The blind panic observed in mentally handicapped individuals is very rarely observed in adult out-patients. It may be that a person with a mental handicap finds it more difficult to control his or her fear rationally in the way a non-mentally handicapped person does. The individual of normal intelligence is influenced by the social restraints of the situation, the physical restraints of the situation and his or her own verbal mediation. It may be that a person with a mental handicap does not have the same ability to attend to these internal and social factors.

Therefore the person who is phobic of escalators may run away, make a tremendous fuss or actually try to jump over the side and off a moving escalator without any thought of the danger of jumping off the escalator, no thought of the social embarrassment they may cause themselves by making a scene in a busy shopping centre and no internal dialogue indicating that these other considerations may be important. The only thought is that they have to get away from the escalator. Given these considerations it may be that treatments designed for individuals who do not have a mental handicap cannot be transferred automatically to people with a mental handicap, but may require some modification.

Conclusions

Some previous authors have been somewhat pessimistic as regards the treatment of anxiety in people with a mental handicap. However, Calamari, Geist and Shahbazian (1987) concluded that their results 'call into question the sometimes held assumption that developmentally disabled persons are not good candidates for psychological treatments involving techniques other than simple behavioural management procedures'. Most recent studies reported here have shown very positive responses to anxiety management training and relaxation procedures.

Finally, there may be ethical considerations in the use of relaxation treatment related to the original problems in definition. While it is beneficial for someone who is extremely worried, anxious and nervous to achieve a measure of relaxation, it is not always possible to establish that such problems are there or that such relaxation processes are occurring. People who have a severe mental handicap find it difficult to report the concepts of anxiety or discuss their feelings and thoughts related to anxiety.

In this way relaxation training could be used as a simple management technique to keep certain individuals quiet and undemanding. Therefore, serious considera-tion should be made when embarking on a programme of relaxation training to whether or not it should be used in conjunction with another programme. This programme might be one to encourage people to engage in more educational or stimulatory activities. It might be included in a programme to help people overcome their fears or phobias. It could be used to help certain individuals become more accessible to their social environment so that they become more easy to talk to and to socialize with. It could also be used to decrease self-injurious or challenging behaviour so that these individuals might become more accessible to other events in their lives. Thus relaxation training would always be used as an enabling technique to allow individuals to access other activities or social opportunities.

The management and treatment of anger

Often problems in anger and aggression are managed rather than treated. By this it is meant that outside agencies impose control on the individual experiencing anger by using restraint; drug therapy or seclusion. This is distinct from treatment where the individual himself or herself is given some means whereby they can control their own anger.

Two initial problems must be addressed when considering the treatment of anger in people with a mental handicap. The first, noted by several authors, is that clients have far less opportunity to control their own anger than other sections of the population. Many clients have been brought up in restricted and indeed restrictive hospital or home environments. Controls are often imposed on their anger and aggression throughout life and this will clearly affect the person's ability to learn how to impose controls upon themselves. Alternatively stimuli which might make the person angry may have been removed through childhood in a protective environment, thus denying the individual opportunities to learn how their own anger works. Therefore they may not have developed coping strategies or ways of managing their anger which other people in the community have learned. As a result, they may have few mechanisms for dealing with the normal frustrations which various living situations cause. This may be more acute when clients are expected to live in the community with the usual pressures that community living exerts.

A second problem concerns the ability of people with a mental handicap to recognize emotion and anger in themselves or others. Gray, Fraser and Leuder (1983) studied two groups of 13 subjects, one with moderate–mild mental handicaps and one with severe–moderate mental handicaps. The subjects looked at six standard photographs representing joy, sadness, anger, fear, surprise and disgust and were told a short story about each. All subjects in the study were less accurate in their perception than non-handicapped people and number of errors correlated with intelligence in that fewer errors were made by the less mentally handicapped individuals. However, the authors looked at the pattern of results in more detail and found simple, pleasant/unpleasant dimensions were recognized by subjects as well as non-handicapped people. As the emotion became more intense the subjects' recognition became poorer and it was particularly poor with anger and fear. Although this is only one study, it was well controlled, and would suggest that the recognition of anger is of special difficulty for people with a mental handicap.

If the client is unable to recognize anger in themselves it may be more difficult to treat. Alternatively if they mislabel other emotions for anger, the result could be a higher incidence of aggressive or withdrawal problems than would be the case if the emotion were labelled correctly.

Anger management training

The treatments for anger-related problems fall into two main categories – self-control procedures which rely on the individual using various cognitive strategies to recognize and control the onset of anger and its consequences; and treatments which employ relaxation as a counter-conditioning measure incompatible with anger.

Novaco (1975) has been one of the most influential writers in the promotion of cognitive self-control procedures for anger. He assumes that the way in which people view their circumstances determines how they will feel. The way we appraise the situation determines whether we are likely to become angry. The thoughts and intentions we attribute to others will affect our anger, as will the self-statements we make to ourselves concerning a situation. These cognitions will affect our arousal and subsequent anger and actions resulting from the anger. In this chapter we have already reviewed the way in which self-statements can affect emotion and performance.

Corresponding to Novaco's views on the development of anger, treatment approaches emphasize cognition, expectations and appraisal of situations. Treatment falls into three stages: firstly the client is taught about the various forms and functions of anger and its behavioural consequences. He emphasizes the individual nature of anger, with personal triggers for anger responses. He also reviews the way in which behavioural consequences of anger can escalate or be exacerbated by a vicious circle of cognition, leading to arousal, leading to behaviour, leading to further cognition, greater arousal and so on.

In the second stage he reviews ways of dealing with cognition and feelings associated with anger. During this phase subjects would roleplay various situations to practise the analysis and alteration of self-statements through self-instructional training and cognitive restructuring. Social skills training would also be employed to teach individuals how to be more appropriately assertive, and in greater control of the behavioural consequences of their anger. During these two stages the client practises exercises in recognition and control of anger.

The final stage is more personal with clients reviewing their own 'anger triggers', practising the recognition of the onset of anger and coping with it once they are feeling the emotion. Towards the end of this stage the client is confronted with the real threatening environment which he or she has previously found anger provoking.

The other approach, employing relaxation treatments, has also been used either on its own or in combination with cognitive techniques. This approach would use regular relaxation exercises (see earlier sections of this chapter) on the assumption that relaxation is incompatible with the response of anger. The person may also be taught cue controlled relaxation so that when they feel the onset of anger they can use the cue words to induce the incompatible relaxation response. Several studies have used this in conjunction with the above methods of cognitive restructuring in an attempt to achieve enhanced treatment results.

Benson et al. (1986) investigated the effects of anger management training with 54 mildly or moderately handicapped adults. They compared four groups employing different aspects of the treatment. The self-instructional training group was taught the difference between positive coping self-statements and negative 'trouble' self-statements. They then practised these during roleplays. A relaxation group was taught abbreviated progressive relaxation and then practised it during unprovoking roleplays. A problem solving condition was taught to analyse and solve anger situations as problems during roleplay. Finally an anger management condition combined all three interventions. Self-report measures and responses to anger evoking roleplays found that anger management training was effective with the subject population. However, there were few differences between the groups and it is a methodological flaw that there was not a no-treatment condition.

Webster and Azrin (1973) used relaxation training and a mild punishment procedure to reduce disruptive behaviour in subjects with a mental handicap and a mental illness. The relaxation was a regular procedure and following a disruptive outburst subjects were required to put on night clothing and lie in bed for two hours. These measures were extremely effective in reducing disruptive behaviour although the relative contributions of relaxation and the reinforcement contingencies are not clear.

Lindsay (1988) reported the reduction of anger and aggressive outbursts in a man with severe mental handicap who displayed constant debilitating obsessive compulsive rituals. The rituals were treated using a response prevention treatment but during this treatment the individual became extremely aggressive. This was successfully treated using cue controlled behavioural relaxation training. In another case study Lindsay (1990) used abbreviated progressive relaxation to treat the aggressive outbursts and self-injurious behaviour of a man with mild mental handicap. The treatment was extremely successful and it was felt that APR was a more useful technique because it is an active rather than passive relaxation approach (see earlier in this chapter on the differences between abbreviated progressive relaxation and behavioural relaxation training). Because the treatment is active it gave the subject something to do when he began to feel aggressive, and this activity was also incompatible with anger.

There is some evidence then, that anger and its behavioural consequences can be controlled in people with a mental handicap using psychological treatments. However, the research literature is extremely sparse and only tentative conclusions can be reached. All we are able to say at the moment is that two main approaches, self-instructional training and relaxation techniques, may both be effective either alone or in combination with the subject group. We know nothing about which conditions may favour either treatment or which aspects of the treatment are particularly effective.

References

American Psychiatric Association (1980) *Diagnostic and Statistical Manual of Mental Disorders*, 3rd edn, American Psychiatric Association, Washington, DC

Benson, B.A., Rice, C.J. and Miranti, S.V. (1986) Effects of anger management training with mentally retarded adults in group treatment. *Journal of Consulting and Clinical Psychology*, **54**, 728–729

Bernstein, D.A. and Borkovec, T.D. (1973) *Progressive Relaxation Training*, Research Press, Illinois

Calamari, J.E., Geist, G.O. and Shahbazian, M.J. (1987) Evaluation of multiple component relaxation training with developmentally disabled persons. *Research in Developmental Abilities*, **8**, 55–70

Fransella, F. and Bannister, D. (1977) *A Manual of Repertory Grid Techniques*, Academic Press, New York

Gowans, F. and Hulbert, C. (1983) Self-concept assessment of mentally handicapped adults: a review. *Mental Handicap*, **11**, 121–123

Gray, J.M., Fraser, W.L. and Leuder, I. (1983) Recognition of emotion from facial expression in mental handicap. *British Journal of Psychiatry*, **142**, 556–571

Helsel, W.J. and Matson, J.L. (1988) The relationship of depression to social skills and intellectual functioning in mentally retarded adults. *Journal of Mental Deficiency Research*, **32**, 411–418

Kazdin, A.E., Matson, J.L. and Senatore, V. (1983) Assessment of depression in mentally retarded adults. *American Journal of Psychiatry*, **140**, 1040–1043

Lindsay, W.R. (1986) Cognitive changes after social skills training with young mildly mentally handicapped adults. *Journal of Mental Deficiency Research*, **30**, 81–88

Lindsay, W.R. (1988) Relaxation treatment to help an extremely obsessional and aggressive man. Paper presented to *The Annual Conference of The British Institute of Mental Handicap*

Lindsay, W.R. (1990) Using abbreviated progressive relaxation for the self-control of aggressive outbursts in man with a mild mental handicap. (Unpublished observations)

Lindsay, W.R. and Baty, F.J. (1986a) Abbreviated progressive relaxation: its use with adults who are mentally handicapped. *Mental Handicap*, **14**, 123–126

Lindsay, W.R. and Baty, F.J. (1986b) Behavioural relaxation training: explorations with adults who are mentally handicapped. *Mental Handicap*, **14**, 160–162

Lindsay, W.R. and Baty, F.J. (1989) Group relaxation training with adults who are mentally handicapped. *Behavioural Psychotherapy*, **17**, 43–51

Lindsay, W.R. and Kasprowicz, M. (1987) Challenging negative cognitions: developing confidence in adults by means of cognitive behaviour therapy. *Mental Handicap*, **15**, 159–162

Lindsay, W.R. and Michie, A.M. (1988) Adaptation of the Zung Self-Rating Anxiety Scale for people with a mental handicap. *Journal of Mental Deficiency Research*, **32**, 485–490

Lindsay, W.R., Fee, M., Michie, A.M. and Baty, F.J. (1988) The effects of cue controlled relaxation on adults with a severe mental handicap. Paper presented to the *IASSMD World Congress in Mental Handicap, Dublin.*

Lindsay, W.R., Michie, A.M., Baty, F.J. and McKenzie, K. (1988) Dog phobia in people with mental handicaps: anxiety management training and exposure treatments. *Mental Handicap Research*, **1**, 39–48

Lindsay, W.R., Baty, F.J., Michie, A.M. and Richardson, I. (1989) A comparison of anxiety treatments with adults who have moderate and severe mental retardation. *Research and Developmental Disabilities*, **10**, 129–140

Lindsay, W.R., Richardson, I. and Michie, A.M. (1989) Short-term generalised effects of relaxation training on adults with moderate and severe mental handicaps. *Mental Handicap Research*, **2**, 197–206

Luiselli, J.K. (1978) Treatment of an autistic child's fear of riding a school bus through exposure and reinforcement. *Journal of Behaviour Therapy and Experimental Psychiatry*, **9**, 1969–1972

McPhail, C.H. and Chamov, A.S. (1989) Relaxation reduces disruption in mentally handicapped adults. *Journal of Mental Deficiency Research*, **33**, 399–406

Marks, I.M. (1981) *Cure and Care of Neurosis: Theory and Practice of Behavioural Psychotherapy*, Wiley, New York

Marks, I.M. and O'Sullivan, G. (1988) Drugs and psychological treatments for agoraphobia, panic and obsessive-compulsive disorders: a review. *British Journal of Psychiatry*, **153**, 650–658

Marshall, S. (1989) A comparison of self-instruction training and modelling in the acquisition of an abstract task. Paper presented to *The Annual Conference of The British Psychological Society, St. Andrews.*

Mayers, A. and Craighead, E. (1984) *Cognitive Behaviour Therapy with Children*, Plenum, New York

Meichenbaum, D. (1974) *Therapist Manual for Cognitive Behaviour Modification*, Unpublished manuscript, University of Waterloo, Waterloo, Ontario

Meichenbaum, D. (1977) *Cognitive Behaviour Modification: an Integrative Approach*, Plenum, New York

Meichenbaum, D. and Goodman, J. (1971) Training impulsive children to talk to themselves: a means of developing self-control. *Journal of Abnormal Psychology*, **77**, 115–126

Michie, A.M. and Lindsay, W.R. (1988) Issues in the assessment of cognition in people with a mental handicap. Paper presented to *The British Psychological Society Annual Conference, Leeds*

Novaco, R.W. (1975) *Anger Control: the Development and Evaluation of an Experimental Treatment.* Heath, Lexington, Massachusetts

Novosel, S. (1984) Psychiatric disorder in adults admitted to a hospital for the mentally handicapped. *British Journal of Mental Subnormality*, **30**, 54–58

Oliver, C. (1986) Self-concept assessment: a case study. *Mental Handicap*, **14**, 24–26

Schilling, D. and Poppen, R. (1983) Behavioural relaxation training and assessment. *Journal of Behaviour Therapy and Experimental Psychiatry*, **14**, 99–107

Schroeder, S.R., Peterson, C.R., Solomon, L.J. and Artley, J.J. (1977) E.M.G. feedback and the contingent restraint of self-injurious behaviour among the severely retarded: two case illustrations. *Behaviour Therapy*, **8**, 738–741

Steen, P.L. and Zuriff, G.E. (1977) The use of relaxation in the treatment of self-injurious behaviour. *Journal of Behaviour Therapy and Experimental Psychiatry*, **8**, 447–448

Webster, D.R. and Azrin, N.H. (1973) Required relaxation: a method of inhibiting agitative, disruptive behaviour of retardates. *Behaviour Research and Therapy*, **11**, 67–78

Wells, K.C., Turner, S.M., Bellack, A.S. and Hersen, M. (1978) Effects of cue controlled relaxation on psychomotor seizures: an experimental analysis. *Behaviour Research and Therapy*, **16**, 51–53

Zung, W.K. (1965) A self-rating depression scale. *Archives of General Psychiatry*, **12**, 63–70

Zung, W.K. (1971) A rating instrument for anxiety disorders. *Psychosomatics*, **12**, 371–379

14

Parents – problems and perspectives

Peter Baker

To a certain extent the relationship between parents and professionals has been somewhat uneasy. Parents may be seen by professionals as demanding, unrealistic and interfering, professionals in turn may be seen as uncaring, elusive and disorganized. Cunningham and Davis (1985) in the description of parents outpourings described three basic categories of complaint:

1. Poor information and guidance.
2. Poor organization.
3. Unsuitable personality characteristics in professionals.

These criticisms can be easily dismissed if we assume that the anger is part of a pathological process that necessarily accompanies the existence of a handicapped member within the family. However, on many occasions such criticism is justified and the parent does not need a therapy oriented approach to deal with this assumed pathology, but rather needs pragmatic help through a more efficient service.

Professionals working with handicapped children cannot fail to note the difficulties and stress caused by the unquestionable burden of the presence of a handicapped child in the family. Several parents have written graphic and moving accounts of their experiences (Boston, 1981; Wonnacott, 1981; Hannam, 1988); these describe in detail the toll taken on parents. 'The daily grind' is a term that arises frequently in the literature in this area and for many sums up their experiences. It is easy to concentrate on this negative side and ignore the fact that many parents cope very well and receive immense enjoyment and fulfilment. Boston (1981) described her reaction to a booklet from the Down Children Association.

> 'It was a great release to me to read the booklet and the training schedules. At last I had something that didn't approach the fact of having a mentally handicapped child as a *tragedy* but as a *reality of life*; a problem, but one which could be better faced with the support of others. It was also seen as a problem which could be, at least partially, solved.'
> (Italics not the authors)

Breaking the news

Individual reports, written accounts and several studies show a great deal of dissatisfaction from a large number of parents about the way in which they were informed about the diagnosis of mental handicap in their child (e.g. Gayton and Walker, 1974; Cunningham and Sloper, 1977; Hannam, 1988). One mother with her child then in her teens, recalled:

'The first we knew that Sarah had Down's syndrome was when a student nurse came in to make the bed the morning after Sarah was born. She started telling me with the best possible intentions, that her brother had Down's syndrome. The implications of what she was saying dawned on me. I felt numb as if I wasn't really there.'

It is likely that the assumption that there is not a way of breaking this sort of bad news and leaving the parents satisfied has led to the perpetuation of bad practice. However, there is now evidence that the high levels of dissatisfaction with this process are not inevitable and there are guidelines for good practice (Cunningham et al., 1984).

Guidelines for the disclosure of diagnosis

1. Parents should be told as soon as possible.
2. Parents should be told together.
3. The child should be present. This conveys the message that it is thought that the baby is valuable.
4. The discussion should be private.
5. The news giver should be a well-informed person, for example the paediatrician concerned.
6. The news giver should explain the facts as simply as possible and be wary of influencing decision making.
7. A subsequent interview should be arranged so that the parents can ask questions and seek practical advice.
8. Follow-up should be arranged at home with a keyworker, usually a health visitor, general practitioner or social worker who can offer continuing support, practical information and advice.

The impact the news has on the parents

The disclosure of the diagnosis of mental handicap will destroy most, if not all, of the expectancies built up about the child. As human beings we naturally need expectancies about the future, albeit with a range of options. When these are destroyed we will immediately seek to construct a new set of expectancies. It is these that are readjusted in the 'process of readjustment'.

Cunningham and Davis (1985) have modified McKeith's (1973) suggestion of a system of classification of common feelings experienced by parents.

Biological reactions

These are fundamental to most people and hence are common to professionals and parents. These will include feelings of protectiveness toward a vulnerable newborn. In the case of handicap this can become over-protectiveness with an increased sensitivity to any implied suggestion of criticism or negativism toward the child. Conversely the protection might extend toward the existing family and result in the rejection of the newborn.

Resentment and revulsion are common feelings toward the abnormality. Many parents may oscillate between these feelings and the apparently conflicting feelings of protectiveness.

Feelings of inadequacy

Serious doubts regarding parents reproductive adequacy can arise, often affecting sexual relationships. There is a fundamental desire in human beings to see their children as an extension of themselves. Their offspring in some way blemished is in a way seen as a blemish on themselves. These feelings of a reproductive inadequacy may affect many other members of the family. Rifts may occur with arguments regarding whose side of the family the handicap is on. Siblings may also be affected with fears about their own reproductive adequacy.

The arrival of a child who is different and who, it would be anticipated, will require specialist skills in rearing, may cast serious self-doubt about the ability to cope. The severity of the child's handicap may well be equated with the degree of difference required from normal child-rearing practices. The more severe the handicap the more specialized the rearing skills and requirements.

Feelings of embarrassment

When parents are forced to 'go public' with their child, they may come across reactions in other people that will only serve to compound their own sense of embarrassment. They may find avoidance in friends and neighbours. Similar reactions may be found in siblings, the other parent and grandparents. Avoidance of prolonged discussion regarding the child may well be experienced from professionals in the paediatric service.

This embarrassment from others communicates to the parents that they have done something wrong. Reaction to this might be to adopt stances of defiance, curtness or even to become apologetic.

Feelings of guilt

These might be related to the embarrassment and feelings of inadequacy. Ideas may surface surrounding blame for the handicap occurring, mothers especially might worry about anything they may have done during pregnancy that might have caused the handicap to occur. For example, smoking, drinking, working too hard, etc. However, it is more likely if these feelings are present that they are related to the belief in the parents that they are not doing enough to help their child, or the other children in the family are suffering. Guilt is usually related to the perception of what has been required in terms of rearing and the related perception of the adequacy of the efforts made.

Feelings of fear

The sudden destruction of expectancies leads to the introduction of many uncertainties. These uncertainties generate fear of what the future might hold for their child. With a sick child with a poor life expectancy parents may be afraid to develop an attachment. They may also be frightened of the power of their own feelings. These emotions may be alien to them, such as feelings of rejection towards the child, bitterness and anger toward others.

Feelings of bereavement
The loss of the 'hoped for child' is often compared to the process of bereavement. This model has proven to be useful to some parents to understand their own reactions. However, its wholesale adoption by professionals has served to perpetuate the ideas of inevitable pathology. It has also encouraged a tendency to dismiss any criticism as part of the anger, denial or guilt stage, whichever is the most convenient explanation.

'Early parent counselling'

The emotional impact of the arrival of a handicapped child is clearly considerable. A period of readjustment will have to occur and this can be aided by appropriate counselling. This is not as Cunningham and Davis (1985) point out the sort of approach required for the minority of parents who suffer severe disruption and depression when given the news of diagnosis. Counselling for the majority of parents should not be viewed as the treatment of a pathology. Rather their reactions should be seen as normal and healthy and they should be given active skilled help. One such scheme is described by Hornby *et al.* (1987) where parents, who themselves have a child with a mental handicap, are given training to support other parents.

Cunningham's (1979) model of psychic crisis at disclosure of handicap is perhaps the most well known and accepted model of adjustment (Figure 14.1).

Although this is essentially a stage model its use is to guide counsellors and should not be imposed on the parents. Many parents will not display all the stages and some might oscillate between phases at different times and in different contents.

Life after diagnosis

A danger inherent in using a bereavement/stages model is the assumption that after all the turmoil in the period immediately following diagnosis, acceptance takes place. This acceptance is characterized by an adjustment to life without undue stress. This is clearly not the case. In studies addressing the family's experience of having a member with a mental handicap there appears to be a consensus that parents, mostly mothers, of children with a mental handicap continue to experience high levels of stress (e.g., Bradshaw and Lawton, 1978; Byrden, 1980; Beckman, 1983; Baker, 1987). Searle (1978) in a description of her experience as a parent called for professionals to discard their ideas of stages and progress and begin to understand the deep lasting changes that life with a child who has a mental handicap brings. She explained that the shock, the guilt and the bitterness never disappear but stay on as a part of the parent's emotional life.

Wikler (1981) categorized potentially stressful experience into two kinds:

1. Those stresses that continue over the lifetime of their child. These she called chronic stresses.
2. Those periodic potential crises, that occur over time in the life cycle of the family and the child.

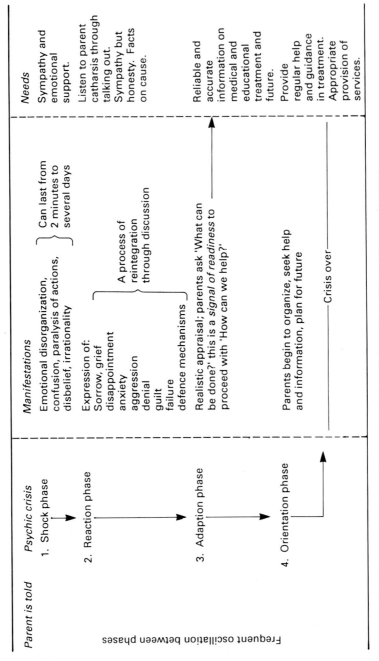

Figure 14.2 Model of psychic crisis at disclosure of handicap (Adapted from Hall and Grunewald, 1977.)

Chronic stresses unique to families with a child who has a mental handicap

Stigmatized social interactions

The public have a tendency to stereotype all people with a mental handicap as completely lacking in social competence. Parents may face reaction from others that are quite hostile. They may also have to readjust their own attitudes, as before their child was born it was likely that their own views were the same as this stereotype described above. As the child gets older the discrepancy between their size and apparent age and their mental functioning may tend to increase, thus making the child more noticeable.

Increased and prolonged burden of care

The burden of caretaking is often increased and more prolonged in a child with a mental handicap. There may be secondary problems associated with the mental handicap which increases the workload for the parents. More severe mental handicaps are often associated with multiple physical handicaps. There is also a higher incidence of behaviour disturbance in children with a mental handicap.

This burden can be seen to be endless; parents of older children cannot look forward with any certainty to relief from the burden of care afforded to parents of normal children. The child's handicap might make respite more difficult to organize. Parents may feel that only a specialized sitting service would be acceptable and the informal baby-sitting networks available to parents of normal children are not an option available to them.

Lack of information

For information and advice most parents rely on their own experiences of being parented, and on advice from friends, relatives and neighbours. These resources are usually inadequate for children with a mental handicap, where more specific information may be required.

Financial concerns

The needs of many handicapped children will have financial implications. Prolonged incontinence will incur extra costs for laundry, bedding, nappies and clothing. Prolonged crawling, hyperactivity or some problem behaviours will also take their toll on clothing. Many severely handicapped children may require a special diet, due perhaps to feeding problems or difficulty in swallowing and digestion. Difficulty and mobility of the child might also result in restricting access to shopping facilities with the 'best buys'. Lack of mobility might also dictate that extra heating is required. The child may require extra stimulation requiring the purchase of extra specialized toys. Travel to clinics will be an extra cost.

It is emphasized here that not all parents will suffer from these financial burdens. Many parents resent the fund-raising events for their children, because of the implication that the presence of a handicapped child in the family means they are in need of financial assistance. The argument for the financial impact on family stress has a tendency to be overstated. Bradshaw and Lawton (1978) examined the effect of the provision of financial assistance through the 'family fund' and found no difference in reported levels of stress.

Periodic potential crises over time

Wikler (1981) hypothesized that ten critical periods are potentially stressful for the parent of a child with a mental handicap. These are based upon times when a discrepancy emerges between what the parents expect of a child's development and parenting and what actually takes place. When these occur the family may experience renewed emotional upheaval, similar to that experienced when presented with the initial diagnosis. They would need to reactivate their coping mechanisms to re-establish family functioning.

Five of her periods are defined by the chronological age of the child and are related to an age which for a normal child is characterized by achieving a major development milestone. The other five are distinctive events not experienced by parents of normal children.

Crisis arising from lack of normal developmental progression

Developmental milestones have greater significance for almost all parents. Expectations of the baby's first steps and first words are strong. Information regarding children's normal development is readily available for anyone who wants to measure their child against normality.

The discrepancy between the child with a mental handicap's rate of development and the norm is an issue focused on for diagnosis and treatment. Consequently, this is the source of stress for the parent. Wikler called these periods 'developmental crises' and claimed that the poignancy lies in the gap between what is expected and what occurs. She identified five such developmental crises on the basis of normal developmental milestones:

1. The child should have begun to walk (ages 12–15 months).
2. The child should have begun to talk (ages 24–30 months).
3. The child should have started normal play groups/schooling (the start of the public labelling of 'difference' with attendance at 'special classes').
4. The onset of puberty (tension between physical appearance versus mental–social ability).
5. The 18th birthday (symbolic of reaching adulthood and independence).

Crises associated with distinctive events not experienced by parents of normal children

Wikler (1981) argued that, in the same way that parents have expectations that are culturally derived about normal development, they also have expectations about the parenting experiences. The events that occur only in the family of the child with a mental handicap could be critical periods in which the discrepancy between what was expected of parenting and what happened was the greatest. She suggested these crises might include:

1. The diagnosis of mental handicap.
2. Parents considering that others might rear their children, e.g., fostering, adoption, long-term residential care.
3. The younger normal sibling performs at a higher developmental level than the child with a mental handicap.
4. Child management necessitating professional involvement, e.g. epilepsy, stereotypic behaviour, health issues unique to children with a mental handicap.

5. As the parents grow older serious discussion about guardianship and the possibility of relinquishing responsibility to somebody outside the family.

At each of these times the parent will be reminded that had their child been normal that this process would have been unnecessary. This will revoke the original emotional upheaval and disappointment. Wikler *et al.* (1981) in a retrospective study asked parents to describe their feelings at each of these stages. Their responses supported the idea that their experiences were not a time-bound adjustment, but rather one of chronic periodic sorrow.

'Coping'

Parents are not merely passive recipients of all this adversity. Although as a group they are more stressed than the normal population there is a large individual difference in their reactions, with the vast majority of parents coping, some coping very well.

To understand this it is important to understand how stress work. It does not work in a way in which an engineer might say that metal in a bridge becomes stressed. In this type of explanation or model of the process the metal in the bridge is simply at the mercy of the elements and is passively bombarded by the forces of wind and rain etc. and eventually gives in. People are not like this; they interact with the things that might stress them and seek to ameliorate the effect of these stressors.

Recent research has acknowledged this complex and interactional nature of stress and coping and has utilized Hill's (1959) ABCX model of family stress (e.g., Wikler, 1986; Cole, 1986). Hill's original scheme begins with the identification of four components of the family's experience of stress:

A – (the demand or stressor event) interacting with
B – (the family's crisis meeting resources) interacting with
C – (the perception and definition made of events) producing
X – the crisis reaction.

A – The stressor event – This is the problem situation that presents itself to the family for solution. For example, financial concerns, stigmatized social interactions, the prolonged burden of care, etc. This would also include the 10 critical periods described by Wikler.

B – The family's resources – These will mediate the adverse effects of the demands made. These are the families capabilities for meeting demands and needs and are characteristics of the individual members, the family unit and their community. These are pre-existing resources like the parenting ability, home management skills, family cohesiveness, friendships and religious involvement. Resources then might be added, strengthened, or developed as a specific reaction to the problem. These would include the involvement of mental handicap services.

C – Family perception – This is the meaning the family gives to the total crisis situation. The definition they have of the stressor and their perception of their resources.

X – Crisis reaction, family stress arises when the members judge that their resources are inadequate to handle the demands. This stress becomes distress, when the family subjectively define the situation as unpleasant or undesirable.

This model dismisses the notion of a direct relationship between the demand (A) and the resulting family crisis (X). It proposes two major buffering variables, family resources (B) and the subjective and meaning assigned (C), protecting the family and enabling coping.

Research using the coping models is still in its infancy and its usefulness remains, as yet, unproven. There is increasing recognition that research should be using this type of model but with the exception of Wikler (1986), very few studies consciously address all of the different aspects of coping and attempt to fit them into a theoretical model. Those studies that do look at coping or resources have addressed only a portion of the whole picture.

'Support systems and networks'
Marital relationships have been examined by Friedrich (1979) as a predictor of successful coping. It was found that marital satisfaction or the security the mother felt within a relationship was the best overall predictor of coping. Various studies have confirmed that the presence of both parents within the home is a significant predictor of coping (German and Maisto, 1982; Beckman, 1983). Social support in general is not significantly related to coping, but was related to maintenance of the child with a mental handicap within the home. The idea that parents of children with a mental handicap have a small, dense network of support to use as a coping strategy has been raised by several authors (Granovetter, 1973; Kazak and Marvin, 1984; Waisbren, 1980). These small, dense networks were found to foster a sense of cohesiveness and support with enhancement of positive feelings about the child, but they also were found to generate stress as they restricted access to other resources. Bryne and Cunningham (1985) suggested that the social networks can be seen as providing feedback about coping. A closed dense network would be inclined to give more reliable feedback as there would be fewer people to disagree, but will be less flexible and not generate as many alternatives. On the contrary, a more open network would be more diverse but less consistent in its feedback.

Studies of religious belief have generally been found not to contribute to family adjustment (Friedrich, 1979; Germand and Maisto, 1982). Although earlier studies, e.g. Farber (1959), suggested that the likelihood of the child being maintained at home was related to strength of religious belief.

Fathers

The role of fathers and the effect of their having a child with a mental handicap has generated much mythology and assumptions but very little good research. It is often assumed that the 'tough unemotional male' image would make devastating news, such as the diagnosis of handicap, harder to manage. McConachie (1982) in a review concludes that the suggestion that the initial impact is worse for father is unwarranted. It is based mainly on the observations of distress (not usually seen openly in men) and on reports by mothers who may be showing their concern for their partners. The discovery of the child's handicap is likely to have an equally profound effect on both parents.

As the child develops fathers have been found to cope less well with children whose handicap is obvious by their appearance (Cain and Levine, 1963). There is also some evidence that fathers are less likely to accept the existence and extent of mental handicap in their sons (Levine, 1966).

Fathers of handicapped children are less likely to develop psychiatric symptoms than mothers. Wing (1975) reported that 20% of fathers had experienced mild or severe psychiatric symptoms at some time since the child was born, compared with 57% of mothers. This is greater than a 2:1 ratio of women to men expected in the general population. The great majority of mothers attributed their symptoms to concern over their handicap child, whereas few of the fathers did so.

Given the greater demands a child with a mental handicap makes on the family, one would expect fathers to be more involved in the work load than usual. However a consistent finding in the research on this area is of poor participation in child care activities (Wilkin, 1979; Ayer and Alaszewski, 1984; Baldwin, 1985). Wilkin (1979) looked at the quality of participation. Only two tasks were found in which more than half of the fathers participated equally with mothers, lifting and baby sitting. Baby sitting was usually carried out when mothers were also at home. He concluded that most fathers should and could have done more. The rate of contribution was not different from most ordinary fathers but the burden of care was significantly greater. This lack of involvement is clearly a problem. To a certain extent the problem is encouraged by the way in which professionals deliver their service to the family. The majority of contact is with the mother, fathers are often not invited. The presence of fathers is often seen by professionals as getting in the way of communication between themselves and the mother. Cummings (1976) pointed out that when fathers are not involved they may continue in unduly pessimistic or optimistic beliefs concerning their child's future, feel diminished competence in handling their child and have little chance to meet and share experiences with other fathers of handicapped children. Clearly involvement of fathers is essential and services should be accommodating and flexible to allow this to happen.

Out-of-home-placement

Parents are often pulled by conflicting social pressures once they decide upon in-home versus out-of-home placements. On one hand current service philosophies dictate that in-home care until the child is 18 or 21 is to be preferred. Yet on occasions the child's presence is perceived as burdensome or proves to create enough stress to interfere with everyday family functioning, thus affecting the rights of those family members. The issue becomes, how to provide for the child's best interest, without sacrificing most of the family's time and energy to the cause.

Cole (1986) suggests the use of the ABCX Model (discussed earlier) in an attempt to understand the parents' experience of deciding for an out-of-home placement.

A – Stressor events

Research would indicate the following stressors which would make an out-of-home placement more likely: disruptive behaviour, stereotypic or self-injurious behaviour, a second handicapped child, absence of the father and the presence of multiple physical handicaps.

B – Family resources

Research has identified lower parental income, unavailability of grandparents, reduced parent–sibling and spousal support, non-use (or non-availability) of respite care, sitter unavailability, absence of friends, neighbours and/or church assistance, as characteristic of families who place their children out of home.

C – Family perception

Parents understanding and attributions of the handicap will to some extent mediate the decision. Perceptions like, 'a challenge to be met', 'God's plan', 'an opportunity for growth, care and empathy', will all make out-of-home placement less likely. Perceptions like 'the final straw' will make out-of-home placement more likely.

Over-simplistic statements that risk stereotyping families who opt for out-of-home placement are to be avoided: 'They are less educated, they have less money, they live in poorer neighbourhoods, they have more handicapped children'. There will always be exceptions to any of these generalizations. It is important to consider all aspects in the process of decision making, not only the demands of the child but also the family's resources and perceptions of their situation.

'Letting go'

So far our discussion has centred around the experience of parents with young children. Current philosophies guiding service provision would work towards the person with a mental handicap leaving home once they have achieved adulthood. Many parents find this position intolerable and continue to exert a great deal of influence over their offspring even when they have reached adulthood. Ferrera (1979) found that although parents supported the concept of normalization and integration for people with a mental handicap, they resisted it in relation to their own offspring.

This reluctance to 'let-go' was investigated by Card (1983). He found in a survey of parents with an adult with a mental handicap living at home, that the vast majority of the respondents supported independent living training but were reluctant for this to apply to their offspring. Nearly all parents intended to keep their offspring at home until age or ill health made this impossible.

Various explanations of this phenomena have been suggested; these all at present remain untested hypotheses. The establishment of independence in normal childhood is determined largely by the child. Adolescents become independent by rejection of certain aspects of their parents. In an adolescent with a mental handicap this may well not occur. Card (1983) suggested that without this rejection they are unable to regard their own offspring as adult and are not prepared to face the pain and loss involved in readjusting to a new and more separate relationship.

Parents may also rely on their offspring. There may be financial advantages for keeping them at home. For some parents their child's care may have occupied so much of their time and energies, that it left little room for anything else. The vacuum that would be created by the removal of their offspring might seem impossible to fill.

Some parents might object to the standard of residential care or accommodation available. These may be well-founded objections.

Those that are providing a service to adults with a mental handicap need to decide who their service is for. Is it for the parents and family or is it for the person with a mental handicap? On occasions the needs of the two will conflict. Parents or professionals need to work together to prevent situations occurring where a person with a mental handicap suffers the double trauma of loss of parents and a hasty, ill-planned admission into residential accommodation.

References

Ayer, S. and Aszewski, A. (1984) *Community Care and the Mentally Handicapped Services for Mothers and their Mentally Handicapped Children*, Croom Helm, London

Baker, P.A. (1987) Measurement of stress in parents with a child with a mental handicap; the influence of residential care. *M. Phil. Thesis*, University of Edinburgh

Baldwin, S. (1985) *The Costs of Caring*, Routledge and Kegan Paul, London

Beckman, P.J. (1983) Influence of selected child characteristics on stress in families of handicapped infants. *American Journal of Mental Deficiency*, **88**, 150–156

Boston, S. (1981) *Will, My Son*, Pluto Press, London

Bradshaw, J. and Lawton, D. (1978) *Tracing the Cause of Stress in Families with Handicapped Children*, York, University of York Publications

Byrne, E.A. and Cunningham, C.C. (1985) The effects of mentally handicapped children on the families – a conceptual review. *Journal of Child Psychology and Psychiatry*, **26**, 847–864

Byrden, R.L. (1980) Measuring the effects of stress on mothers of mentally handicapped infants – must depression always follow? *Child Care, Health and Development*, **6**, 111–125

Caine, L.F. and Levine, S. (1963) *Effects of Community and Institutional School Programmes on Trainable Mentally Retarded Children*, Research and Monograph, Series B, No. B-1, Council for Exceptional Children, NEA

Cole, D.A. (1986) Out of home placement and family adaptation, a theoretical framework. *American Journal of Mental Deficiency*, **91**, 226–236

Card, H. (1983) What will happen when we've gone? *Community Care*, **28 July**, 20–21

Cummings, S.T. (1976) The impact of the child's deficiency on the father – a study of fathers of mentally retarded and chronically ill children. *American Journal of Ortho-psychiatry*, **46**, 246–255

Cunningham, C.C. and Davis, H. (1985) *Working with Parents: Frameworks for Collaboration*, Open University Press, Milton Keynes

Cunningham, C.C., Morgan, P. and McGucken, R.B. (1984) Down syndrome – dissatisfaction with disclosure of diagnosis inevitable? *Development Medicine and Child Neurology*, **26**, 33–39

Cunningham, C.C. and Sloper, P. (1977a) Parents of Down syndrome babies: their early needs. *Child Care, Health and Development*, **3**, 325–347

Farber, B. (1959) Effects of severely mentally retarded child on family integration. *Monographs of the Society for Research in Child Development*, **Z4** (Z serial No. 71)

Ferrara, V.M. (1979) Attitudes of parents of mentally retarded children toward normalisation activities. *American Journal of Mental Deficiency*, **84**, 145–151

Friedrich, W.N. (1979) Predictors of the coping behaviour of mothers of handicapped children. *Journal of Consultant and Clinical Psychology*, **47**, 1140–1141

Gayton, W.F. and Walker, L. (1974) Down syndrome – informing the parents. *American Journal of Disabled Children*, **127**, 510–512

German, M.L. and Maisto, A.A. (1982) The relationship of perceived family support systems to the institutional placement of the mentally retarded child. *Education and Training of the Mentally Retarded*, **17**, 17–23

Granovetter, M. (1973) Strength of weak ties. *American Journal of Sociology*, **78**, 1360–1380

Hannam, C. (1988) *Parents and Mentally Handicapped Children*, 3rd edn, Classic Press, Bristol

Hill, R. (1959) Generic features of families under stress. *Social Casework*, **39**, 139–156

Hornby, G., Murray, R. and Jones, R. (1987) *Child: Care, Health and Development*, **13**, 277–288

Kazak, A.E. and Marvin, R.S. (1984) Differences, difficulties and adaptation: stress and social networks in families with a handicapped child. *Family Relations*, **33**, 67–77

Levine, S. (1966) Sex role identification and parental perceptions of social competence. *American Journal of Mental Deficiency*, **70**, 822–824

McConachie, H. (1982) Fathers of mentally handicapped children. In *Fathers: Psychological Perspectives* (eds Beail, N. and McGuire, J.), Junction Books, London

McKeith, R. (1973) The feelings and behaviour of parents of handicapped children. *Developmental Medicine and Child Neurology*, **15**, 24–27

Springer, A. and Steele, M.W. (1980) Effects of physicians early parental counselling on the rearing of Down syndrome children. *American Journal of Mental Deficiency*, **85**, 1–5

Waisbrain, F.E. (1980) Parents reactions after the birth of a developmentally delayed child. *American Journal of Mental Deficiency*, **84**, 345–351

Wikler, L.M. (1981) Chronic stresses of families of mentally retarded children. *Family Relations*, **30**, 281–288

Wikler, L.M. (1986) Family Stress theory and research of families of children with mental retardation. In *Families of Handicapped Persons* (eds Gallagher, J.J. and Vietze, P.M.), Brooks Baltimore, London

Wikler, L.M., Wasow, M. and Hatfield, E. (1981) Chronic sorrow revisited, parent v professional depiction of the adjustment of mentally retarded children. *American Journal of Orthopsychiatry*, **51**, 63–70

Wilkin, D. (1979) *Caring for Mentally Handicapped Children*, Croom Helm, London

Wing, L. (1975) Problems experienced by parents of children with severe learning retardation. In *Right from the Start* (eds Spain, B. and Wigley, G.), National Society for Mentally Handicapped Children, London

Wonnacott, L. (1981) The parents. In *Right from the Start, 81* (ed. Shennan, V.), Report of conference proceedings, MENCAP, London

15

Contemporary developments in mental handicap

15.1 Microcomputers

Phil Odor

Introduction

Since the late 1970s, it has been possible to manufacture cheap, small, self-contained computers which are able to create colour graphics, make sounds, and (sometimes) speak. A home, business and school mass market came into being. One side-effect of this was that teachers and therapists began to apply such microcomputers to the special needs of handicapped children, whilst Health and Education administrators have taken advantage of inexpensive office systems originally aimed at commercial office users.

Inevitably, these new systems and techniques have migrated away from school and therapeutic settings into hospitals and day care centres. Nursing staff will increasingly come into contact with microcomputers used by other professionals, and applications will arise in the care of mentally handicapped patients which are under the direct control of nurses themselves. This chapter outlines some of the applications which are being developed today. Our aim is not to show the inner details of particular systems (which will differ from machine to machine), but rather to give a framework for understanding the techniques in use, so that nursing staff can take advantage of new systems for their own work, and help other professionals in theirs.

What use is a microcomputer to carers?

Four areas of application will be considered, as follows:

1. Microcomputers used in administration (which, since the focus is not on direct use with patients, will not be dwelt on).
2. Microcomputers as aids to teaching, therapy and learning.

3. Their uses in assessing patient performance.
4. Their uses as aids to communication (including writing, reading and drawing).

Administrators are faced with a central problem of storing, retrieving, sorting through and selecting from large quantities of (usually textual) information, and preparing reports based on these. This is an area in which computer systems excel, and therefore many commercial packages have been designed to allow easy manipulation of texts. Where information is well structured (such as patient records), administrators usually use *databases*: these are programs that store and retrieve tables of information, and are powerful in searching through these tables for specific information. Where the information is unstructured (such as in the writing of descriptive reports), *word processors* offer a convenient way both of generating and easily editing new printed documents, and for re-using parts of old ones.

Microcomputers are powerful enough to undertake both of these tasks, and to store large amounts of information. It is therefore tempting to try to set up local databases (perhaps within a ward or particular department) to serve local administrative needs, and to use word processors for local report writing. As far as word processing is concerned, this is a reasonable ambition: once word processing skills are learned, the effort involved in creating neat and legible reports is much reduced. However, setting up large databases is not a trivial task and the work involved in maintaining the information, ensuring that it is properly structured, and is usable by all concerned, should be left to central computing services (who can also worry about the legal niceties of the confidentiality of the patient records, their security, and other essentials). Most databases, especially in hospital settings, are most useful when shared with a large number of people. A warning should be given against the creation of local databases at great expense, and the nurse should be encouraged instead to develop word processing skills, which will be a much more productive exercise. The remainder of this chapter concerns itself with direct application to patients.

Because its ability to store and test information allows the microcomputer to engage in a kind of limited teaching dialogue with a learner, and because the ways in which it can present that information can be engaging and motivating, much effort has gone into producing computer-based learning packages. These packages have been particularly interesting to special education teachers, since the handicapped learner perceives the microcomputer as being a teacher with infinite patience which can repeatedly go over a difficult area with absolute regularity and precision (thus avoiding confusion), and which often can be made available for one-on-one work when a human teacher with other responsibilities could not. However, casting the computer in the role of teacher sets it tasks which it cannot perform too well: the difficulties and limitations will be discussed later, as will other roles the computer can be put to in the teaching/learning process. In one such role, computers simulate real-world or imaginary situations, which can then be explored either by the learner alone or by the learner and teacher. Another uses the computer as a tool for the learner's own problem solving. For any of these approaches to work, a learner must be in a position both to understand what is being displayed by the machine, and to make selections and choices which the computer can interpret. Clearly, for a lot of mentally handicapped patients, text and keyboard are non-starters: therefore, alternative input and output methods will be discussed.

Much of therapy and teaching is aimed at understanding current knowledge, abilities, and limitations of a learner. Embedded into much computer-based learning therefore are methods for assessing his or her performance whilst they are engaged in the task. Again, the nature of computer-based assessment, including systems that simply test, will be described, rather than those that test and teach.

Finally, computers can be used to help overcome physical, communication, and cognitive difficulties, in a more direct way than by acting as teachers of new skills. Computer-based augmentative communication systems, aids to writing, and drawing systems can function as prostheses where remediation has failed. Systems used in these ways will be discussed briefly.

Microcomputers have moved from being esoteric oddities to commonplace, almost household articles. As with a motor car, it's helpful, if you use one, to know enough about the components to discuss your requirements with a salesman, or your problems with a garage mechanic. At the same time, it's not necessary to know the internals of those components in any detail. Therefore, what makes up a microcomputer system will be outlined.

Computer systems

The chameleon-like nature of microcomputers makes them appear more mysterious than they are. Computers slavishly follow sequences of electronic instructions (programs) which are held in electronic memory. The instructions in these programs dictate when text is to be displayed, or a picture is to be drawn; when the sound circuits are to play music or to recreate speech; or when to pause the sequence of execution to wait for the person using the system to enter a command. These commands may come from various 'input devices'. The most common is a keyboard, but since this is a complex and confusing object for many handicapped people, other alternatives have been created. The computer program might for instance expect input from a joystick (like the ones used in video games); or one or more switches; or from a drawing tool.

It is this large variety of controls and displays that makes the microcomputer such a potentially engaging and motivating tool for learning. However, such *hardware* is essentially passive: it is the *program* (sometimes called the *software*) which defines how creatively the controls and displays are used.

Since a single computer may run many different programs (hence its apparently changeable character), there has to be a way of permanently storing the instructions so that they can be transferred into the computer and run at will. The sequences of instructions are usually stored as magnetic patterns on small discs. Transfer into the computer is called 'loading' or sometimes 'reading'. The converse process of making a permanent record of information currently in the computers is termed 'saving' or 'writing'. Programs on the disc are thus a little like music on a cassette: both are magnetically stored and both need conversion into a different form to be usable. Playing a cassette is a little like loading a program. Recording a cassette is similar to saving data.

We are now in a position to see what makes up a running microcomputer system. There will be *programs* on *discs*, one of which will be *loaded* into the computer's *memory*. The computer interprets each program's step to determine how and when to produce *output* (on colour displays, through printed text or using sound), and when to demand *input* (from *keyboards*, *switches* or other such devices). Some programs deal exclusively with text (such as *word processors* and *databases*). These programs display characters and interrogate the keyboard. Others (like drawing packages) handle *graphics*, expecting input from drawing tools and putting out pictures to the screen and printer. Programs written for special needs handle even more varied inputs and outputs.

With this stereotype in mind, we can now turn to how the computer can be used in teaching.

How are computers used in teaching, therapy and learning?

As discussed above, to use a computer effectively, one needs to *control* it with commands which the program understands, and to *understand the response* which the program has the computer make. For most people with severe learning difficulties, physical limitations, or perceptual problems, most of the appeal and power of microcomputers in teaching comes from the richness and range of specialized input and feedback methods which overcome the limitations of textual displays, and conventional keyboard. It is this variety that allows teachers and therapists to construct specialized learning and communication environments for handicapped people, and the options will be returned to repeatedly in what follows. What are the alternatives for control and feedback?

Inputs

The learner can make the most basic choices or responses via single or multiple switches. The simplest of these are flat plates (which can be marked with colour, pictures, textured surfaces, icons or whatever else makes sense to the learner in the context of the task, including sticking real objects to the switch as signifiers). However, there are many alternatives – large pads (which can withstand a strike from a limb, being walked on in location tasks, or being rolled on to encourage whole-body activities); grunt switches (to detect and help shape sounds); non-contacting switches (which sense body proximity, and therefore do not need accuracy); mercury switches (which can be used to capitalize on semi-random limb or head movements), and many more. Choosing the right switch is an art in itself: for more details, see Webster *et al.* (1985).

Joysticks can be used to select a direction, whereby the learner can explore the relationship between hand movement, and chosen function. Joysticks are sometimes referred to as 'pointing devices', because they are usually used in conjunction with programs which allow selection to be made by displaying the options on the screen, and using the pointing device to move a screen marker to the chosen item. Note in passing, the abstract nature of this idea: much work may be needed to make plain the relationship between movement and screen activity. Other pointing devices include the mouse (used by moving it around on a flat surface, whereupon the screen marker mirrors the hand movement), light pens (which maintain the impression that one can 'draw' on a TV screen); touch screens (where pointing directly to the screen identifies the choice to the program) and others.

Sometimes, switches are grouped together into a more flexible unit. One such is a collection of 128 switches in a rectangular, flat array which comes in the size of A3 or A4 paper. The British version is called a Concept Keyboard – because the idea is to draw conceptually meaningful pictures on a piece of A3 or A4 paper, and overlay the keys with this more immediate set of controls. Of course, the switches know nothing of the overlay diagrams, but each overlay has its own interpreting program, which responds appropriately. Concept Keyboards are often used as a 'half-way house' for marginal text users. In such circumstances, the overlay might contain whole phrases or whole words, the selection of which could be an attainable task where letter by letter construction is not.

Outputs

Understanding the machine's output is also considerably easier if the hardware and software designers offer other options than screens full of characters. Speech output is simple and cheap (although the quality is not yet as good as it could be), and usually involves buying an external box. Pictures are relatively easy to handle (though care needs to be taken if concessions to machine limitations are not to produce cartoon-like results which are difficult to understand), and limited animation is also possible. Music, or other sound prompts, are well within the scope of the unadorned microcomputer.

However, the nurse may also come upon microcomputers whose outputs are not directed at sound, speech, pictures, or text, but at control of some physical object which engages the learner. The simplest of these involves the control of one or more toys, or, via appropriate safety circuits, the control of mains operated household items such as radios, lights, and so on. (For guidance on safety issues, see Nisbet, 1989.) More complex possibilities exist: several computer-controlled wheelchairs and similar vehicles have been created, which motivate through mobility rather than symbology.

How are these tools used by the designers of computer-based teaching and therapy packages?

Computer-aided instruction: the computer as a teacher

Directly 'replacing' a teacher by a computer is the aim of Computer Aided Instruction (CAI) Programs. The motives for using it include:

1. Economic gains (machines are cheaper than humans).
2. CAI's potential for lengthy and repetitive training without teacher fatigue; failure of temper, and variability.
3. A belief (particularly amongst those offering behavioural programmes) that the CAI methodologies closely mirror their own, and are thus good delivery vehicles.

In CAI packages, the program first delivers a piece of information or an example; then poses a problem and waits for a response. Normally this takes the form of accepting a single selection from a fixed set of choices (sometimes overt, such as the display of a set of pictures, sometimes hidden, as when the learner has to type a word, or draw a picture). Once the learner has made a choice, this is compared with the pre-stored expected answer. 'Right' answers are rewarded and further information and problems presented: 'wrong' answers result in either repetition of the problem, or finer explanations or examples, depending on the underlying teaching theory and the programmer's efficiency.

The kinds of information and 'questioning', and the sorts of response, depend upon the needs of the learner, drawing on the repertoire of computer input and output options described above. There are many permutations: voice prompted problems with picture choices displayed on a touch screen, or animated figures on a screen 'asking' for the correct response by pointing to each in turn. In the former, the choice is made by pointing to the screen: in the latter, the learner selects by hitting a switch at the right time. (Note how critical are the sub-skills of visual scanning, motor abilities, understanding of cause and effect, and many other aspects of individual competence – if the wrong assumptions are made, then CAI constitutes a more complex, not a simpler learning environment.)

Such CAI programs offer many assessment aids. The most obvious is the position reached in a program – the further through, the more has been assumed to have been learned. Another indication is the number of failed attempts *en route*, and where they were; and yet another is the time taken on each.

However, CAI programs have been increasingly severely critized in recent years (Self, 1985). The main problems are, firstly, in the program collecting enough information from its interaction with them to make sound judgements of the abilities of learners; and, secondly, how to write programs of sufficient complexity and depth to respond appropriately to these abilities. To get an insight into the first problem, consider a human teacher observing a learner – taking in cues from posture, facial expression, spoken language, and many other facets of communication: few of these are available to a machine. For example, although computers can easily *generate* speech, they are still very poor at *understanding* language – even if it is typed in, much less spoken. To get a feel for the difficulties involved in the second problem (that of creating good instructional material), try writing (in English!) instructions on how to get from your front room to your place of work. What happens at traffic lights? At an accident? In the dark? On public transport on Sundays?

Nursing staff will be involved in skill training, and sometimes CAI will be an appropriate tool. Matching the abilities of the person to the CAI package style is crucial, and requires careful consideration not only of the particular task to be learned, but whether the interactive demands of packages on offer are too complex, or the teaching style too restrictive.

Complete replacement of teacher or therapist by machine is an extreme measure. Much more powerfully, it is possible to use computers as an extra collaborative partner in the teacher/learner group, and we turn to this approach next.

Games, simulations, and construction kits: the computer as plaything

Much can be learned from carefully constructed play environments (see, for example, Musselwhite, 1986). Microcomputers make for remarkably powerful playthings. Many toys, while having appropriate levels of complexity and motivational power, are inaccessible because they need fine manual dexterity, or are unforgiving about speed of response, or require planning or memory skills which are out of range of the handicapped person, even though the underlying 'play-idea' might be within grasp. The wide range of inputs and outputs of the microcomputer, together with its ability to provide prompts and cues to help in planning and memorization, make it a good vehicle for setting up either alternatives to standard toys, or better means of control over them. Moreover, the computer-playthings can be easily adapted to new circumstances. Similar help is available to Occupational Therapists (Cromwell, 1986).

The differences between computer-based-play and computer-based-instruction is not so much that the latter is heavily structured, whilst the former is not, but rather that the structuring in play environments *is up to the learner and teacher/ therapist*. As with any other playthings, computer-based play can be free-flowing (relying on the adaptive inventiveness of the teacher to avoid degeneration into meaningless or repetitive behaviour), or can be made part of very controlled and predetermined programmes. What does differentiate the two approaches is a philosophy of how to assess performance. CAI emphasizes *measurement* and *testing*, against implicit or explicit norms. Play environments emphasize *observation* and *teacher analysis*. The teacher or therapist will set up a play environment which stimulates and exposes the activities he or she need to observe and encourage. These environments can be considered under two headings: content/access, and style.

Content/access

The rich repertoire of computer controls creates opportunities to devise systems which encourage many aspects of performance of interest to therapists and teachers. For example, *perceptual-motor skills* are easily targeted by highly specific games (and the degrees of accuracy necessary for success can be tailored easily to provide positive, motivating experiences). Similarly, if emphasis is to be placed on *postural training*, the control system can be sited to operate when the person is properly positioned. If awareness of *cause and effect* is the content area to be learned, then very precise and obvious 'causes' can be set up (usually switch based), with 'effects' tailored to the person's known or hypothesized areas of interest. Bright screen displays, music, or even control of a vehicle have all been used, encouraging *exploration* and *problem solving*, and training *mobility*. *Communication* training will be discussed later. For more details, see Hawkridge (1985), Goldenberg (1979) and Goldenberg *et al*. (1984).

Style

Although the curricular content of play is infinitely variable, it helps to distinguish two styles of playful learning: exploration, and construction.

Exploration – Here the computer is programmed to simulate a small 'world'. This can be as simple as a set of hidden objects which have to be uncovered or discovered. Or it can be as complex as animated adventure, in which the central character is controlled by the learner, who guides the animation in (safe) investigations of (simulated) dangerous, or difficult missions. Simulations exist at every level of complexity, with many forms of input and feedback. In all cases, however, both teacher and learner can be involved, with rich opportunities for observation. Just as importantly, the computer simulation can be re-run again and again, to try different tactics and strategies: reality rarely offers such options.

Construction – In contrast to exploring and playing in someone else's world (analogous to playing with a doll's house), children learn by building their own toys (using, for instance, Lego). Computers can also be used to build things. The distinction is that the objects are usually simulated, or the constructs are symbolic. At one extreme, people with poor motor control can instruct the computer to assemble pictorial representations of real-life objects: wrongly assembled, these objects collapse or don't 'work'. Or at the other extreme, much simplified programming languages, like Logo, allow learners to put their own sequences of instructions together, and test their expectations of what might happen against the real actions of the computer (see, for example, Weir (1987) for how such approaches can be used with different children: her own early work was with autistic children). Such 'programming' can be achieved without text, using simple Concept Keyboard overlays or switch-boxes.

Observation here involves not only attending to the process of play, but analysing the product: flaws in construction can reveal much of the thinking and perceptual processes involved.

To maximize on the benefits of each style of play, both from the learner's *and* the observer's perspective, there needs to be active involvement of an able partner during the (sometimes extended) periods of play, and this work may well be shared amongst several professionals.

Strengths and weaknesses of computer-based learning

Computers are rich in interactive modes, and a careful programmer will render them patient, non-pejorative deliverers of highly structured skill-training materials (provided that controlling the *computer* is not a task so complex that it interferes with accessing the *learning program*: an issue that can only be resolved by careful pre-assessment). However, there are several weaknesses in using computers as teachers:

1. They are not as perceptive as humans, being unable to detect or interpret much human language or behaviour.
2. Programmers still cannot deal with the combinational explosion of complexity which arises when trying to take into account variables such as learning style, boredom thresholds, memory problems, and language levels.
3. Assessment is reduced mainly to variants on numerical scoring, which may or may not be objective.

In contrast, using computers as tools for play opens up new styles of assessment through observation and opportunities for tailoring play environments. Used well, this approach maximizes the strengths of human and computer, but has the disadvantage that it usually requires new learning on the part of staff as well as handicapped person, and forces the invention of truly individualized programmes of work, which makes heavy demands on staff time.

What role can computers play in assessment?

In many ways, the roles microcomputers play in assessment closely relate to how they are used in learning. (Again, we leave aside the administrative application of computers to recording of results on Databases.) In one group of applications, computers are used in the delivery and automatic marking and analysis of structured tests. These might be reaction times, visual or auditory discrimination tests, multiple choice tests of non-verbal or verbal reasoning, and so on. This is reminiscent of computer-aided-instruction. Material is heavily structured and pre-organized; other humans are taken out of the testing situation; the machine is responsible for scoring and analysis; and (as with CAI), the full repertoire of specialized inputs and outputs can be brought to bear in order to overcome particular problems a patient might have. Microcomputers are also used to select highly tailored tests from large banks of well-checked test questions (the process known as 'Item Banking'). You can think of both such dedicated testing tools as being CAI without the instructional part, since no information is given (except, perhaps, in memory tests). What remains is the interactive question and answer session, with its attendant choice of next appropriate question, followed by machine-based analysis and report. CAI merely embeds such testing into the teaching process.

In contrast, the observational techniques used in assessing exploration, construction, memory and problem solving in play are stylistically very different to CAI and other computer-based tests. When a teacher sets up a computer-based play environment (say, a switch bank controlling a bank of sound sources), she or he is simultaneously setting the stage for specific observations: of bid-ability, self-assertion, inquisitiveness, understanding of cause-effect pairings, understanding of signifier/sound pairings, concentration, memory, and so on. The discipline of rigorously defining what is to be tested, and how the results are to be interpreted, is not abandoned with such observational styles of assessment, but is instead moved outwith the computer program, and rests with the observing team. The computer's role here is to ensure repeatability; record interactions; and to provide the optimum mix of complexity and attainment which will maximally engage the handicapped person.

How a computer is used to help those with communication, writing, and drawing problems

Communication aids

Section 6.1 described some of the augmentative techniques used with those people whose speech or language problems prevent them being understood as well as their cognitive potential might allow. The strategies available range from letter boards and word banks for those who are at least minimally text-able, through structured iconic systems such as Bliss, on to pictographic systems like Rebus. For the communication impaired person, these manual systems raise several difficulties:

1. Many of them are essentially 'closed group' systems. That is, that they are only usable when communicating with another person who has learned to interpret the specialized symbology employed. Microcomputers offer the possibility of mediating between one symbology and another: for example, taking inputs from switches labelled with Bliss or other pictographic symbols, and translating them into text or directly into speech, thus opening up the group.
2. There is the problem of communication speed. Even for an able-bodied person, it is difficult enough to keep up appropriate conversational gambits when communication is mediated by pointing at symbols, and interrupted while waiting for their interpretation. For a person whose handicaps include physical disability, this problem gets much worse, to the point where the whole nature

of communication opportunities changes, and the communicator becomes frustrated or worse, passive. In extreme cases of physical handicap, it may not be possible to indicate the symbology directly at all. In both cases, computer-based communication aids can help by firstly storing complete phrases under single keys which can be readily retrieved, and in the second case by allowing menu driven systems to be used by those who can only manage to operate one or two switches.

3. All manual communication systems suffer from having a too restricted space on a manageable-sized communication board on which to display a reasonably extended choice of words and phrases. Computer-based systems, by displaying the choices on the screen, can overlay many more layers of phrases: the usual limiting condition is how well able the person is to remember how to get to a particular wanted phrase.

4. Finally, most iconic or even textual systems suffer from the disadvantage that in a world of spoken language, they are secondary, silent, partners. Being assertive with a communicatioan board is a very difficult art to learn. Speech synthesized communication aids can restore the balance of initiation in favour of the speech impaired person.

Dedicated communication aids necessarily have to be portable. Those based on mains driven computers are only usable as training devices and unless they can be backed up by a personal, portable communication aid, they merely serve to frustrate even more when the person is no longer allowed access to them. Dedicated portable aids include Canon Communicators or Memowriters, or Churchill Lightwriters (all of which are designed for people who can understand text); TouchTalker, LightTalker, IntroTalker, and similar voice synthesized systems are able to store a wide variety of messages, alterable to suit individual users, and are accessed in a variety of ways ranging from direct selection (as on other, normal keyboards), to the use of single or double switches. These systems do not necessarily rely on text for display of choices.

In addition to such dedicated equipment, communication systems are also being devised which run on the newer portable (sometimes called laptop) computer systems.

Assessment for the right communication aid is a difficult and sometimes protracted exercise. The cognitive abilities of the communication impaired person may not be well understood until some communication aid has been put in place: once that communication aid is working and a better assessment of a handicapped person's capabilities is made, it may be that radical re-consideration is needed of the communication system, the aid, or both. Take for example the case of a speech impaired and physically handicapped person. The issues to be considered when choosing a communication system include:

1. Choosing the right symbology.
2. Choosing an input device appropriate to the physical disability.
3. Choosing a control strategy which is within the cognitive and perceptual capabilities of the person.
4. Negotiating appropriate initial language for the communication system which will be meaningful and useful to the person concerned, and will motivate them to use that system.
5. Setting up and evaluating the aid and training the person in its use in realistic settings.

In this latter context, the crucial role of the day-to-day carers cannot be over-stressed. If a person is to be encouraged to make use of computer-based communication aids, then those aids have to be demonstrated as effective to the user. For this to be seen to be true, the person and their newly installed aid must be included in conversations, attended to when interjecting, and treated with consideration and respect. It is vital in this evaluation and subsequent training to attend carefully to the content of the communication, not the act. Since nursing staff will be in the front line of personal contact during this phase, it is important that they familiarize themselves with the particular system which is being developed for the handicapped person and ensure that they are able to set it up for use, and can understand the range of language presently embedded within it.

In some cases, the communication aid will be producing text, and a nurse should be attentive to the content of messages, and should make time to respond appropriately. In other cases, the computer system will be generating speech: in the present State of the Art this may be rather crude in quality, and again some effort on the part of the able communicating party is needed to make best use of such systems.

We said above that communication aids need to be personal and portable. Nonetheless, training in the skills necessary to operate such an aid can take place on a mains powered microcomputer system. Here we return to what might be taught using computer-based learning. Computer programs are available to encourage visual tracking (necessary to handle menu choice systems); to develop an understanding of the symbol system (both the vocabulary and the syntax); and yet others are used to determine which are the best control sites for switches and other input systems. The process of transition from training and assessment using the workstation to control of a portable communication aid can be confusing to the onlooker: it is not always clear when, for example, a computer is being used as a computer-based learning tool, and when a pre-communication aid. However, unless the patient is absolutely bedridden and immobile, it can safely be assumed that a move will eventually be made on to a portable system.

Up to now we have assumed that the handicapped person will be using their augmentative communication skills to talk to other human beings. In fact, this is only a part of the story. The same tracking, selection, and communication skills that are built up to allow the use of an augmentative system are gateways to technological partners as well as human ones. For example, a communication aid which can be used to select phrases and speak them for human listeners, can also pass those same strings of characters to another computer, there to interact with, say, a computer-based learning package. Equally, a physically handicapped person who has learned to scan and select from a menu of choices of phrases, can also scan and select from a menu of choices of environmental controls. And, as we said above, increasing sophistication in the design of wheelchairs even allows high level communication with these mobility systems when the person's physical abilities are not up to low level control of a joystick (Nisbet, Loudon and Odor, 1988). Because learning one set of skills provides such a wide-ranging increase in personal power, the route to better communication may go via the encouragement of mobility or environmental control; or computer-based learning; or play activities, first. Thus simple toy controllers operated by switches and elementary scanning menus may provide the motivation to learn a skill which can then be transferred into control of an augmentative communication aid. Equally, control of personal mobility for a multiply handicapped individual may be the stimulation necessary to catalyse interest in broader issues of personal control, in particular control of communication and learning.

In a well-defined programme for a multiply handicapped communication impaired person, there will be several professionals operating in concert. Teachers and speech therapists will be devising common curricula which will seek to identify what motivates the person. They will use this knowledge firstly to set up play, mobility, or control activities which develop confidence in and refine targeted skills, and thence through more and more structured stages apply those skills on the one hand to the control of the communication aid, and on the other to accessing broader educational opportunities. This will be both through the communication aid itself, and through control of computer-based learning. It is important for the nursing team to be aware of the aims of these activities as they progress from relatively unstructured to highly structured, and to make appropriate and increasing use of communication strategies as they emerge through improved use of the communication aid.

Writing

It would be wrong to assume that there is a sharp distinction between text-able and illiterate people. There is a continuum of ability, and sometimes surprising peaks and troughs in the profile of competences. When we say that a person cannot write, we are making a very broad statement which covers a multitude of problems ranging from being physically unable to form letters, through a lack of understanding of the phonetic relationships between letters and sounds, to a problem with accurate spelling (but, nonetheless, perhaps an ability to form interesting sentences), and so on. Microcomputers can help both in learning to write, and in writing itself. As with communication aids, there is no clear distinction between those programs used for assessment and learning, and those that might be used as a writing prosthesis: at some point one makes the decision to transfer from computer-based learning to pencil and paper, or to remain with the computer as a permanent aid. There should be no shame in the latter choice.

The simplest way in which a computer can help is in the formation of letters. Provided that a person can recognize letters sufficiently to operate a keyboard (and this may not be a conventional typewriter layout, but rather a more conveniently arranged selection of switches on a Concept Keyboard), then the computer can generate neat typed copy which can be presented with pride. Perhaps just as importantly, the ability to view what one has typed, and make corrections and changes before committing to paper breeds another kind of confidence: the confidence to try, in the knowledge that no permanent record of failure will be made should errors occur. This piece of understanding is a highly abstract concept, and may take a long time to develop. Making a mark on a piece of paper is an immediate (if irrevocable) act which is relatively easily understood. The relationship between pressing a switch and a mark appearing on a TV screen is more tenuous. That the mark can be removed by another switch is even more difficult to grasp. To go beyond that, and understand that words on the screen may be pushed about or removed in order to change what one has written can be a very complex notion. For this reason, word processors used for encouraging writing in mentally handicapped people, tend to be highly simplified, and often have a series of staged progressions in which the more complicated editing tools are suppressed and hidden.

Many schemes for teaching reading and writing adopt whole phrase and whole word strategies, in which the learner is encouraged to select from a repertoire of words or phrases to build the sentence he or she wants to make. Word processors with banks of words built into them can be used in a similar fashion. The advantage of using a microcomputer rather than strips of carboard is that the resulting prose can be saved, loaded again later to be revised, and can be printed out: pieces of cardboard create no permanent record.

These and other techniques can be enhanced by the use of the same repertoire of alternative inputs and outputs which we have already pointed out make CBL and communication aids powerful and motivating. For example:

1. Word processors can be attached to speech synthesizers. These can then read back the words selected or the text produced, giving another channel for independent self-evaluation by the writer of the text he or she has produced. Note that the speech output here is for the handicapped person, not the rest of the world.
2. Physically handicapped writers can use single switch, double switch, joystick, and other aids to selection where they may not be able to use a conventional keyboard.
3. Concept Keyboards can be overlaid with supplementary pictographic material to help recognize and differentiate between textual characters or words.
4. Systems can be set up which mix iconic and textual displays for those in transition between an augmentative system and a textual one.

Once again, careful appraisal of appropriate inputs and feedback mechanisms is an essential prerequisite to using computer-based writing tools, and tailoring of initial language in the word banks mirrors the careful choice of language used in communication aids. Indeed, in some circumstances, it is not easy to distinguish between the efforts put into pre-training for a communication system, and the efforts put into pre-training for using a writing tool.

Drawing

We take for granted the use of pictures and drawings in much early and remedial teaching. Many psychometric instruments tacitly assume that pictorial understanding is unimpaired and base tests of other faculties on that assumption. Yet some people find great difficulty in drawing even vague approximations to real objects or recognizing spatial relationships. We would perhaps be more suspicious of this difference in performance between picture comprehension and picture production, were there better tools for exploring where the limitations actually lie. In the past, drawing abilities have been a rather all-or-nothing competence: rather in the way that some potential writers become log-jammed at their inability to form letters, so some potential artists become log-jammed at their inability to control the production of shape. That there may be artistic skill without physical control sounds paradoxical until it is realized that microcomputers can offer tools for editing drawings which are as powerful as the ones we have now come to accept as commonplace in the editing of text. So, for example, pre-stored shapes may be put into shape banks and selected from (just like word stores and phrase stores can be used in sentence making): these shapes may be manipulated independently, and enlarged, distorted, moved and removed later at will; grouped together, saved and loaded, and printed just as text fragments may be altered and rearranged at great length before the final piece is printed. These kinds of 'drawing prostheses' offer yet one more potential dimension of insight into remaining abilities, and one route to development which would be difficult to emulate without using microcomputers. Once again, the usual range of enhancements is possible: in particular, control of the drawing process through alternative input devices makes it possible to develop these artistic skills with little reliance on manual dexterity, hand-eye coordination, or any of a range of other normally limiting factors.

Science fiction (and to some extent computer salesmen) promote the image of the computer as a human replacement. I have suggested in this chapter that a much more appropriate role for them to play in the lives of multiply handicapped people is that merely of a tool. Sometimes the tool is used as part of a three-way interaction between therapist, nurse, or teacher; handicapped learner; and computer, where all three collaborate in learning or assessing a new skill. Sometimes the tool is a personal prosthesis for a handicapped person: a communication aid, or writing aid, or an aid to drawing or mobility. The major task facing those who wish to use tools in this way with their patients is that of matching the skill repertoire of the handicapped person against the repertoire of special inputs, outputs, and associated control software which are now available on affordable microcomputers, and tailoring chosen systems to meet the developmental aims for the handicapped learner.

I have made references to further reading above. However, in this particular area, there is no substitute for actually trying some of the computer packages, and the interested nurse should aim for hands-on experience if at all possible.

References

Cromwell, P. (1986) *Computer Applications in Occupational Therapy*, Haworth Press, New York

Goldenberg, P. (1979) *Special Technology for Special Children*, University Park Press, New York

Goldenberg, P., Russel, S.J. and Carter, C.J. (1984) *Computers, Education and Special Needs*, Addison Wesley, London

Hawkridge, D., Vincent, A.J. and Hales, G. (1985) *New Information Technology in the Education of Disabled Children*, Croom Helm, London

Musselwhite, C.R. (1986) *Adaptive Play for Special Needs Children: Strategies to Enhance Communication and Learning*, Taylor & Francis, London

Nisbet, P.D. (1989) *Microcomputers for Special Needs – Safety Considerations*, CALL Centre Information Sheet 7

Nisbet, P.D., Loudon, A. and Odor, J.P. (1988) *The CALL Centre Smart Wheelchair*, CALL Centre Research Paper 7

Self, J. (1985) *Microcomputers in Education: a Critical Appraisal of Educational Software*, Harvester Press, New York

Webster, J.G., Cook, A.M., Tompkins, W.J. and Vanderheiden, G. (eds) (1985) *Electronic Devices for Rehabilitation*, Chapman and Hall, London

Weir, S. (1987) *Cultivating Minds, a Logo Casebook*, Harper & Row, New York

15.2 Advocacy

Mary Holland

Advocacy for people with a mental handicap is fairly new in Britain. There are a number of forms of advocacy – self-advocacy, citizen advocacy, legal advocacy and collective/class advocacy. None in itself is sufficient to safeguard the interests of vulnerable people, but each provides a way of representing and upholding the rights and interests of people who have been excluded from or ignored by society.

Self-advocacy

The origins of self-advocacy by people with a mental handicap were in Sweden in the late 1960s, and in 1970 a 3-day conference was held, with 50 representatives from all counties in Sweden. News of this spread and in 1972, Campaign for Mentally Handicapped People (CMH) set up the first national conference of people with mental handicap in Britain under the title *Our Life*. Twenty-two people with mental handicap attended the 3-day conference. In a report of the proceedings, Ann Shearer described the degree of handicap of the delegates:

'The group fell well within the middle to top range of people we call mentally handicapped. Two of the participants found it particularly hard to follow the thread of a discussion and express themselves clearly even when asked a direct question; one needed help with washing and dressing; one was incontinent at night. Several had epilepsy; one delegate was nearly blind, one deaf and two others had additional physical handicap. None, however, found it impossible to contribute to the discussions about the way they lived and worked and saw people around them.'

(Our Life, 1972)

Four types of self-advocacy groups have been described (Washington People First, 1984):

1. An 'autonomous' or 'ideal' group is one that is independent in organization, finance and time from professional services or parent bodies. The group will have an independent advisor. Such a model frees group members from direct conflict of their interests with those of parents or professionals. They are free to speak about the services they receive without embarrassment or fear of recrimination, but this independence is at a price: the group must be able to support itself and take responsibility for its actions and decisions from the

beginning. The People First self-advocacy group in London is an example of this model.

2. The 'divisional' self-advocacy group is formed as a special section/division of an existing parent or professional organization. The Participation Forum, a section of the London Division of MENCAP is an example. The major advantage of this is that the larger organization (parent/professional body) usually provides resources, e.g. a meeting place, use of telephones, photocopying, paper and, in some cases, a small grant. It will also provide opportunities for the self-advocacy group to educate parents/professionals and to make an impact on the work of the larger body. The major disadvantage is the potential for conflict of interest.

3. The 'coalition model' brings together people with different types of disabilities to form one self-advocacy group. Under this structure, members with mental handicap have their own section, but join together with other sections for specific events and in determining policies. A larger and more diverse group adds legitimacy, increases political power and improves ability to generate funding. However, people with mental handicap may need to progress more slowly than other members, and they can become restricted in their involvement or can be overpowered by more articulate members.

4. The 'service system' model, like the divisional model, has the advantage of providing resources. As the setting is based at the service (e.g. ATC/SEC), there are no transport problems. In Britain, the major growth in self-advocacy is within service settings.

What have ATC/SEC self-advocacy groups achieved? In 1986/87, a survey undertaken in adult training centres (ATCs), social education centres (SECs) and mental handicap hospitals in England, Wales and Scotland found that 60% of ATCs and SECs had established groups in which people could speak up for themselves. In hospitals, the picture was not so rosy. Only 27% had self-advocacy groups, and almost half of these were restricted to one ward only. The main achievements of these self-advocacy groups were:

1. Those resulting in general changes, e.g. in leisure activities, dining arrangements, equipment, etc.
2. Those resulting in change within self-advocates. Many individuals were reported to have improved their skills and developed greater self-confidence through involvement within the group.

The groups experienced problems as well. Mainly these were to do with members not having necessary skills and not having enough support from staff. Indeed, 50% of the ATC/SEC self-advocacy groups that had stopped functioning had done so because of problems relating to staff. Maintaining a self-advocacy group in a 'service setting' (ATC/SEC or hospital environment) can result in undue influence of staff over the group. One means of maintaining independence can be for the group to have the help of an outside adviser who is independent of the service setting.

People First of London is completely independent of services. It was established following a visit to the First International Self-Advocacy Leadership Conference in 1984 in Seattle, USA. Nine self-advocates who attended the conference decided to form their own People First group, and since 1984 the group has met once a month at the King's Fund Centre in London. The group's advisor is not linked to any service. Members of People First are often called upon to address professional and parent bodies. In the summer of 1987, People First organized a successful weekend conference for self-advocates from England and Wales. In 1988, they were hosts of the Second International Self-Advocacy Leadership Conference. The two main difficulties facing People First are:

1. Insufficient time from an advisor. Although members carry out all the tasks themselves – responding to letters, managing bank accounts, writing speeches, making visits, planning conferences – they need support.
2. The distance that some members have to travel to attend meetings.

Other self-advocacy groups are semi-independent. They are linked to services in some way – for example, because of transport. The most well-established semi-independent group is the Lothian Rights Group, which has met in Edinburgh since 1981. The Group meets in an ATC in the evening, when staff and clients are no longer there. Members come from a variety of settings – some are ex-hospital residents, others have always lived with their families. They are not all members of one ATC, but are in contact with a variety of services. One of their major achievements, through direct action, was to save a transport service for people with physical disabilities which was under threat of closure.

Self-advocacy is still in its infancy, but it is clear that it is fundamental to the fight for equal rights, equal dignity and equal opportunities for people with mental handicap.

The Avro ATC Students' Council (self-advocacy group) emphasizes these fundamental principles in its Constitution, which concludes:

'. . . The most important of these is our right to respect for our human dignity. We will fight until everyone knows this and understands this. We are on the move towards a better understanding, and nothing placed in our way will stop us.'

Citizen advocacy

Citizen advocacy is carried out by trained, selected volunteers and coordinating staff working on behalf of people who are unable to exercise or defend their rights as citizens. Citizen advocates are individuals who are independent of those providing direct services to the people for whom they advocate. The fundamental principles of citizen advocacy can be applied to all people who have been overruled or ignored. These principles developed from the treatment of one group in particular – people with mental handicap, who have been excluded from education, employment, political activity and leisure opportunities, denied access to quite basic human rights, and, too often, ridiculed when trying to exercise choices which would be regarded as quite unexceptional in other sectors of society.

The first citizen advocacy scheme in the United Kingdom was established in 1981 by five national voluntary organizations – MENCAP, MIND, The Spastics Society, The Leonard Cheshire Foundation and One-to-One – when they joined together to form The Advocacy Alliance. (Today, The Advocacy Alliance is known as National Citizen Advocacy, and it runs a national resource and advisory centre.) The Alliance set up pilot schemes to introduce citizen advocates to residents of three long-stay mental handicap hospitals in south-west London.

The hospitals' agreement to open their doors to independent volunteer advocates must not be underestimated – especially when it is remembered that two of the hospitals, St. Ebba's and Normansfield, had been the subject of serious public enquiries.

Citizen advocacy enables people to exercise choices which society takes for granted, but which have been denied to many. Kit, an advocate with National Citizen Advocacy, acts for Molly, who lives in Normansfield long-stay mental handicap hospital. In speaking about being Molly's advocate (National Citizen Advocacy, 1988), he said:

'I have introduced Molly to the concept of choice. You see, she doesn't have much opportunity to choose. She doesn't choose her clothes, her food, her companions or her accommodation. It's quite a big thing for her to choose coffee instead of tea, a red dress instead of a blue one.'

In 1984, a similar citizen advocacy scheme was started in Sheffield, working not only in hospitals but with people living in the community in local homes, hostels or with their families. Since that time, more citizen advocacy schemes have been set up throughout the country, in London, Hereford, Worcester, Nottingham and Avon. Citizen advocacy is a partnership between two people – one who has a mental handicap (disability) and another, who does not. The independence of the advocate is essential. To ensure this, advocates should be:

1. Supported by, but independent of, the advocacy office.
2. Independent of the agencies and settings which provide services for the individual with mental handicap (e.g. independent of local authority, hostel, etc.).
3. Independent of the individuals' families, if the family interests are different from those of the individuals.

An advocate's primary loyalty must be to their individual partner. Many people with mental handicap are more dependent on services and on their families than others. Sometimes the needs of service providers, or even families, can distort those of the individual.

One of the key figures in the citizen advocacy movement in the USA is John O'Brien. He describes a citizen advocate as:

'A valued citizen who is unpaid and, independent of human services, creates a relationship with a person who is at risk of social exclusion, and chooses one or several of many ways to understand, respond to and represent that person's interests as if they were the advocate's own, thus bringing their partner's gifts and concerns into the circles of ordinary community life.'
(*Citizen Advocacy: A Powerful Partnership* 1988, p. 3)

It is important that advocacy is not seen as a job by the advocate or by the individual. The aim of citizen advocacy is to increase the number of people who choose to relate to a person with mental handicap without being paid for that relationship. Long-term commitment is an important part of citizen advocacy. Far too often, people with mental handicap have large numbers of people who come and go in their lives. To be effective, the advocate needs to understand and explore the needs and interests of the individual. This cannot be done overnight. It requires time, care and commitment.

Advocates must be flexible to develop new roles as individual needs and circumstances determine them. These roles can be wide and varied, ranging from acting as the spokesperson, guide to practical learning, information aide, financial advisor, friend/companion, defender/upholder of cultural and ethnic identity.

Legal advocacy

Legal advocacy is carried out by lawyers and other legally trained individuals, who assist people in exercising or defending their rights. This form of advocacy can require casework, negotiation, scrutiny of legislation and regulations, assessment of service requirements, representation before administrative tribunals and agencies (including civil and criminal courts), and monitoring compliance with laws and regulations which pertain to the rights of their 'clients'. A citizen advocate could, however, apply to become an individual's Appointee and thus be able to make claims for and receive DSS benefits on behalf of that individual.

Collective/class advocacy

Collective/class advocacy is when a group of people join together to campaign on issues that affect more than one individual. They may employ someone to pursue the campaign on their behalf. Organizations such as Mencap and CMH take up issues at a national level, scrutinizing parliamentary activities, lobbying for new legislation, and making representations on behalf of their 'client' group.

The Disabled Persons Act 1986

The Disabled Persons (Services, Consultation & Representation) Act 1986 breaks new ground for advocacy for people with disabilities. It gives people over the age of 16 the right to appoint someone to represent their needs (an authorized representative) regarding the provision of local authority social services. Disabled people under the age of 16 cannot appoint a representative themselves, but this may be done by their parent or guardian or, if they are in care, by the local authority. A parent or guardian may appoint him/herself as their child's representative. A local authority may appoint a representative for a disabled person who appears to them to be unable to do so by themselves by reason of any physical or mental incapacity. The authorized representative has a right of access to the disabled person at all reasonable times, regardless of whether they are living in hospital/residential accommodation or hostels.

Although the Act provides that the authorized representative may act only in relation to local authority social services, there is a provision that at a future date the Secretary of State may extend the role of the authorized representative to services provided by health authorities and to other services. Unfortunately, despite the fact that this Act has been on the statute books for 4 years, the sections providing for authorized representation have not yet been implemented.

Conclusion

The 1978 review of the Mental Health Act stated:

'. . . The most important factor in safeguarding the position of vulnerable patients and ensuring their rights are upheld is personal contact between the patient and someone whose job it is to explain the position from the patient's point of view. . . .'

A vigorous and vocal advocacy movement is essential if the rights and interests of the some 30 000 people still living in long-stay mental handicap hospitals are to be upheld.

Equally, advocacy is fundamental to successful care in the community. Without advocacy, people with mental handicap will remain a people apart.

References

Citizen Advocacy: A Powerful Partnership (1988) National Citizen Advocacy, 2 St Paul's Road, London N1 2QR

Constitution of the Avro Adult Training Centre Council. Avro ATC, Avro Road, Eastwood, Southend on Sea, Essex

Our Life (1972) Conference Report of the Campaign for Mentally Handicapped People. Available from VIA, Oxford House, Derbyshire Street, London E2 6AG

Review of the Mental Health Act 1959 (1978). Cmnd 7320, HMSO, London

15.3 Sexuality

Ann M. Green

Introduction

'All human beings have a sexual drive. This sex drive exists in children and continues into old age... we all of us have a sex life in whatever way it may be constituted – heterosexual relationships, homosexual relationships, masturbation... this is as true of the mentally handicapped as anyone else, for they are human too.' (Rea, 1973).

Until the 1970s the sexual and emotional needs of people with mental handicaps were rarely discussed and seldom the cause of action (Shearer, 1972). The reluctance to see people with intellectual disabilities as sexual beings may relate to a number of commonly held myths (see Craft and Craft, 1978); the relative comfort for parents of promoting a Peter Pan syndrome in relation to sons or daughters with significant handicaps; and the over-emphasis placed on mental age (as opposed to chronological age) by some professionals and many members of the public at the time.

Two decades of service developments, influenced by the philosophy of Normalization (Nirje, 1969; Wolfensberger, 1972), have increased awareness of people with disabilities as sexual beings (Kempton, 1976; Greengross, 1976). The acceptance of the rights of people with mental handicaps, the associated growth in the Advocacy movement (see Section 15.2) and the implementation of the policy of Care in the Community have similarly pointed to the need for sex education and counselling for people with mental handicaps.

Programmes of sex education have been developed which emphasize the need for individuals to have a basic understanding of their bodies (e.g. Kempton, 1978), stress the need for appropriate inter-personal and sexual behaviours (e.g. Dixon, 1988); and highlight the importance of assertiveness (saying 'no') in protecting individuals from exploitation (e.g. Blum, 1985). Craft and Craft (1985) have summarized the need and the rationale as follows:

1. The vast majority of those with a mental handicap will develop normal secondary sexual characteristics. They need more help, not less, in making sense of these changes and the accompanying strong emotional feelings.
2. They need knowledge that will protect them from exploitation and from unwittingly offending others.

The focus of sex education and counselling has therefore been that of enabling or empowerment; the promotion of positive sexual expression; and the avoidance of behaviour that may impede participation in community based lifestyles and activities.

The development of sex education packages for clients has in turn generated a growing awareness of the training needs of staff and carers in relation to sexuality and mental handicap. Many staff have been ill equipped by their qualification training, or in-service programme, to meet the needs of clients for sex education, or for sexual counselling.

A range of staff training programmes and packages have emerged both in local services (see for example Green, 1988) and under the auspices of various training agencies (Family Planning Association, BIMH, etc.).

The curricula of staff training programmes have typically included examination of staff attitudes; expansion of staff knowledge of sex and sexuality; communication and counselling skills; sex education programme design (including format, content and teaching methods); case studies; and use of resource packs and other instructional materials (see for example Dixon, 1986). The main objectives of such courses have been to encourage staff to meet the sexual and relationship needs of people with mental handicaps by providing them with opportunities to examine and clarify their own feelings and attitudes; to acquire skills which promote comfort and confidence in the subject area; and to defuse the sensitivity of the issues by adopting a problem-solving approach in the context of recognition of the 'valued' client.

As sex education and counselling became integrated into special education, further education, day services and residential settings, managers gained a greater understanding of the social and professional sensitivity of the work and the potential vulnerability of staff working directly with clients.

Many agencies have drawn up policies that underpin activities and innovations in service development in the area of sexuality and mental handicap; and that support and describe the practice orientation or framework for staff. In addition, managers, professionals and groups of care staff have developed procedural guidelines that describe the rights and responsibilities of clients; the role and responsibilities of staff; the networks of support; and the legal framework (Hounslow Social Services Department, 1983; Chamberlain, 1984).

The implementation of sex education and sexual counselling, which began in a somewhat selective manner (e.g. preparation for discharge from hospital, or crisis intervention in the community) is now more widely available and more sophisticated in approach. Instruments to assess the sexual knowledge or attitudes of clients are more frequently used to determine a baseline and permit more accurately targetted training and intervention (Fischer et al., 1980; Wish et al., 1980; Watson and Rodgers, 1980). Practitioners have adapted training programmes and resources to meet the needs of clients with greater degrees of intellectual impairment. In this context Ann Craft (Craft and Craft, 1985; Craft, 1986) has suggested that it is important to identify separately 'what specifically we want the student to *understand*' and 'what specifically we want the student to *do*'.

She indicated that the 'do' component is always likely to be the more important and that clarifying the limits of the goal, in relation to 'understanding', may prevent staff from being overwhelmed by the enormity and complexity of some parts of the sex education curriculum. Some training packs originally designed for adolescents and adults with only mild or moderate levels of handicap, possibly presenting within the framework of educational impoverishment or social deprivation, have been re-designed in a format adapted for the special needs of people with severe and profound mental handicaps. In general, educational programmes and training materials have become more explicit and unambiguous, with greater emphasis placed on practical aspects through the use of role play and behavioural rehearsal.

Staff training packages have also developed a more customized approach to the differing needs of staff working at a direct or indirect level with adults, or involved in the management or support of services. The range of training currently available includes basic introductory courses aimed at raising participants awareness of the issues of sexuality and mental handicap; advanced workshops offering 'skills to mastery' level training for staff who will become educators or counsellors of clients; and 'training-the-trainers' packages designed for managers, senior staff and training officers who wish to implement a cascade approach to training groups of staff within human service organizations. The curricula of staff training programmes has similarly expanded to cover staff support systems, supervision, and aspects of monitoring and evaluation.

In the early eighties, Sebba suggested that social attitudes to sexuality and mental handicap had reached the 'tolerance' phase of Kempton's elimination–tolerance–cultivation scale (Sebba, 1981). She also indicated that much remained to be done before people with mental handicaps could exercise their rights to fulfil their sexual and emotional needs to the same extent as other people (Sebba, 1985). Two new areas of concern have emerged which may have considerable impact on the progress that will be made in the nineties. Firstly, the growing awareness of the problem of sexual abuse in the child-care field has significant implications both for children and for adults in the field of mental handicap. Secondly, the spread of AIDS and HIV-related conditions has had a marked effect on the impetus to teach about sexuality and has also impinged on the practice of enabling, or supporting, the sexual behaviour of clients.

Sexual abuse

The incidence and prevalence of sexual abuse within the mental handicap sector is not reliably known.

Within the general population estimates of the prevalence of sexual abuse vary between studies (e.g. in the USA and Britain) and according to the survey methodology and definitions used. Russell (1986) has suggested a prevalence rate of 38% of adult women; Finkelhor (1986) and Taylor (1989) have both quoted rates varying from 6% to some 60% for females in the USA.

In Britain Baker and Duncan (1985) have reported 12% of females and 8% of males having been sexually abused before they were 16 years old.

Surveys of children or adults with mental handicaps have yielded similarly alarming figures. Chamberlain et al. (1984) reporting on an American study of 87 females aged between 11 and 23 years found that half of those with mild handicaps, 32% of those with moderate handicaps and 9% of those with severe handicaps had experienced sexual intercourse; one third of the young women with mild handicaps and a quarter of those with moderate handicaps had been victims of rape or incest. In a recent letter to the *British Medical Journal*, Cooke (1990) indicated that she had evidence of the widespread nature of abuse of adults with mental handicaps. She reported information obtained from Consultants in the psychiatry of mental handicap which suggested that the overt prevalence of abuse was about 4–5% but that there was likely to be a higher prevalence of undetected abuse, and that sexual abuse was much more common than physical abuse or neglect.

Even taking a conservative view of the hard data currently available, and acknowledging that suggestions of higher rates of undetected or unreported sexual abuse can at best remain soft indicators, it would appear that young people with mental handicaps may be open to a similar, or perhaps greater, risk as their counterparts in the general population.

It has been suggested that people with mental handicaps may be vulnerable to increased risk for sexual abuse because of their own characteristics (Schor, 1987); the motivations of perpetrators (Finkelhor, 1984; Longo and Gochenour, 1981); characteristics of their environments, e.g. relative social, and sometimes geographical, isolation, with fewer situational safeguards (Schor, 1987); and factors related to the delivery of service by caregivers (Brown and Craft, 1987).

A picture emerges of a 'safe victim': who may look like an adult but will not make adult demands on a relationship; who may be pliable, acquiescent and eager to please; who may be overly responsive to attention and affection; who may have communication difficulties or possess no sexual language, minimizing the risk of disclosure; who may have received little or no sex education which would inform and thereby protect; who may live in large settings (e.g. hospitals) where supervision is difficult, or small settings which are socially isolated; who may require intimate, physical care which lowers the normal boundaries of personal space; who may be cared for by staff with little training in prevention or intervention in recognizing, reporting or investigating circumstances which may be abusive; and whose care or support may be planned and managed by staff unaware of the risks involved.

The advances made in the area of sexuality and mental handicap in the 1970s and 1980s have provided a framework in which sexual abuse may begin to be addressed. However, much of the work requires revision and development to meet a more demanding challenge. Agency policies and procedural guidelines need to be drawn up in relation to the specific parameters of sexual abuse and people with mental handicaps; clearer data are required on the incidence and prevalence of sexual abuse in this client group; staff training programmes need to expand their curricula to include aspects of prevention of abuse, handling of suspicions and allegations, and therapeutic interventions (including long-term support); client educational programmes need training methods and materials designed to reduce the vulnerability factor and maximize protection; and information about sexual abuse needs to be more widely available to parents, carers, staff, advocates, and members of the public.

Much can be learned from the child-care field; and potentially much can be generalized to other groups of disabled people. It has been argued that people with intellectual disabilities have a special vulnerability: although the specific mix of characteristics may vary, people with physical handicaps, people with sensory impairments and elderly people may be equally, though differently, vulnerable. It may be that work in child sexual abuse will become a model for developments in a range of other care groups.

At present the whole issue of sexual abuse and mental handicap remains sensitive and under-resourced. The complexity of cases; the lack of skills, systems and procedures; and the potential for publicity and litigation create a minefield for carers, professionals and service managers alike. Brown and Craft (1989) highlighted the many outstanding tasks in this area and suggest that progress will only be made:

'If services are able to contain the anxiety they provoke and create structures which can withstand the tension between enabling people to live as independently as possible while protecting them from abuse or exploitation.... Meanwhile services are pressured into colluding in the dynamics surrounding sexual abuse by keeping it "secret" and sweeping it under the carpet....'.

AIDS and HIV

During the first half of the 1980s concern about the spread of AIDS and HIV-related conditions, especially among gay men and intravenous drug users, resulted in a growth of media campaigns and health promotion or preventative education strategies. These, together with the impact of deaths within the most 'at risk' groups, led to some changes in sexual behaviour – particularly in respect to homosexual men. The effects on the heterosexual population appeared to be less marked. More recent campaigns aimed specifically at heterosexuals and young people have similarly failed to achieve the desired degree of behavioural change. (Consumers Association, 1989). Little is known of the impact of such campaigns on people with mental handicaps.

Jones (1987) has pointed out that people with mental handicaps are not in general a high-risk group in terms of contracting AIDS. Nevertheless the special vulnerabilities (described above) may place clients at risk; and Kastner *et al.* (1989) have suggested that an increased risk of HIV infection may exist for some individuals who display high-risk behaviours. They cite two case studies which they identify as the first published reports of individuals with mental handicap who have become infected with HIV. In both cases the infection was transmitted from homosexual individuals with HIV to their sexual partners with mental handicaps.

The spread of HIV infection potentially affects the field of mental handicap in two ways. First, children contracting HIV congenitally through maternal infection may become developmentally disabled (Ultman *et al.*, 1985; Special Children, 1987). Second, infection with HIV can impose additional difficulties in the care of people with existing mental handicaps.

The number of people with pre-existing intellectual disabilities who have subsequently become infected with HIV is unknown. Kastner *et al.* (1989) suggested that clients in institutional care may be least likely to be infected with HIV because they may be less sexually active than clients in community settings. They further note that the prevalence of HIV in the general population is probably higher than among people with mental handicaps who reside in the community. The case could also be made to suggest that people with mental handicaps in some controlled institutional settings (e.g. prisons) may be more likely to be infected with HIV than people residing in hospitals. Offenders with borderline or mild intellectual disabilities, moving between prison, hospital and social service settings, if infected with HIV may introduce a greater risk to previously lower risk settings.

The testing of people with mental handicaps for HIV is fraught with difficulty; can a person with a mental handicap fully comprehend the implications of the test? If not, should the test be carried out? If consent is given for voluntary testing, will the person have the emotional coping skills to deal with a positive result? Will the person have the intellectual capacity to understand the implications of a positive result?

The general screening of individuals who have not consented to testing for HIV is considerably controversial (Johnson and Griffiths, 1989).

The case for screening people with mental handicaps for HIV is based on the need:

1. To obtain more accurate data on prevalence.
2. To target education, counselling and support to at risk groups.
3. To protect uninfected clients.
4. To protect staff who provide services and care.

The case against screening rests on the ethical and legal considerations: the need to avoid additionally stigmatizing the client group as high risk; and the need to avoid prejudice which may compromise community integration and introduce discussions about segregation to prevent transmission.

As suggested in relation to sexual abuse, client training packages, staff training programmes, agency policies and procedural guidelines need to be adapted and extended to cover AIDS and HIV. Kastner *et al.* (1989, 1990) have clearly expressed the need for human service agencies in the mental handicap sector to develop policies that address issues and concerns about:

1. Client education and training.
2. Testing policy and procedure.
3. Residential care of people with mental handicaps who are infected with HIV.
4. The management of sexual and aggressive behaviours.
5. Hygiene and transmission of HIV.

Jones (1987) has suggested an outline strategy for education about AIDS. He noted that carers and educators have a specific responsibility to teach clients with mental handicaps the message about AIDS in an appropriate and understanding form: first, clients who are sexually active may be at risk; and second, some clients are likely to have experience of media campaigns, health education leaflets or general coverage of AIDS and HIV and may be confused and anxious. (It may be worth noting that some of the posters and TV campaigns may look like advertisements for sexual intercourse to someone with limited comprehension and poor verbal ability.)

Resource materials for education about AIDS and HIV within staff training programmes are readily available (Health Education Council, 1988; CCETSW, 1989). At present there is less available for direct use with people with mental handicaps, but the Family Planning Association has been collaborating with BIMH to produce a series of booklets on AIDS and people with learning difficulties.

Sex education and counselling for people with mental handicaps began to develop in the context of normalization, integration and community care. The challenge for the next decade may be to maintain further developments, in relation to sexual abuse and AIDS, within this framework. If the desire to protect vulnerable clients, or the urge to segregate people who may pose a risk, becomes too strong much progress will be reversed.

References

Baker, A.W. and Duncan, S.P. (1985) Child sexual abuse: A study of prevalence in Great Britain. *Child Sexual Abuse and Neglect*, **9**, 457–467

Blum, G. (1985) *Feeling Good About Yourself* (Video), Concord Films Ltd., Ipswich

Brown, H. and Craft, A. (1987) The Big Secret. *Community Care*, **22**, 18–19

Brown, H. and Craft, A (eds) (1989) *Thinking the Unthinkable*. Papers on sexual abuse and people with learning difficulties, F.P.A. Education Unit, London

CCETSW (Central Council for Education and Training in Social Work) (1989) *Living and Working with HIV*. A training pack for staff of the personal Social Services, CCETSW, London

Chamberlain, A., Rauh, J., Passer, A., McGrath, M. and Burket, R. (1984) Issues in fertility control and mentally retarded adolescents: I. sexual activity, sexual abuse and contraception. *Paediatrics*, **73**, 445–450

Chamberlain, P. (1984) *Personal Relationships and People with Mental Handicaps*, Kings Fund, London

Consumers Association (1989) AIDS Advertising – are we becoming immune? *Which Way to Health*, Feb., 29–32

Cooke, L.B. (1990) Abuse of mentally handicapped adults. *British Medical Journal*, **300**, 193

Craft, A. (1986) Sexual, social and emotional development in people with Down's syndrome. *Mental Handicap*, **14**, 34–36

Craft, A. and Craft, M. (1985) Sexuality and personal relationships. In *Mental Handicap: A Multi-disciplinary approach* (eds Craft, M., Bricknell, J. and Hollins, S.), Balliére Tindall, Eastbourne

Craft, M. and Craft, A. (1978) *Sex and the Mentally Handicapped*, Routledge and Kegan Paul, London

Dixon, H. (1986) *Options for Change: A Staff Training Handbook on Personal Relationships and Sexuality for People with Mental Handicaps*. Part 1 Methods and Part 2 Materials. FPA Education Unit and BIMH Publications, London

Dixon, H. (1988) *Sexuality and Mental Handicap: An Educators Resource Book*, L.D.A., Cambridge

Finkelhor, D. (1986) *A Sourcebook on Child Sexual Abuse*, Sage. Beverley Hill, Ca.

Fischer, H.L., Krajicek, M.J. and Borthwick, W.A. (1980) *Sex Education for the Developmentally Disabled*, University Park Press, Baltimore

Green, A.M. (1988) Sex education for people with mental handicaps: a staff training package. In *Clinical Psychology in Action* (eds West, J. and Spinks, P.), Wright, London

Greengross, W. (1976) *Entitled to Love: The Sexual and Emotional Needs of the Handicapped*, National Marriage Guidance Council, Rugby.

Health Education Council (1988) *Aids Resource List*, HEC, London

Hounslow Social Services Department (1983) *Sexuality of People with Mental Handicap: Guidelines for Care Staff*

Johnson, M.A. and Griffiths, P. (1989) Screening for HIV. *British Journal of Hospital Medicine*, **41**, 119

Jones, C. (1987) AIDS and people with mental handicaps. *Mental Handicap*, **15**, 163–165

Kastner, T.A., Hickman, M.L. and Bellehumeur, D. (1989) The provision of services to persons with mental retardation and subsequent infection with human immunodeficiency virus (HIV) *American Journal of Public Health*, **79**, 491–494

Kastner, T., De Lotto, P., Scagnelli, B. and Testa, W.R. (1990) Proposed guidelines for agencies serving persons with developmental disabilities and HIV infection. *Mental Retardation*, **28**, 139–145

Kempton, W. (1976) Sexual rights and responsibilities of the retarded person. *Official Proceedings of the 103rd Annual Social Welfare Forum*, National Conference on Social Welfare, Washington DC. Columbia University Press, New York

Kempton, W. (1978) *Sexuality and the Mentally Handicapped*. (Nine sets of slides). Concord Films Council, Ipswich

Longo, R.E. and Gochenour, C. (1981) Sexual assault of handicapped individuals. *Journal of Rehabilitation*, **47**, 24–27

Nirje, B. (1969) The normalisation principle and its human management implications. In *Changing Patterns in Residential Services for the Mentally Retarded* (eds Kugel, R.B. and Wolfensberger, W.), President's Committee on Mental Retardation, Washington DC

Rea, N. (1973) Point of view. *British Journal of Mental Subnormality*, **36**, 3–6

Russell, D.E.H. (1986) *The Secret Trauma: Incest in the Lives of Girls and Women*, Basic Books, New York

Sebba, J. (1981) Sexuality and mental handicap – a report of the Winifred Kempton Workshops. *Apex*, **8**, 116–118

Sebba, J. (1985) Sexuality and Mental Handicap: A Review. In *Current Issues in Clinical Psychology* (ed. Karas, E.), Plenum, New York

Shearer, A. (1972) *A Right to Love*, Mencap/Mind, London

Schor, D.P. (1987) Sex and sexual abuse in developmentally disabled adolescents. *Seminars on Adolescent Medicine*, **3**, 1–7

Special Children (1987) AIDS: fear of mental handicap in children. *News*, **8**, 4

Taylor, S. (1989) How prevalent is it? In *Child Abuse and Neglect: Facing the Challenge* (eds Stainton Rogers, W., Hevey, D., and Ash, E.), Batsford, London

Ultman, M.H., Belman, A.L., Ruff, H.A. *et al.* (1985) Developmental Abnormalities in infants, and children with AIDS and AIDS related complex. *Developmental Medicine and Child Neurology*, **27**, 563–571

Watson, G. and Rodgers, R. (1980) Sexual instruction for the mentally retarded and normal adolescent. *Health Education Journal*, **39**, 88

Wish, J.R., McCombs, K.F. and Edmondson, B. (1980) *The Socio-Sexual Knowledge and Attitudes Test*, Stoetling Company, Chicago

Wolfensberger, W. (ed.) (1972) *Normalisation: The Principle of Normalisation in Human Services*, National Institute on Mental Retardation, Toronto, Ontario

16

Community integration

Roy McConkey

'Our goal is to see mentally handicapped people in the mainstream of life, living in ordinary houses, in ordinary streets, with the same range of choices as any citizen, and mixing as equals with the other, mostly non-handicapped, members of their own community.'
(*An Ordinary Life*, King's Fund, 1981)

For the past 200 years or more, people with a mental handicap have been isolated from the rest of society. Families felt the stigma of having an imperfect child and cut themselves off from their neighbours as a way of hiding their shame. Or the infant was 'put away' into institutional care in settings which were geographically isolated and self-contained. The public rarely ventured in and the patients had no need to go out.

Even when attitudes changed and services shifted from care towards training, the isolation continued. Special schools and centres were provided exclusively for the 'mentally handicapped'. Although such services could address this group's special needs, the inevitable consequence was that children with this disability continued to be isolated from their non-handicapped peers. Adult persons in particular were given few opportunities to share in the working or leisure life of their community.

Such a state of affairs still seems normal, even unavoidable. The reason for it is confidently stated – their disability demands it. These citizens have neither the intellect nor the social competence to cope with normal society. Hence the attitude that 'it's better for them to be sheltered with their own kind'.

This reasoning soon becomes a self-fulfilling prophesy. The people are judged to be socially incompetent and they are then kept apart from society; which of course ensures that they have no opportunity of becoming socially competent! It's like blaming a non-swimmer for his incompetence having banned him from ever using the swimming pool!

Social isolation produces handicaps

But more than that, instead of the disability causing the social isolation it is likely that some of the handicaps these people experience actually *result from* the social isolation which these people have had forced upon them. This viewpoint has been consistently argued by Zigler (and many others) from the 1960s onwards. His careful research into the effects of institutionalization showed clearly the depressing effects it had on the residents' performance on cognitive and social tasks (Zigler, 1969). Removing the social isolation should – and does – reduce their handicaps.

Gold (1975) tried to capture this thinking in his new definition of mental handicap. His starting point is to view this disability as part of the human condition and to dispense with hypothetical concepts such as intelligence to explain their differences from 'normal' people. Instead he argues that what distinguishes them is their 'level of functioning which requires from society, significantly above average training procedures and superior assets in adaptive behaviour, manifested throughout life.'

In short, it is society's response that determines whether or not a person with this disability becomes handicapped. Hence the emphasis in modern services on individual training and the need for greater community involvement.

The right to an ordinary life

Arguably though, the most effective challenge to the social isolation of disabled people has come NOT from specialists or service providers – often they have a vested interest in maintaining the status quo – but it has come from parents and the disabled people themselves. Their case was simple; these human beings have the same rights as any other.

The International League of Societies for Persons with a Mental Handicap succeeded in persuading the United Nations to pass a resolution (No. 2856) on the declaration on the rights of mentally retarded persons (20 December 1971) which states in its preamble, 'the necessity of assisting mentally retarded persons to develop their abilities in various fields of activities and of promoting their integration as far as possible in normal life.'

Subsequent American and British legislation has opened up more opportunities for integration, in education for example, while the rise of parent groups and self-advocacy movements internationally has increased the pressure for community initiatives in housing and employment.

A new service philosophy

Community-integrated services are not merely an alternative way of providing help to clients. Rather they are based upon a different set of principles which have been summarized best by the 'ordinary life' group of the King's Fund Centre (Towell, 1988) as follows:

1. People with learning difficulties (mental handicap) have the same human value as anyone else and the same human rights.
2. Living with others within the community is both a right and a need.
3. Services must recognize the individuality of people with learning disabilities.

Years of tradition cannot be unwound quickly. Community integration of people with mental handicap has taken root and it promises to become the dominant service philosophy in the early decades of the next century. Yet much remains to be done in order to make it a reality for everyone with this disability, irrespective of where they live in the United Kingdom. Equally important, the non-handicapped community needs to be prepared for life with a disabled person.

In this chapter we describe the extent of the social isolation experienced by people with mental handicap, outline ways whereby the community can become more accepting of persons with this disability and explain new styles of services in the community, including family support services, which aim to give people who are mentally handicapped a greater involvement in society. The implications for staff roles and the management of services are also discussed.

A life apart

This section reviews the numbers of people who continue to live in institutional care; the social isolation that can be experienced by people with mental handicaps while living in the community and the reactions of the general public to mental handicap.

Institutional care

Although the majority of persons with a mental handicap now live in the community, the number of adult persons residing in special institutions ('hospitals') remains unacceptably high despite governmental intentions to shift the balance of care towards the community. The latest figures suggest that 31 400 persons in England and 1640 persons in Wales are in institutional care while in Scotland the figure stands at 5400. A national survey undertaken in Scotland in 1984 of all adults persons in receipt of services (Baker and Urquhart, 1987) estimated that there were proportionately 42% more people in hospital care in Scotland than in England and 62% more than in Wales.

The Scottish survey describes the mental handicap hospitals as being situated on large campuses, on the outskirts of towns or cities or even deep in the country. They therefore tend to be relatively inaccessible to such features of daily life as shops as well as to training, leisure and recreational facilities. The hospitals ranged in size from 20 to 1070 beds with a median of 172. At the time of the survey some 96% of hospital residents were living in sex-segregated ward settings. Seventy-six wards in 16 hospitals had 30 or more residents; the largest ward had 60 persons. The average length of time residents had been in hospitals was 18 years; but over 1000 had lived there for 30 or more years with some exceeding 60 years – a lifetime apart. A similar picture has been painted of institutions elsewhere in Britain (Alaszewski, 1986).

Such living conditions make it virtually impossible to overcome the residents' social isolation. The solution – in part at least – is their transfer to community living settings which should meet the criteria set out in the Jay Report (1979); namely 'the accommodation we provide should be, in terms of size, design and location, as much like the accommodation we ourselves would wish to live in.'

The advent of special financial benefits – Board and Lodging allowances – from central government has increased markedly the numbers of people now residing in ordinary houses within the community. In addition to the benefits of living in a more homely environment, such houses offer the residents many more opportunities for sharing in the life of the community. However as we shall see, community placement does not mean community integration.

Living in the community

Nearly all British children with a mental handicap now grow up in an ordinary family home; mostly with their natural parents, others with foster or adoptive parents. Likewise when they become adults, they often continue to live at home and to attend day centres (e.g. adult training centres). If an out-of-home placement becomes necessary, parents would prefer for their son or daughter to live with another member of the family or in a supervised ordinary house in the community (McConkey and Concliffe, 1989). Admission to a special hospital is the least preferred option.

But solving the problem of geographical isolation does not guarantee the handicapped person's social integration. Surveys of teenagers with Down's syndrome in Hampshire (Buckley and Sacks, 1987); of teenage pupils in special schools (severe learning difficulties) in Manchester (Cheseldine and Jeffree, 1981) and of young adults in Ireland (McConkey and Conliffe, 1989) highlight their dearth of friends and lack of involvement in community activities even though all were living at home with families.

'We would describe most of the teenagers as socially isolated, with few real friends or social activities outside school. While they had the normal range of teenage interests they were rarely able to actively pursue them by going to discos or playing sport out of school. Most of their time was spent in passive and solitary activity.'
(Buckley and Sacks, 1987, p. 138)

The young people are equally aware of their isolation. 'I had friends when I was small, friends down the road. They are grown up now, they are working .... They have families and are gone out of my life.' (Roche, 1981).

Likewise, merely locating services such as day centres or hostels in the community has not produced social integration. Surveys in Dublin (McConkey, 1987) and London (Locker, Rao and Weddell, 1981) found that only one in twenty of the immediate neighbours of a community residence had ever been inside it and only one in fifty had been visited in their homes by a resident from the home. In fact, more than half the neighbours had never even talked to one of the residents although they had seen them around the area.

When Atkinson and Ward (1987) talked to 50 people in Somerset who had been relocated in community dwellings from a mental handicap hospital they found wide variations in the different kind of social relationships that had developed from 'very, very happy' to 'very, very lonely'. Although most were relatively happy with their new situation, only five of the 50 had moved on from acceptance in the community to becoming active participants in the network of neighbourhood relationships.

Community contact with mental handicap

If people with a mental handicap are isolated from the local community then the converse is equally true: people in the community have been isolated from those with a disability. National opinion polls bear this out. At best one in eight people report regular contact with a person who has a mental handicap and over half have never met anyone with this disability. Such isolation is the prime breeding ground for myths and stereotypes to develop – they're violent; sexually promiscuous.

More pertinently, it can lead to people being reluctant to have contact with the 'stranger' who has a mental handicap. A MORI opinion poll carried out in Britain for Mencap (1982) found that one of the main concerns people expressed at the prospect of having two adults with a mental handicap move in next door to them, was that 'they would feel awkward in their presence'. A Birmingham woman expressed her thoughts thus, 'We don't know how to cope with them. We're not used to their ways. But if they were integrated into society more then we would learn to cope with them, instead of them being shut away in places.'

If half the population are uncomfortable or embarrassed at meeting a person with mental handicap, as this poll suggests, then it is likely they will avoid being in their company. More pertinently, they could mobilize opposition to having community services sited in their locality.

. An Irish national survey explored this issue in detail (McConkey, 1990). The opinions of people living in the vicinity of nine staffed group homes for people with a severe mental handicap were contrasted with those of people from a comparable housing estate in which there was no group home. People who had experienced living beside neighbours with a mental handicap reported many fewer problems arising than those anticipated by people living in areas where there was no group home (Table 16.1).

The people in the community who were found to be most apprehensive about the effect the home would have on the community tended to be over 60 years of age; they had had no local contact with a person who had a mental handicap and they had resided in that area for less than 5 years.

But even in areas where a group home had been running successfully for 2 or more years, the two main problems reported by at least one in five of the neighbours interviewed, were not knowing how to react when they met a person from the home and the feeling that the residents of the home were isolated and kept to themselves. The people with mental handicap may be living in the community but they are not always part of it.

The lesson is clear; community integration can never come about solely as the result of preparing the person with disability for living 'independently'. His or her new neighbours also need opportunities for overcoming their fears and anxieties

Table 16.1 Percentage of people perceiving problems arising from a group home in their locality

	No group home (N=615)	Group home (N=426)
Problems for the person with mental handicap:		
They would be teased	46	16
They would be victimized/picked on/ taken advantage of	30	7
Isolated/kept to themselves	37	22
Inadequate professional care and supervision	13	5
Problems for the neighbourhood:		
People embarrassed/don't know how to react	36	22
A danger/threat to children	11	1
Mentally handicapped people violent/irresponsible	10	2
Property value of houses would fall	9	1
They would be noisy/create disturbances	9	1

if they are to be prepared for a life together. It is ironic that so little has been done to address this issue. The reason will probably become clear as we explore it further; community education is proclaimed to be everyone's responsibility and hence it is nobody's!

Educating the community

Educating the public on how to get on with disabled people is not easily done. These people differ greatly in personality, abilities and interests. There is therefore no correct way of interacting with them. Moreover disputes exist among professionals and parents as to what is best for people with disabilities. Some say they need only love and care in the security of familiar surroundings, whereas others maintained that they need to get out and about, doing as much as they can for themselves.

But perhaps the most telling argument against giving the public directives on how they should act towards disabled people, is that it would emphasize how different they are and could unwittingly create an even greater barrier! We don't do it for other groups in society – immigrants, old folk, itinerants – so why pick on the disabled?

Yet research has shown that once people find they can get on with disabled people, they are much more positively disposed towards them. Rokeach (1973) has proposed that the attitudes we hold towards other people, are in fact reflections of our own self-concept. If we feel badly about ourselves – for example 'I'm afraid of meeting mentally handicapped people' – then our attitudes towards them will be coloured accordingly. But, he argues, if people's self-concepts can be changed for the better – 'I can get along with mentally handicapped people' – more positive feelings will be expressed to this group. Change has first to occur in the person, before there is a shift in attitudes.

This viewpoint flies in the face of traditional wisdom that attitude change results from giving people lots of information about the disability; hence the call for more television programmes, radio advertising and poster displays! If Rokeach is right then these ventures are a waste of money. They remain attractive to many because they are an easy option and because they help to confirm the beliefs of the converted – parents and staff. Yet there is little evidence that they result in changes in people's behaviour; an outcome also found in many health education campaigns.

Changing people to change attitudes

One consensus from the international research into the factors that produce an attitude change towards disabled people is the experience for the able-bodied of actively interacting with peers who are handicapped. They note too that it is the *quality* of contact rather than the quantity of contact that is important and they warn that certain contacts may actually increase rather than decrease the public's negative impressions.

The features that have produced positive changes in attitudes can be summarized as follows.

Planned personal contact – In many instances mentally handicapped people are their own best ambassadors. They win people over if the meeting proves enjoyable and non-threatening. This is more likely achieved if:

1. They meet in ordinary places rather than in specialist centres. Hence in an adult education programme on mental handicap, participants met the residents from a group home in the local pub (McCormack and McConkey, 1983).
2. The people should share an activity together rather than relying solely on conversation. For example, teenagers who joined in physical activities and cooperative games with handicapped peers showed changes in attitudes (Salend, 1981) whereas participation in class discussions had no effect (Siperstein, 1977).
3. The people from the community may need an opportunity to prepare themselves for the meeting. One way of doing this is to show them a video of people like themselves interacting with mentally handicapped people similar to the ones they are likely to meet (Dowrick, 1983).
4. It is best if people's first contact is with individuals with whom they can communicate relatively easily. As their confidence increases they can be introduced to more severely handicapped people.

Contrast these guidelines with most people's introduction to mental handicap – a guided tour of a mental handicap centre. Research in the USA suggests that such tours rarely change people's attitudes and they may in fact reinforce people's negative beliefs (LeUnes, 1975).

Tours do *not* allow members of the public to meet people with disabilities at a personal level. They do not allow them to share a common activity and little preparation is given to reduce the apprehensions of the tourists other than the assurance that the staff will be on hand to 'protect' you.

Afterwards the tourists often enthuse about the facilities and the dedication of the staff and perceive them in a more positive way, but invariably the tour only serves to emphasize the disabilities, not the personalities, of the people observed. They leave with their own inadequacies highlighted, 'I could never do that work', and as Rokeach predicted, thinking less well of the handicapped people. Of course, tours of centres need not be like that, if some thought and effort were put into them. But too often staff are so preoccupied with getting the work done that the tours have to be completed as fast as possible.

Fortunately the solution is simple; it is much better for meetings to occur in community settings where the public can feel more at home. For instance, an education programme about mental handicap aimed at fifth year pupils in secondary schools, involved a group of young adults from the local training centre visiting the school for a club and sports session. Afterwards the pupils showed marked increase in their confidence at meeting a person with mental handicap, and these improvements were maintained 3 months later (McConkey, McCormack and Naughton, 1983).

Target groups

The second key to more successful community education is to direct the message to target groups rather than the community in general. That is key people who could have a particular influence on the lives of people with a mental handicap. This would include shop assistants, clergy, police and local politicians. The educational inputs can then be attuned to these people's particular interests and concerns and can be put over concisely.

For example, here are some of the strategies which have been suggested for educating neighbours of proposed or newly established group homes (Hogan, 1986):

1. Give the 'new' neighbours the opportunity to visit similar residences and to meet people with a mental handicap there.
2. Have the prospective residents already engaged in some pursuits within the district before they move in, e.g. doing voluntary work or using the leisure facilities.
3. Organize presentations and workshops for civic, community and church leaders with people who have a mental handicap as panellists.
4. Neighbours from a group home in another area could be invited to share their experiences either via video or by talking at a group meeting.

Community education of this sort does require extra efforts. But these are much less intensive than the preparation required to prepare the person with a handicap for life in the community. If only some of that effort were to be directed at local people, the prognosis for community integration would be so much better.

Here we come to an impasse. The staff in services for people with mental handicap are rarely given the opportunity to spend time meeting the community whereas those who are presently engaged in community work have little understanding of the needs of people with mental handicap. This vacuum cannot continue if the goal is to be community integration; an issue to which we will return later.

Care by the community

Thus far we have described ways by which the community can become more tolerant of people with a mental handicap. But in itself that is but a prelude to community integration. The next step is to explore the possibility of some people from the community becoming helpmates of a person with a mental handicap; providing some of the support and guidance which they frequently need, at least in the early phases of community life.

This is radical thinking. Over the years, but especially since the establishment of the Welfare state in Britain, the 'community' has enlisted and paid an increasing number of special people to do the job of looking after the handicapped; nurses, teachers, auxiliaries etc. Latterly the professional ranks have been swollen by an influx of new specialisms and teams. No one can dispute the tremendous contribution they have made but as financial restrictions take hold, it is evident that there never will be sufficient professional staff to meet the needs.

Nor would it be desirable. As the Independent Development Council for People with Mental Handicap (1982) observed 'excessive reliance on separate, specialist services is both expensive and wasteful and serves to segregate people with mental handicap from community life.'

The alternative is to explore other sources from which help could come. The most obvious has been the services provided for the community as a whole. In the main this has meant educational and related services. The pros and cons of integrated education will be debated for many years to come but two areas have been particularly successful in accommodating to the needs of people with mental handicaps.

1. *Integrated pre-schools* – Parents value greatly the social benefits of children attending neighbourhood playgroups. The Preschool Playgroups Association actively encourages their members to enrol children with disabilities and

provides excellent literature and training courses. Likewise an increasing number of nursery schools cater for these children, so much so that the proportion of pre-schoolers in specialist services has dropped markedly.

2. *Further education* – The opportunity in recent years for young adults with a mental handicap to continue their education through Colleges of Further Education has increased their opportunities of participating in courses alongside their age peers. Openings are now also available on Government Training Schemes.

But society does not provide comparable services to meet the other needs of people with mental handicaps – housing, employment and leisure. So what is to happen when no community service exists or if it does, it is frequently overworked and under-resourced?

Person-to-person services

First we need to be clear about the type of service that best suits these people. Four features have been emphasized in recent years:

1. *Individualized* – Services should be organized to meet the needs of the individual rather than to cater for groups of people. A great deal of emphasis is now placed on having Individual Programme Plans for clients. The home-based teaching services which are now widely available to families soon after the birth of a handicapped baby are one of the major success stories of modern services (Pugh, 1981).
2. *Personalized* – The person's social and emotional needs must not be overlooked. Also the people providing the service are more significant than the building in which the service is located. There is now a greater consciousness of the need to assess a person's quality of life and to look at their total lifestyle.
3. *Localized* – The service should be available in the client's neighbourhood so that there is a greater chance of them remaining part of their community. Bussing children across the city to special schools and adults to training centres has invariably fractured their social contacts. Moreover the service does not in any sense 'belong' to that community in that few if any of the local people avail of it. It is not surprising then if contacts with local people are few.
4. *Normalized* – In the sense that disabled people are provided with a range of experiences which are commensurate with those of their able-bodied peers and wherever possible, they should use existing general services with extra help as they need it. Service evaluation tools such as PASS (Wolfensberger, 1972) have highlighted the devaluing practices of much current service provision.

A service based on these four attributes is far removed from that on which services have been traditionally organized – schools, day centres and hospitals. Moreover it is very unlikely that these systems will ever be able to adapt to these new ideals. The constraints of precedent, management structures and staffing conditions are not easily broken. Rather, new models of services are needed.

Family care

The most effective model to date is care within the family. Parents provide the individualized and personal care that professional staff find difficult to emulate. It is community based and most strive to make their family life as normal as possible.

What is often forgotten is that such care is provided by people who are untrained (and unpaid) and who before the child was born, had little or no prior experience of mental handicap. These ordinary men and women from the community have not only learnt to cope but they have become the child's teacher, nurse and therapist as well.

We must not underestimate the stresses which some parents have to cope with – double incontinence in a multiply handicapped teenager; children who suddenly scream and kick in public places or the overactive child who knows no dangers and needs to be constantly watched. As one mother put it, 'I belt to the loo and belt back down again because he'll have done something naughty in the space of time it takes me to get up and come down again. It is the constant attention ... you have to be there. During the holidays and weekends he sends me up the wall.'

The brunt of care falls on mothers. Various surveys have come up with strikingly similar results in terms of the proportion of fathers who never help – for example 94% don't help with washing and ironing; 71% with toileting the child; and 44% with baby-sitting. Nor can men use work as the excuse; unemployed fathers provided the least support. Rather the reason has more to do with the traditional sex roles in our society (Wilkin, 1979).

The majority of mothers also receive little help from neighbours or other family members; the most commonly given reasons being that they didn't need it or they had never looked for it. Said one mother, 'I'm too proud, I wouldn't ask anyone. I have four sisters and I never asked and none of them offered to take her.' Another instance of how society's attitudes affect families.

Family support services

A priority in community care services must be to support families in caring for their handicapped offspring. There is widespread agreement internationally as to the form these supports should take (WHO, 1985):

1. *Short-term breaks* – The child or adult is cared for outside of the family to give the parents a break. This could occur regularly, say one week in four, or for a set period each year while the family take a holiday. When a respite care service was implemented in Exeter the number of requests for admission to full-time residential care dropped markedly (Brimblecombe, 1983). Mental handicap hospitals and hostels have provided these facilities in the main but in recent years they have been supplemented by fostering schemes and by voluntary agencies.
2. *Day care* – Although most developed countries provide schooling for children with special needs, the same opportunities are not always available to families in the adult years. Hence the provision of out-of-home facilities is most important especially when the adult has behavioural or intensive care needs.
3. *Counselling and advice* – Families need access to medical and psychological advice both in regard to their child and their own well-being. In addition therapists and social workers can provide much useful practical guidance and assistance. A 'named' person or 'key worker' gives the family a defined link with services.
4. *Financial support* – The additional costs of rearing a child with a disability are well established – in clothing, medicines, diet, laundry, etc. A range of benefits

are now available to families both from the state and from charities, such as the Rowntree Trust. These can cover alterations to the home and the provision of special equipment.

Family care is the most cost-effective community service. The danger is that it is taken for granted and families are left to struggle on with little or no assistance in times of financial stringencies.

Leaving home

A second danger is also becoming apparent. Ageing parents are still expected to care for their sons and daughters who may be into their forties and fifties. Although many do so willingly, it may restrict the handicapped person's options and prevent them developing a life of their own. It may also mean a painful transition when their parents die (Richardson and Ritchie, 1986).

Hence parents may need to be encouraged to plan for their sons and daughters leaving home just as happens with their non-handicapped brothers and sisters. But it is not easy for them to do this. One mother expressed the dilemma thus, 'I don't want them to think I'm pushing my child on ... I don't want them to think I'm saying, "Please will you take her?".'

Others are confident that they offer a better life; 'We can give her a lot more love than she can get outside. Home life is much more stable.'

Card (1983) points out that the onus in our culture is for adolescents to break away from the parents' protection. As this initiative is usually not taken by teenagers and adults who are mentally handicapped, 'the parents are not prepared to face the pain and loss involved in readjusting to a new and more separate relationship with their adult offspring'. Richardson and Ritchie (1986) found that many elderly parents were isolated and had no one among the family or friends with whom they could explore these issues and little help was forthcoming from professional sources.

However, those families who used short-term care regularly were more disposed to contemplating a move away from home, having been reassured that their son or daughter could live happily elsewhere. Thus the family supports listed earlier are applicable to all families. The immediate challenge must be to extend them throughout the community to all families caring for a handicapped member.

Foster-care

But what if families are no longer able or available to cope? Could it be that other people from the community, rather than professional staffs, might undertake to help in similar ways? The answer is an unequivocal yes. The growth throughout Britain of foster-care and adoption schemes for children with mental handicaps is clear evidence that there are people willing to share their lives in this most constant and intimate way. Of course such schemes require diligent planning and monitoring by specialist staff to safeguard the individual's interests, and special fostering allowances are usually paid. Indeed it is essential that all the supports offered to natural parents are made available to foster families.

These new 'residential' services have been a huge success – not only in the quality of care which the families provide but also in the value for money which they offer. It can be four times more costly for a child to live in a special centre than with a foster family.

In recent years fostering has been extended to cover teenagers and adults with a mental handicap. Barnardo's in Liverpool have found foster-homes for youngsters with profound and multiple handicaps while their Fred Martin project in Glasgow has placed with families ex-residents in their late teens and twenties from a mental handicap hospital. Similar schemes for adult persons are well established in the USA (Sherman, Frenkel and Newman, 1984).

Finally, many more people have volunteered to provide short-term – 'respite' – care for children with handicaps. These schemes give the family a chance to have a break while the child is cared for in a family setting rather than being admitted to a hospital-type environment. Their potential too for effective community education should not be overlooked. One foster mum told Walsh (1986):

> 'Yesterday at the zoo was the most emotionally draining experience I have ever had. How do you cope with the way people stare? I was not embarrassed; I just didn't know how to deal with their lack of tact.'

In recent years these care schemes have developed into many other variants, such as looking after the child for variable lengths of time, even just part of day, or a person going to stay in the child's home when the parents are away.

All these schemes embody the four essential attributes noted earlier – they provide a service that is individual, personal, local and normal. Nor is it care *in* the community; it is care *by* the community.

A caring community

Given the success of fostering schemes, is it possible that ordinary people could be recruited to provide other forms of help which in the past have been done by specialist staff? The experience from numerous 'demonstration' projects suggests that it is viable. Here are examples of other 'person-to-person' schemes now operating in Britain and Ireland:

1. *Home teaching* – Volunteer 'teachers' have been recruited to visit the child or adult at home to give individual tuition with language skills (in liaison with a speech therapy service) or to help with reading and writing, along similar lines to adult literacy schemes.
2. *Home aides* – People have been recruited to help families in the care of their handicapped son or daughter. They attend when the person returns from the day centre or school and they may stay until bedtime. In addition to helping with the general caring chores at home – feeding, bathing – they may accompany the person for leisure activities.
3. *Open employment* – The Pathway scheme developed by Mencap facilitates the placement of adults with a mental handicap in open employment by recruiting a 'helper' from the workforce who undertakes to keep an eye on the new employee and to smooth his or her integration with the other workers. Under these arrangements there has been a dramatic increase in the number of sustained placements in open employment.

   Similarly an Irish scheme recruited volunteer helpers to train adults with severe mental handicaps on-the-job for work in local services, such as fast-food outlets. Once the person became more familiar with the job, the trainer gradually withdrew (de Lacey, 1988).

4. *Evening classes* – Adult persons with a mental handicap have been able to join in a range of evening classes through having a specially recruited 'companion' with similar interests enrol in the class with them. The helper provides extra assistance for the student and reassurance that the class tutor does not have to cope alone.
5. *Befriending schemes* – These can take many forms. A pool of people can be recruited and paired with a person with mental handicap to accompany them for leisure pursuits and thereby increase their involvement in community activities. Other schemes have sought to introduce the person with a handicap to a particular hobby or sports club. The idea being that just as these people need extra help in looking after themselves at home or in education, so too they need help at making acquaintances and developing friendships (Walsh, 1986).
6. *Independent living* – University students living away from home share accommodation with handicapped adults, who are fairly competent at looking after themselves but benefit from having somebody around in case they get into difficulties. This arrangement eliminates the costs of employing staff.

Likewise, a person with mental handicap might continue to live on in the family home after the death of a parent with a neighbour providing a home-help service (Shennan, 1983).

As this listing demonstrates, schemes of this sort can address many of the needs which traditional services have ignored. Through them it has become possible for the person with mental handicap to gain employment, develop friendships and to take part in leisure pursuits. The goal of an ordinary life has started to become a reality, albeit for a few.

Making these schemes work

All these schemes involve a new type of volunteer helper. Out goes the image of the 'do-gooder' to be replaced by that of a 'benefactor', Edgerton's term for people in the community who befriended ex-patients of institutions and who were 'very successful at providing affection with respect'.

These helpers often receive payment for their work; although rarely is it sufficient to become a living wage. However, it recognizes the worth of their work and enables contractual arrangements to be drawn up that overcome the unreliability associated with voluntary commitment.

Five key features underpin all these schemes:

1. *Person-to-person commitment* – In all of them the first priority is to establish a link between the helper and an individual person or family, rather than with a centre or building.
2. *Support and back-up is readily available* – Professional staff have often been the instigators of these services and they have shouldered the job of advertising, recruiting and selecting the helpers. But their job cannot end there. The helpers must have a professional confidant, guide and supporter. This relationship is crucial. They need time to get to know one another and for trust to develop. The flow of information should be two-way and the supporter should take responsibility for maintaining contact rather than leaving it to the helper.
3. *Phased selection of helpers* – The need for helpers can be widely advertised without committing a service to taking on board all those who apply. Complete

openness is essential when it comes to describing what the helpers are expected to do. They must be under no illusions about what they are letting themselves in for. A useful approach has been to phase the selection over a number of weeks, so that those who are not keen to continue can opt out. This period of time also gives the professional staff an opportunity to detect unsuitable candidates and redirect them elsewhere.

4. *Time-limited commitment* – The helper's initial commitment should be limited to a stated period of time or to a number of visits. If at the end of this time they do not want to continue, they can bow out gracefully knowing they have fulfilled their undertaking and nobody has been let down. Equally if they want to continue, a new 'contract' can be entered into, which could redefine the amount of commitment the helper will give.

5. *Assumed competence* – None of the helpers receive prolonged training. Rather it is presumed that their 'commonsense' is sufficient and by-and-large this has proved to be the case. Opportunities need to be provided though for the helpers to discuss and share the problems they encounter. More formal training opportunities, with an emphasis on practice rather than philosophy, have also proved beneficial.

A feasible alternative?

The presumption thus far, is that people from the community will be found in sufficient numbers to make it possible to instigate and sustain such schemes throughout the country. Unfortunately we lack the experience as yet to pinpoint the circumstances which ensure both the success of these schemes with a range of clientele and the provision of a dependable and permanent service. We do, however, have a number of useful pointers.

First, there is evidence that as many as one in four people would be receptive to an invitation to help. A national survey in Ireland quizzed over 1000 people about their willingness to help adults with a mental handicap who lived in their immediate neighbourhood. The characteristics which most distinguished the willing from the unwilling were that they had had past experience of doing voluntary work with people who had a mental handicap; they were married with children under 16 years of age; in the past they had regular contact with people who had a mental handicap; they had a relative living in their neighbourhood; they were under 40 years of age and they were female (McConkey, 1990). Hence these people's interest was not just based on altruism but they had experience to draw upon. These findings also reinforce the need for personal contacts as a central plank, in community education.

Second, many of these schemes were set up outside of existing service structures using special funds, e.g. Urban Aid grants. The great risk is that once such funding finishes the new schemes may have to fold. Hence secure funding is an obvious prerequisite to ensuring continuity and such schemes must be integrated into health and social service budgets.

Third, the schemes are very time-intensive to set up and may show little pay-off in the initial stages. Often the personnel running the scheme have had to carry other responsibilities while gaining expertise in new areas, such as getting to know the local communities and effective advertising. Personnel will need to be recruited to develop and support such services.

The widespread establishment of these types of community involvement schemes has profound implications for the roles of professional staff within mental handicap services and for how such services are presently structured. We shall examine each of these in turn.

New styles of services

The shift towards care in the community has left unchanged many of the management and staffing structures found in institutional settings. The community hostel can be run as a mini-hospital and the adult training centre as an extension of social service bureaucracy. Indeed the worse features of institutionalization are associated more with staffing practices and roles than with the physical locations of services (King, Raynes and Tizard, 1971).

Staff roles

Successful community-based services in housing, employment, education and leisure have helped to define new roles for professional staff. In summary these are:

1. Staff are assigned to work with particular individuals with whom they are encouraged to build up a relationship; e.g. as keyworkers. The numbers of people assigned to any one staff member will be small but they are responsible for identifying that individual's particular needs and working towards meeting them.
2. Staff are not employed on the basis of their qualifications but rather on the functions they fulfil. Thus the title 'home leader' is used in community residences rather than 'staff nurse'. As we have seen, many people can successfully fulfil helping roles without any prior qualification.
3. The staff are dispersed over a range of community settings rather than gathered into specialist centres. Although this has the danger of staff feeling isolated, adequate support and advisory structures can mitigate this problem. The chief advantage is the scope it gives staff for furthering integration through informal (or formal) community education initiatives.
4. The staff (and their clients) are given a major say in how the service functions. Decision-making is devolved with management fulfilling a supportive rather than directive role.
5. The full-time staff of services can be supplemented by part-time paid workers (such as family aides) and voluntary helpers. Hence the total numbers of people involved in service provision can be large and demands particular skills in people management and the coordination of service inputs.

This profile of staffing is very different to that found in many existing services. The transition can prove difficult; particularly for staff who were recruited for a particular job which they fulfilled satisfactorily for many years but now that job no longer exists.

This issue highlights the need for ongoing staff development within services; a much-neglected area. Mansell (1988) rightly argues for the small-scale incremental approach in which the good ideas of a few people are nurtured and sample projects encouraged so that people see examples of new, and good, practices and the benefits which flow to clients and staff alike. 'Thus attempts to clarify and reinforce particular views and attitudes (about service philosophies) follow, rather than precede, involvement in new ways of working'.

Staff training also has to break away from the narrowly defined areas of skill acquisition or attitude change aimed at front-line personnel and become embedded in the whole process of service development that spans planning, management and delivery. Consequently training will probably be on a multi-disciplinary, multi-agency basis and with an agenda derived from the needs of clients in that particular area. The Open University course, 'Patterns for Living' is an example of this style of training.

An unresolved issue is the role of pre-service training, such as a nursing or social work qualification in community services. At present promoted posts often depend on people having such a qualification. This disadvantages staff who have shown their competence through working in the service and who, perhaps because of family commitments, would never be able to undertake full-time training courses.

'Distance learning' packages on a modular basis, which could be combined with supervised practice to give a nationally recognized qualification, is one possible solution. Pre-service training would then become less important.

Management of community services

It will not be easy to develop a new style of service management. The long-term dependency of these clients makes them unique in our society. The variations among individuals is very great and ideally the service should be attuned to each person's needs and be sufficiently responsive so that as their needs change, so too does the service. Moreover a range of services are needed to cover the diverse needs of this client group for accommodation, employment, education and leisure.

Management structures used in hospitals, education or industry are unlikely to prove suitable for this task and yet up to the present that is all we have had to go on. At this point in time it is easier to describe the attributes which the management of services has to attain than to prescribe how it can come about:

1. Comprehensive local services will have to be planned and managed by different agencies – health, local authorities and voluntary bodies. Appropriate methods have to be devised for collaborative work at different levels from the top down.
2. At a regional level, 'a strategic framework should be developed to provide leadership on the policies relating to the direction and rate of change; resource allocation; planning and management arrangements, manpower developments and support for innovation' (Towell, 1988).
3. A high emphasis must be placed on consultation and participation with service users; families and the local communities. Among other things, this will necessitate decentralizing operational management to a local level so that a high degree of personal contact is possible between managers and 'consumers'.
4. Service structures need to clearly specify job roles and reporting responsibilities and include mechanisms for reviewing progress and ensuring the quality of service delivery.

Throughout Britain there is a great deal of variation among services in the way community developments are managed. In time, we will be able to identify the critical features of effective management but for the present we may have to tolerate and forgive the mistakes made – provided the managers learn from them.

Nor should we under-estimate the challenge which lies before us. Mansell (1988) argues that the effectiveness of services can be measured by the kind of lifestyle they enable people to have. 'Good services enable people, whatever their disabilities, to participate in a full range of household and community activities, to continue to develop their expertise and confidence ... and to build up and maintain a network of supportive friendships and relationships'. Barely a generation ago, such words would have been pious hopes. Today they have become the reality for some. Who knows what the future will bring?

References

Alaszewski, A. (1986) *Institutional Care and the Mentally Handicapped: The Mental Handicap Hospital*, Croom Helm, London

Atkinson, D. and Ward, L. (1987) Friends and neighbours: Relationships and opportunities in the community for people with mental handicap. In *Re-assessing Community Care* (ed. Malin, N.) Croom Helm, London, pp. 232–248

Baker, N. and Urquhart, J. (1987) *The Balance of Care for Adults with a Mental Handicap in Scotland*, ISD Publications, Edinburgh

Brimblecombe, F.S.W. (1983) *Honeylands Progress Report, Paediatric Research Unit, Exeter*, Royal Devon and Exeter Hospital

Buckley, S. and Sacks, B. (1987) *The Adolescent with Down's Syndrome: Life for the Teenager and for the Family*, Portsmouth Polytechnic, Portsmouth

Card, H. (1983) What will happen when we've gone? *Community Care*, **28**, 20–21

Cheseldine, S. and Jeffree, D.M. (1981) Mentally handicapped adolescents: their use of leisure. *Journal of Mental Deficiency Research*, **25**, 49–59

de Lacey, E. (1988) Developing community involvement in services. In *Concepts and Controversies in Services for People with Mental Handicap*, (eds McConkey, R. and McGinley, P.), Brothers of Charity, Galway; pp. 277–298

Dowrick, P.W. (1983) Self-modelling. In *Using Video: Psychological and Social Applications*, (eds Dowrick, P.W. and Biggs, S.J.) London, Wiley, pp. 105–124

Edgerton, R. (1967) *The Cloak of Competence*, University of California Press, Berkeley

Gold, M. (1975) *An Alternative Definition of Mental Retardation* (Unpublished paper, Institute for Child Behaviour and Development), Urbana-Champaign

Hogan, R. (1986) Gaining community support for group homes. *Community Mental Health Journal*, **22**, 117–126

Independent Development Council for people with mental handicap (1982) *Elements of a Comprehensive Local Service for People with Mental Handicap*, King's Fund Centre, London

Jay Committee (1979) *Report of the Committee of Enquiry into Mental Handicap Nursing and Care, Vol. 1*, Cmnd 7468-1, HMSO, London

King's Fund (1982) *An Ordinary Life: Comprehensive Locally-Based Residential Services for Mentally Handicapped People*, 2nd edn, King's Fund Centre, London

Kings, R.D., Raynes, N.V. and Tizard, J. (1971) *Patterns of Residential Care: Sociological Studies in Institutions for Handicapped Children*, Routledge and Kegan Paul, London

LeUnes, A. (1975) Institutional tour effects on attitudes related to mental retardation. *American Journal of Mental Deficiency*, **79**, 732–735

Locker, D., Rao, B. and Wedell, J.M. (1981) Changing attitudes towards the mentally handicapped: The impact of community care. *Apex: Journal of the British Institute of Mental Handicap*, **9**, 92–93, 95, 103

McConkey, R. (1987) *Who Cares? Community Involvement with Handicapped People*, Souvenir Press, London

McConkey R. (1990) A national study of community reactions to groups homes: Contrasts between people living in areas with and without group homes. In *Key Issues in Mental Retardation Research* (ed. W.I. Fraser) Methuen, London

McConkey, R. and Conliffe, C. (eds) (1989) *The Person with Mental Handicap: Preparation for an Adult Life in the Community*, St Michael's House, Dublin

McConkey, R. and McCormack, B. (1983) *Breaking Barriers: Educating People about Disability*, Souvenir Press, London

McConkey, R., McCormack, B. and Naughton, M. (1984) Preparing young people to meet mentally handicapped adults: A controlled study. *American Journal of Mental Deficiency*, **88**, 691–694

McCormack, B. and McConkey, R. (1983) Changing attitudes to mental handicap through an adult education course. *Public Health*, **97**, 352–362

Mansell, J. (1988) Training for service development. In *An Ordinary Life in Practice: Developing Community Based Services for People with Learning Disabilities* (ed. Towell, D.) King Edward's Hospital Fund, London, pp. 129–140

Market and Opinion Research International (MORI) (1982) *Public Attitudes Towards the Mentally Handicapped: Research Study Conducted for Mencap*. Mencap, London

Pugh, G. (1981) *Parents as Partners: Intervention and Group Work with Parents of Handicapped Children*, National Children's Bureau, London

Richardson, A. and Ritchie, J. (1986) *Making the Break: Parents' Views about Adults with a Mental Handicap Leaving the Parental Home*, King's Fund Centre, London

Roche, F-Lundstrom (1981) *Our Lives*, Irish Committee for the International Year of Disabled People, Dublin

Rokeach, M. (1973) *The Nature of Human Values*, Free Press, New York

Salend, S. (1981) Cooperative games promote positive student interactions. *Teaching Exceptional Children*, **13**, 76–78

Shennan, V. (1983) *A Home of Their Own*, Souvenir Press, London

Sherman, S.R., Frenkel, E.R. and Newman, E.S. (1984) Foster family care for older persons who are mentally retarded. *Mental Retardation*, **22**, 302–308

Siperstein, G. (1977) Effects of group discussion on children's attitudes toward handicapped peers. *Journal of Educational Research*, **70**, 131–134

Towell, D. (ed.) (1988) *An Ordinary Life in Practice: Developing Community Based Services for People with Learning Disabilities*, King Edward's Hospital Fund, London

Walsh, J. (1986) *Let's Make Friends*, Souvenir Press, London

Wilkin, D. (1979) *Caring for the Mentally Handicapped Child*, Croom Helm, London

Wolfensberger, W. (ed.) (1972) *The Principle of Normalization in Human Services*, National Institute on Mental Retardation, Toronto

World Health Organisation (1985) *Mental Retardation: Meeting the Challenge*, WHO, Geneva

Zigler, E. (1969) Developmental versus difference theories of mental retardation and the problem of motivation. *American Journal of Mental Deficiency*, **73**, 536–556

17

Resettlement

P.A. Woods and P.J. Higson

Resettlement is a term that has generally come to mean the transfer of residents from large residential institutions (e.g. mental handicap and mental illness hospitals) to alternative residential provision outside of those large institutions, in community living arrangements. Unfortunately, definitions seem to be very unclear in this area as exemplified by the ill-defined boundaries between institutional care, residential care, and community care (Sinclair, 1988). Resettlement programmes have recently been said to '. . . involve considerable change in the way that welfare bureaucracies organize their resources' and to be driven by a moral imperative 'which is . . . about including the excluded in the process of everyday life' (Burton, 1989).

In this chapter we want to examine some of the issues in the process of resettlement from *institutional care* to *community care* and, in particular, we will focus on the two key elements of type of residence and the nature of associated care and support services that people move into. Other major issues concerned with the *process of change* and the ramifications of large hospital contraction and closure have been examined and discussed elsewhere (e.g. Korman and Glennerster, 1985) and will not be covered in this chapter.

Philosophies, policies and practice

Until the 1960s people with a mental handicap in the UK either lived at home with their families (often in intolerably stressful circumstances for all involved) or in long-stay custodial care institutions. The latter were predominantly large mental handicap hospitals, many of which are still with us today. However, in the 1960s and early 1970s, in the wake of the *deinstitutionalization* movement in the USA (Bruininks *et al.*, 1981), a number of experimental projects were initiated in different parts of the country which attempted to develop alternatives to the large long-stay institutions. The Wessex Experiment (Kushlick, 1970), for example, made use of 25-bedded community units and demonstrated that smaller scale residential care, even for people with severe and profound mental handicaps, could be provided in towns and villages amongst local communities.

The growth of board-and-lodging and nursing homes took place in this period also, a trend supported by authors such as Craft (1976), who promoted the transfer of residents from a mental handicap hospital to such alternative custodial care environments. Some of the common themes of the boarding-out, community-unit and other *ad hoc* schemes included:

1. A reduction in the average number of people who lived together.
2. A move away from isolated locations to accommodation in the midst of local communities.
3. An attempt to provide a style of life which approximated that of 'the normal population' more than life in a large institution.

The term *community-based* was frequently used to describe schemes that demonstrated these themes but as Blanch, Carling and Ridgway (1988) have commented, 'Policymakers of the time defined *community-based* as anything other than state hospitals'. National policy guidance was clearly set in the direction of *community care* with the publication of the 1971 White Paper, *Better Services for the Mentally Handicapped*. However, as Atkinson (1988) noted, its interpretation of that concept differed from those taken in more recent policy documents as it advocated the development of 25-bedded local authority hostels as part of this policy. Indeed, that size of residential provision was recommended throughout the 1970s and into the early 1980s by the National Development Team whose favoured model of service revolved around 24-bedded *community units* (Simon, 1980).

In the last 10 years the average size of *progressive* community care accommodation has gradually reduced through averages of six (e.g. Mathieson and Blunden, 1980; Mansell *et al.*, 1987) to that of two or three unrelated people in *shared-living* arrangements in an *ordinary house*. On the way there have been a variety of *core-and-cluster* models, half-way houses, and more recently life-sharing schemes (Harper, 1989) for individuals with a mental handicap have been experimented with.

Least restrictive environments

Since the early 1970s, a concept that has guided the development of services for people with various disabilities in the USA has been the principle of the least restrictive environment (LRE). Its origin was a proposal by Reynolds (1962) for a continuum of placements in an ordered sequence that vary according to their degree of restrictiveness. It is generally presented as a hierarchical rank-ordering of facilities and services running from the most to the least restrictive alternative (e.g. Sehalock, 1983). Degrees of restrictiveness are generally correlated with integration, normalization (see Chapter 0), and the level and intensity of staffing support (see Taylor, 1988). An example of an LRE continuum of residential provision for people with a mental handicap in the UK might look like that shown in Figure 17.1.

Much of the legislation passed in the US Congress in recent years concerning people with disabilities implicitly endorsed the LRE principle and veered policy towards a traditional model which assumed that every person with a disability could be located somewhere on the LRE continuum according to an assessment of their skills and individual needs. If and when the person developed additional skills, and reached a degree of proficiency, the criterion was met for *transition* to a less restrictive placement (Hitzing, 1987).

However, major criticisms of the underpinning assumptions associated with the LRE principle have been levelled in relation both to services for people with psychiatric disabilities (e.g. Blanch *et al.*, 1988) and to people with mental handicaps (e.g. Taylor, 1988). Bronston (1980), for example, noted the confusion in the LRE concept between a person's need for appropriate accommodation and

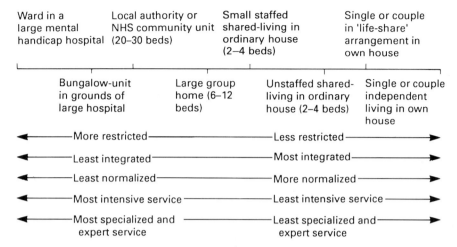

Figure 17.1 A residential care continuum for people with a mental handicap in the UK

their need for care and support. The LRE principle confuses segregation/ integration with intensity of services by assuming that the least restrictive, most integrated settings are incapable of providing the intensive support services needed by people with severe disabilities (Taylor, 1988). In so doing, it directs attention to physical settings rather than to the services and supports that people need to be integrated into local communities.

Because the LRE principle contains a presumption in favour of the least restrictive environment, it legitimates more restrictive environments by implying that there are circumstances under which they would be appropriate. It considers that a person should *be prepared* before they move to a less restrictive environment. Durand and Neufeldt (1980) noted that '...the continuum places an emphasis on creating opportunities that allow the handicapped person to graduate from a segregated to a progressively more integrated setting, to move from a controlled and sheltered environment to one that is progressively less sheltered ... and from a state of dependence to increasing independence' (p. 289). However, more reviews of the literature do not support the assertion that the more restrictive placements prepare people for least restrictive environments; institutions do not prepare people for community living (e.g. Wilcox, 1987), segregated day programmes do not prepare people for competitive work (e.g. Bellamy *et al.*, 1986), and segregated schooling does not prepare pupils for integrated schooling (e.g. Brown *et al.*, 1983).

Integration in non-restrictive environments

In recent years there has been a growing opposition to the LRE principle which is characterized by an unconditional commitment to full integration for all rather than merely a presumption in its favour. Leading protagonists such as Hitzing (1980, 1987) have proposed the placement of people in *natural settings* with an array of support services (of varying degrees of intensity and expertise) determined by their needs. This shift in emphasis to providing *non-restrictive environments* for all, has been contrasted with the LRE principle as moving (Taylor, 1988, p. 51):

1. From the development of facilities and programmes into which people must fit to the provision of services and supports necessary for people with severe disabilities to participate fully in community life.
2. From neighbourhoods to typical homes, from regular school buildings to regular classes, and from vocational models to typical jobs and activities.
3. From professional judgement as a basis for determining community involvement to personal choice.
4. From a presumption in favour of integration to a mandate to provide opportunities for integration.
5. From a conditional ('to the extent necessary, appropriate, feasible') to an unconditional commitment to integration.
6. From requiring individuals to change in order to participate in the community to requiring service systems to change.
7. From restrictions applied categorically as a condition for receiving services to opportunities available to non-disabled people.
8. From disability labels as a factor in determining community participation to a recognition of common human needs.
9. From independence to community belonging.
10. From placing people in the community to helping them become part of the community.

In the UK the thrust towards an unconditional commitment to full integration for all has found expression in policy initiatives such as the King's Fund Centre's *Ordinary Life* proposals (1980), and the *All Wales Strategy* (Welsh Office, 1983). These and other contemporary policy documents emphasize the basic human rights of people with a mental handicap and include three fundamental principles which can be summarized as:

1. A right to lead a life that is 'ordinary' in terms of the 'norm' for the locality in which he or she lives, and the culture that he or she embraces.
2. A recognition that within all local communities and cultures there will be variations from the 'norm' in terms of aspirations, interests, wishes, aptitudes, values and a range of idiosyncrasies that all individuals have to varying degrees. The right to the range of choices that are usually open to people in all aspects of life should also be made available to people with a mental handicap.
3. A recognition that simply providing opportunities to participate in ordinary life activities in local communities, even when a full range of choices that reflect individual preferences, etc., are provided, though necessary, is not sufficient to ensure that people with a mental handicap will be able to participate fully and derive feelings of fulfilment, satisfaction and self-esteem, etc., generally associated with a good quality of life. They will need to receive additional support, training, reassurance and guidance from others to help them acquire practical 'competencies' which in turn will lead to greater confidence, independence, acceptance, integration and the development of a range of positive relationships with significant other people.

Throughout the 1980s community care politics in England have predominantly been manifested as large hospital closure programmes with *resettlement into ordinary houses in the community* being stated as the principal vehicle to achieving this objective. The sheer scale of some of these exercises has been vast compared with the pilot schemes of the 1970s (such as the Nimrod scheme (Mathieson and Blunden, 1980) and the Andover project (Felce *et al.*, 1984)).

However, closer examination of the English hospital closure programmes reveals that claims that they are part of the broad *community care* developments fall short of the mark. Wertheimer (1986) surveyed all NHS mental handicap hospitals and units in England whose complete closure had been approved between May 1979 and March 1985. She found that less than 6% of the ex-hospital residents had moved into *community living in staffed or unstaffed ordinary houses*, but a startling 68% had been transferred to other hospitals, and 17% to NHS hostels or community units! Similarly, Williams (1987) reported that the closure of Starcross Hospital in Exeter had been achieved with only 18% of the former residents moving into community living arrangements: 40% had been transferred to other Exeter hospitals and 36% had been *repatriated* to hospitals in their *area of origin*.

Korman and Glennerster (1985, 1990) provided detailed accounts of the planning and implementation processes involved in closing the 1000 bedded Darenth Park Hospital in Kent. They provided statistical details of the alternative living arrangements to which the former residents of the hospital transferred, amongst which were several 24 bedded hostels and *residential centres* catering for as many as 77 and 80 places! It has to be conceded that several English regions are genuinely trying to achieve their hospital closure plans entirely through resettlement into community living schemes in ordinary houses, but from our vantage point behind Offa's Dyke, we count our blessings that *repatriation* and *24 bedded residential units* do not feature in the *All Wales Strategies* for mental handicap (Welsh Office, 1983) and mental illness (Welsh Office, 1989).

The facility-based approach: staffed group homes

A range of housing arrangements have been employed in the various relocation programmes, but the majority of community living schemes have used staffed and unstaffed group homes. Gathercole (1981) described a staffed group home as '. . .an ordinary domestic scale house in which not more than five or six people who are mentally handicapped live together, cared for by a number of paid staff.' A summary of the main features of the housing and care and support staffing arrangements that are now in common practice in the English resettlement programmes is as follows:

1. There is an emphasis on resettlement to 'areas of origin' which is related largely to regional health authority policies involving transfer of resources on a geographical basis. Although there are no explicit requirements for hospital residents to return to their areas of origin (and indeed there are many examples of where this has not been the case) in the vast majority of cases, the resettlement opportunities that have been 'offered' have been limited to those areas.
2. A range of care and support service providing agencies can be involved including: (a) local authority social services, (b) health authorities, (c) voluntary organizations, and (d) private organizations. Sometimes these support service agencies also provide the housing and sometimes they form a partnership with a separate housing providing agency (e.g. a housing association). In very few situations are the residents the legal tenants or owners of their own houses.

3. In an attempt to maximize the financial resources available to cover the costs
   of both housing provision (e.g. to pay rents, mortagages, etc.) and support staff,
   many of the group homes have been registered as Residential Care Homes or
   Nursing Homes, thus accessing the higher DSS benefits that are available. A
   consequence of this arrangement is that it is the support service providing
   agency (a local authority, health authority, voluntary or private organization)
   or a housing partner agency (e.g. a housing association or housing trust) that
   owns or rents the accommodation. As such it is the agency who controls who
   lives there, and with whom, rather than the residents.

Racino (1988) and Taylor, Racino and Rothenberg (1988) have criticized the
commonly adopted *facility-based* approach to community living, which is still
widespread throughout Britain, on the grounds that there is a tension, and at times
a conflict, between genuine individual needs planning and the funding regulations
and constraints for community living arrangements. To some extent this argument
parallels what the Griffiths Report (1988) referred to as the *perverse incentive* that
DSS Residential Care Benefits provide, in which the funding is tied to the facility,
not the individual and his/her care needs. Amongst the disadvantages to *individual
service users* listed by Taylor *et al.* (1988) were:

1. 'Since providers own or rent the residential setting, they ultimately control who
   lives there.'
2. 'Staff are employed by and accountable to the agency, rather than the people
   receiving the services. The staff's relationship with people is defined by the
   conditions of employment created by the agency and staff.'
3. 'As a good general rule, people in the group [home] receive the level of
   supervision required by the person with the most intensive needs. To the extent
   that an individual has more or less intensive needs than others, he or she may
   not "fit into the program".'
4. 'In order to receive care and support services from a provider, people must live
   at the provider's facility … . Funding is based on the needs of the facility rather
   than the individuals [which]… does not allow for or extend to a person's
   transition into his or her own home.'

Flexible and individualized community living arrangements

In contrast to the facility-based approach is what has been termed the individualized or *person-centred approach* to community living. A key feature of this
approach is the *separation of housing and support*. The importance of this
separation was presented in a manual prepared by Options in Community Living
(a community support agency in Madison, USA) as follows:

'. . . One agency should not provide both housing and support services. While
we often advise and assist clients in funding, renting and furnishing their
apartments, Options no longer becomes the leaseholder or the landlord for client
apartments. We want our clients to feel both control over and responsibility for
their own living spaces. We also believe that receiving Options' services should
not affect where clients live; our clients have a greater choice of living situations
and know that beginning, ending or changing their relationship with us will not

put them under any pressure to move. This policy also frees us from the time-consuming responsibilities and sometimes conflicting relationships involved in being a landlord.'

(Johnson, 1986)

Racino (1988) lists the key elements of a person-centred approach to community living, in which the housing and care support components are separated, as providing:

1. *'Choice in housing* – The person can select from a variety of housing choices, depending on his or her particular circumstances.'
2. *'Choice of home location* – The person can choose where he or she wants to live, including the specific neighbourhood.'
3. *'Choice of living alone or with others* – Because the location and number of people is not predetermined, there is greater flexibility in determining how many people will live together.'
4. *'Choice of room-mate [house-sharers]* – The person can have greater choice of with whom he or she will share living arrangements.'
5. 'Ownership and leasing [tenancy] have both legal and personal ramifications. [It] means that it is the person's home first and foremost. It is a place where staff, rather than the person, can be asked to leave.'
6. *'Individualized supports* – Unlike the typical approach of fitting a person into existing programmes, individualization in this situation means tailoring to or developing the supports that will best match the person and his or her current life circumstances. . :. The individualized nature of the support is typically accomplished through the establishment of an array of possible supports/ services that can be accessed by the person – in any combination.'
7. *'Flexible supports* – Flexibility means the supports must be able to be adjusted in a timely way both in kind and in intensity. Thus . . . when a person needs more [,less,] or different supports, he or she can continue living in the same place, but the supports can be changed.'

A person-centred approach in post-Griffiths Britain?

As noted previously, most of the resettlement schemes that have been developed in the UK through the 1980s have followed the facility-centred approach and thus denied service users many of the advantages of a person-centred approach to community living listed above. Group homes have been both owned (or leased by) *and* staffed by health authorities, local authorities, private (for profit) organiza-tions, voluntary organizations (e.g. Mencap Homes Foundation), and in some cases by Housing Associations and Housing Trusts. To a large extent, though not totally, this state of affairs has been determined by the pressures to maximize funding and the consequent constraints placed upon funding arrangements. Flexibility in care support provision, for example, has been virtually impossible to achieve for a variety of reasons, but principally because our funding and service delivery systems are often not designed to adapt and change at the pace that people's needs change.

The Government response to the Griffiths (1988) and Wagner (1988) reports, *Caring for People: Community Care in the Next Decade and Beyond*, was published in November, 1989. The main proposals outlined in this White Paper (DOH, 1989, p. 4) are that:

'The Government believes that for most people community care offers the best form of care available – certainly with better quality and choice than they might have expected in the past. The changes outlined in this White Paper are intended to:

● Enable people to live as normal a life as possible in their own homes or in a homely environment in the local community.
● Provide the right amount of care and support to help people achieve maximum possible independence and, by acquiring or reacquiring basic living skills, help them to achieve their full potential.
● Give people a greater individual say in how they live their lives and the services they need to help them do so.'

The White Paper adds in the same section (DOH, 1989, p. 5) that:

'The Government therefore believes that the key components of community care should be:
● Services that respond flexibly and sensitively to the needs of individuals and their carers.
● Services that allow a range of options for consumers.
● Services that intervene no more than is necessary to foster independence.
● Services that concentrate on those with the greatest needs.'

The White Paper then describes the main changes in the funding arrangements and organization of service delivery, together with changes in agency and staff responsibilities which are needed to achieve the objectives listed above. It is clear that this policy is guided by two main aims: the need to achieve better value for money from the current amounts expended through the Department of Social Security, the National Health Service and Local Authorities on community care; and the need for an increase in the cost benefits (i.e. the quality) derived from this public expenditure.

This shift in emphasis is not unique to community care and is characteristic of changes being brought about in every area of public spending. In the context of 'Caring for People' it is intended to achieve this change by clarifying the process of identifying the needs of *vulnerable* individuals and making a distinction between the purchasers of services and the providers. Whilst recognizing that many agencies will for the time being undertake both activities, the longer term objective is to achieve a clear split.

It is also clear from the White Paper that there will not be any substantial increase in the total amounts of public expenditure made available for community care and there will be a greater emphasis upon the wider involvement of the whole range of public and private sector agencies than hitherto. Whilst it would appear therefore that the Government intends to put in place new funding and organizational arrangements which will help to achieve a more individualized and person-centred approach to community care, this has to be offset against a very real attempt to cash limit these services. This tension will inevitably effect the decisions which *purchasers of care* and *case managers* will have to make. A recent economic evaluation of the costs of closing mental handicap hospitals and transferring people to community care (Glennerster, 1990, p. 142) concluded that

'. . .planners should expect the costs of new small scale facilities to be higher than the costs of hospital care'.

How therefore within this new scenario will the person-centred approach to resettlement fare? Most professionals (and consumers!), we are sure, would subscribe to this approach, but with 30 000 people with a mental handicap still resident in long-stay institutions, can this be achieved within the resource constraints which will continue to exist no matter which 'colour' the Government is? The choice seems to be clear – to either progress with a person-centred and thus potentially expensive approach, or to reach a compromise way forward without prejudicing the basic principles of such a philosophy of care. Put another way – can we afford to sustain a 'Rolls-Royce' approach while thousands of people continue to live in the twentieth-century equivalent of workhouses? What should our priorities be within the context of this reality?

If we are not to return to the facility-based approach then some practical framework has to be arrived at to translate the person-centred approach into a reality and thus guide these decisions. One approach might be to re-examine the notion of an ordinary life. If we look around us we see an almost infinite variety of living arrangements which people have *chosen* for themselves, although in most instances these choices are limited by available disposable income and also reflect our society's changing pattern of values towards issues such as marriage and parenthood. Hitherto the ordinary life approach to resettlement has been directed towards some notion of an ideal existence which may or may not reflect the actual real world. Of course professionals seek the best outcome for their clients and no one would advocate placing people in less than suitable accommodation, but it is unclear what actually does guide these decisions other than an implicit set of ideals.

It might be more useful to set out a framework, however crude, to assist these decisions in an attempt to maximize the gain for the greatest number of clients in the new post-Griffiths world. Such a possible framework could be derived from an examination and assessment of the local social and housing structure of any target resettlement area. At the very least this would provide a backdrop against which individual needs assessments could be set in reading decisions about the most suitable (not necessarily the most ideal) resettlement solution for a client. This information is readily available in statistical form from local authority planning departments as they too need these data to guide decisions about housing, schools, roads, etc. Local authorities have to make decisions continuously about public expenditure and reconcile competing priorities, all of which affect people's lives. Furthermore, the availability of this information might also aid the emergence of more innovative solutions to resettlement and integration as outlined in a recent Audit Commission report on developing community care for adults with a mental handicap (Audit Commission, 1989).

The same type of methodology might also be useful for informing decisions about the level and type of support each individual will receive after leaving institutional care. Here again any realistic attempt to achieve a person-centred approach must be within the context of what ordinary people do in their daily lives and what expectations they have of the community around them. Some real information about real communities is urgently needed to provide a framework for decision making.

Already we can hear the protests that any less than 'ideal' outcome for an individual with a mental handicap represents a compromise to be avoided as it implies a cost cutting or saving approach to care. Meanwhile 30 000 people continue to live in long-stay institutions and the resources available for resettlement are cash limited. Do we not also have a responsibility to achieve a better way of life for them in their lifetimes, even though it might mean some radical re-thinking about the resettlement process, but without returning to facility-based types of solution?

Conclusions

In this chapter we have tried to review the changes in thinking that have taken place in recent years with respect to resettlement, while at the same time acknowledging that to a great extent this process is determined by the availability of public expenditure. We have also attempted to reconcile the cash limited reality of our services with the need to do the most good for the most people – a timeless dilemma which is becoming much more explicit within the new framework set out in *Caring for People*. We recommend that within a person-centred approach to community care there needs to be a set of ground rules concerning how decisions about resettlement are made and that these should be derived from accurate information about the current social structure, nationally and locally, rather than from a nebulous set of ideals about an ordinary life. In this way we might just be able to improve the quality of life available to all people with a mental handicap in the foreseeable future rather than a small minority, as is the case at present.

References

Atkinson, D. (1988) Residential care for children and adults with mental handicap. In *Residential Care: The Research Reviewed* (ed. Sinclair, I.), HMSO, London

Audit Commission (1989) *Developing Community Care for Adults with a Mental Handicap*, HMSO, London

Bellamy, G.T., Rhodes, L.E., Bourbeau, P.E. and Mark, D.M. (1986) Mental retardation services in sheltered workshops and day activity programs: Consumer benefits and policy alternatives. In *Competitive Employment Issues and Strategies* (ed. F. Rusch) Paul H. Brookes, Baltimore, pp. 257–272

Blanch, A.K., Carling, P.J. and Ridgway, P. (1988) Normal housing with specialized supports: A psychiatric rehabilitation approach to living in the community. *Rehabilitation Psychology*, **33**, 47–55

Bronston, W. (1980) Matters of design. In *Towards Excellence: Achievements in Residential Services for Persons with Disabilities* (eds Apolloni, T., Cappuccilli, J. and Cooke, T.P.), University Park Press, Baltimore, pp. 1–17

Brown, L., Ford, A., Nisbet, J., Sweet, M., Donnellan, A. and Gruenwald, L. (1983) Opportunities available when severely handicapped students attend chronological age appropriate regular schools. *Journal of the Association for the Severely Handicapped*, **2**, 195–201

Bruininks, R.H., Meyers, C.E., Sigford, B.B. and Lakin, K.C. (1981) *Deinstitutionalization and Community Adjustment of Mentally Retarded People*, American Association on Mental Deficiency, Washington DC

Burton, M. (1989) *Australian Intellectual Disability Services: Experiments in Social Change*, King's Fund Centre, London

Craft, M. (1976) The North Wales Guardianship Scheme. *Apex*, **4**, 19–21

Department of Health and Social Security (1971) *Better Services for the Mentally Handicapped*, Cmnd. 4683, HMSO, London

Department of Health (1989) *Caring for People: Community Care in the Next Decade and Beyond*, HMSO, London

Durand, J. and Neufeldt, A.H. (1980) Comprehensive vocational services. In *Normalization, Social Integration, and Community Services* (eds Flynn, R.J. and Nitsch, K.E.), University Park Press, Baltimore, pp. 283–298

Felce, D., Mansell, J., de Kock, U., Toogood, S. and Jenkins, J. (1984) Housing severely and profoundly mentally handicapped adults. *Hospital and Health Services Review*, **80**, 170–174

Gathercole, C.E. (1981) *Group Homes – Staffed and Unstaffed*, British Institute of Mental Handicap, Kidderminster

Glennerster, H. (1990) The costs of hospital closure: reproviding services for the residents of Darenth Park Hospital. *Psychiatric Bulletin*, **14**, 140–143

Griffiths, R. (1988) *Community Care: Agenda for Action*, HMSO, London

Harper, G. (1989) Life Sharing. *Community Living*, **2**, 6–7

Hitzing, W. (1980) ENCOR and beyond. In *Towards Excellence: Achievements in Residential Services for Persons with Disabilities* (eds Apolloni, T., Cappuccilli, J. and Cooke, T.P.), University Park Press, Baltimore, pp. 71–93

Hitzing, W. (1987) Community living alternatives for persons with autism and behaviour problems. In *Handbook of Autism and Pervasive Developmental Disorders* (eds Cohen, D.J. and Donnellan, A.), John Wiley, New York, pp. 396–410

Johnson, T.Z. (1986) *Belonging to the Community*, Options in Community Living and the Wisconsin Council on Developmental Disabilities, Madison, Wisconsin

King's Fund Centre (1980) *An Ordinary Life: Comprehensive Locally-based Residential Services for Mentally Handicapped People*, King's Fund Centre, London

Korman, N. and Glennerster, H. (1985) *Closing a Hospital: The Darenth Park Project*. Bedford Square Press/NCVO

Kushlick, A. (1970) Residential care for the mentally subnormal. *Royal Society of Health Journal*, **90**, 255–261

Mansell, J., Felce, D., Jenkins, J., de Kock, U. and Toogood, S. (1987) *Developing Staffed Housing for People with Mental Handicaps*, Costello, Tunbridge Wells

Mathieson, S. and Blunden, R. (1980) Nimrod is piloting a course. *Health and Social Service Journal*, **25**, 122–124

Racino, J.A. (1988) Supporting adults in individualized ways in the community. *TASH Newsletter*, **March**, 4–7

Reynolds, M. (1962) A framework for considering some issues in special education. *Exceptional Children*, **28**, 367–370

Schalock, R.L. (1983) *Services for Developmentally Disabled Adults*. University Park Press, Baltimore

Simon, G.B. (1980) *Modern Management of Mental Handicap: A Manual of Practice*, MTP Press, Lancaster

Sinclair, I. (1988) Residential care: Common issues in the client reviews. In *Residential Care: The Research Reviewed* (ed. Sinclair, I.), HMSO, London

Taylor, S., Racino, J. and Rothenberg, K. (1988) Individualization and flexibility in community living arrangements. *TASH Newsletter,***December** , 4–5

Taylor, S.J. (1988) Caught in the continuum: A critical analysis of the principle of the least restrictive environment. *Journal of the Association for Persons with Severe Handicaps*, **13**, 41–53

Wagner, G. (1988) *Residential Care: A Positive Choice*, HMSO, London

Welsh Office (1983) *All Wales Strategy for the Development of Services for Mentally Handicapped People*, Welsh Office, Cardiff

Welsh Office (1989) *Mental Illness Services: A Strategy for Wales*, Welsh Office, Cardiff

Wertheimer, A. (1986) *Hospital Closures in the Eighties*, CMH, London

Wilcox, B. (1987) Why a new curriculum? In *A Comprehensive Guide to the Activities Catalogue* (eds Wilcox, B. and Bellamy, G.T.), Paul H. Brookes, Baltimore, pp. 1–10

Williams, C. (1987) Dissolution of the monasteries: An analogue for community care. Presented at *The Annual Conference of the British Psychological Society, Brighton*

18

Ageing and mental handicap

Joze Jancar

Introduction

Fifty years ago patient mortality was considerably higher in all age groups of the mentally handicapped than in the general population; the difference now is relatively small. These changes have been most marked during the past 25 years because of better medical care, introduction of new antibiotics and anticonvulsant drugs, as well as better diet, care and environment for the mentally handicapped. Longevity in patients with Down's syndrome has increased by an average of 40 years and in other handicapped patients by more than 30 years (Carter and Jancar, 1983).

A recent study by McLoughlin (1988) (Table 18.1) reflects increased mean age at death of the mentally handicapped from studies of the hospital population since 1966.

Table 18.1 Mean age at death of the mentally handicapped

Source	Males	Females
Primrose (1966)	38.5	39.6
Richards and Sylvester (1969)	45.7	52.6
Carter and Jancar (1983)	58.3	59.8
McLoughlin (1988)	62.3	66.2

The increased longevity of the mentally handicapped is bringing with it additional mental and physical disorders and diseases associated with ageing and new problems for the families, carers and planners. Until quite recently the field of ageing of the mentally handicapped was rather neglected.

At the fourth Congress of IASSMD in Washington DC in 1976, it was stated in the paper on Psychiatric Aspects of Mental Retardation:

'With greater life expectancy of the mentally retarded we are faced with new problems of dementia in these patients, in particular senile, cerebral arteriosclerotic and presenile dementia. Patients with Down's syndrome appear to be showing with an increased frequency signs and symptoms of a premature form of senile dementia. Because of the great importance of this topic and sparsity of the literature on the subject, it was suggested to the organizing Committee of the next IASSMD Congress that they include in the programme a Symposium on Senescence and Mental Retardation.'

At the same congress a paper on 'Cancer and Mental Retardation' was presented and reported the increase of cancer in the ageing mentally handicapped (Jancar and Jancar, 1977).

At the Congress of IASSMD in New Delhi in 1985 and in Dublin in 1988 there were symposia on ageing included in the programme and many very relevant papers presented.

During the congress in New Delhi, the World Health Organization released a publication, 'Mental Retardation: Meeting the Challenge' in which one of the chapters highlights the magnitude of the problem of the ageing mentally retarded:

'Little attention has so far been given to the needs of the ageing and elderly mentally retarded. The mentally retarded in developed countries now live longer than previously, mainly as a result of improvements in both general health care and specific health care. This has resulted in there being many more elderly mentally retarded people than were expected by the earlier service planners. Little is known about the process of ageing in the mentally retarded, but it is likely that the range of individual variation is even greater than among the non-retarded population. For example, many younger adults with Down's syndrome have been reported to show symptoms of pre-senile deterioration compatible with a diagnosis of Alzheimer's disease.'

(WHO, 1985)

During the eighties a number of papers on the subject of ageing appeared in the world literature including two books and a monograph: *Ageing and Developmental disabilities – Issues and Approaches* (Janicki and Wisniewski, 1985), Monograph on Medical Aspects of Ageing in the Mentally Handicapped (Jancar, 1987) and Ageing in Mental Handicap (Hogg *et al.*, 1988). A detailed clinical study of the elderly mentally handicapped in Northgate Hospital was published by Day in 1987.

In 1987 a National symposium, *Ageing in the Mentally Handicapped – A Multidisciplinary Approach*, took place in Bristol where 24 professionals presented the papers. The parents and carers also participated.

There has been much debate in the literature about what age should be used to denote ageing of the mentally handicapped population. The majority of workers agree that the line should be lower than for the non-handicapped population. Some authors have suggested lowering the age criterion to 40 years (Day, 1985; Aitchison *et al.*, 1989; Jancar, 1989); while Janicki (1984) and Hogg *et al.* (1988) are in favour of including all people over 50 years of age. A number of authors are retaining the statutory age boundaries (60–65 years) which apply to the non-handicapped population.

The evidence of premature ageing, particularly in Down's syndrome, osteoporotic bone changes in the pre-menopausal and menopausal periods in females and other physiological and neurological changes in some cases, warrants caution not to accept arbitrary criteria of the ageing index until a general agreement is reached, but to look for early signs and symptoms of ageing in the individual adult patient.

It is well established that, in the general population, females live longer than males. The pattern appears to be substantially the same in the mentally handicapped population (Primrose, 1966; McCurley *et al.*, 1972; Carter and Jancar, 1983). A review in 1984 of the total mentally handicapped population in the Stoke Park Group of Hospitals in Bristol revealed an interesting sex distribution. Under 40 years of age there were 189 males and 131 females (total 320) and over 40 years of age 366 males and 365 females (total 731) – females living longer (Figure 18.1).

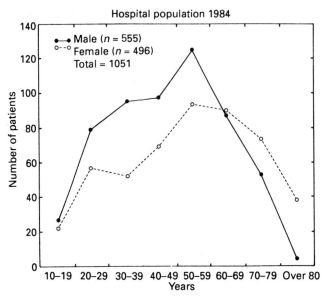

Figure 18.1 Total population in four hospitals in 1984 (Reproduced by permission of the editor of the *British Journal of Mental Deficiency Research*)

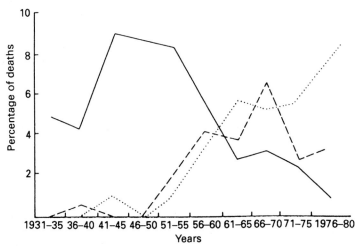

Figure 18.2 Three types of sudden death, 1930–1980: . . . . = myocardial infarction; ---- = cerebrovascular accident; ——— = status epilepticus

In the same year the first female reached 100 years of age. In 1987 there were 36 females and 10 males who were over 80 years of age and three females over 90 years of age.

Apart from increased longevity, the Stoke Park survey shows a marked change of causes of death over the past 50 years. Although tuberculosis is no longer a major cause of death, other terminal respiratory tract infections are still prevalent in the mentally handicapped. Deaths from status epilepticus have decreased, but deaths due to carcinoma, myocardial infarction and cerebro-vascular accident have increased (Carter and Jancar, 1983) (Figure 18.2).

Physical and mental disorders and diseases associated with ageing

Psychoses and neuroses

In 1977 Heaton-Ward undertook an investigation of psychiatric illness occurring in the 1251 mentally handicapped adults at the Stoke Park Hospitals. The prevalence of psychosis and neurosis combined in his survey was 10%. The age of onset of the manic-depressive cases was in the third, fourth and fifth decades in males, and in the fourth, fifth and sixth decades in females. Other surveys have shown an incidence of psychiatric disorders as high as 60% of the hospitalized handicapped population. The differences in percentage depend on the diagnostic criteria, degree of mental handicap and age of the population surveyed.

In 1979 Jancar studied organic causes of mental illness in the same group of patients and noticed that, in quite a few of them, the onset of psychiatric disorder took place after 40 years of age.

In a retrospective survey of two groups of mentally handicapped patients 40 years of age or older, Day in 1985 found that 30% of the long-stay hospital patients surveyed had psychiatric disorders, as did 20% of patients admitted from the community. He concluded that some of the more idealistic proposals for the development of community care ignore the need for specialist facilities and staff. Neurotic disorder is also a significant problem in mildly mentally handicapped middle-aged and elderly people living in the community, and its occurrence is likely to increase as changes in hospital lifestyle and more importantly the implementation of community care exposes more and more mentally handicapped people to the stresses and strains of everyday living.

In 1986 James studied psychiatric and behavioural disorders among the older severely mentally handicapped in one of the Stoke Park Group of Hospitals. Of the 347 in-patients, 28 of the 50 older patients had received psychotropic medication at some time during the last 20 years.

There was a surprisingly high incidence of affective disorders in this group. In fact, this was due to the persistence of manic-depressive disorders continuing into middle life, and in fact due to new cases of manic depression arising in later life.

Behavioural problems such as aggression and overactivity improved with age in some, but not all, patients.

Cognition and behaviour

Hewitt et al. in 1986 reported a study of 148 patients aged between 65 and 88 in the Stoke Park Group of Hospitals who were psychologically tested over a period of 50 years. They found ongoing intellectual development in adulthood until late middle age, usually followed by a decline in intellectual functioning which became significant in 18% of patients whose intellectual deterioration was associated with deficient self-care skills, poor orientation and staff reports of deterioration. This was not related to previous ability levels or prolonged hospitalization. For the entire sample, competence in self-care skills was high, though behaviour disturbance was present in about half. Results are relevant to the work and training of the elderly mentally handicapped.

Down's syndrome

The suggestion that individuals with Down's syndrome age prematurely is not new. More than a century ago Fraser and Mitchell (1876), in reviewing causes of death in 62 cases of Down's syndrome, commented '. . .phthisis caused a large majority of deaths. In not a few instances, however, death was attributed to nothing more than a general decay, a sort of precipitated senility'.

The first neuropathological evidence of senility in Down's syndrome was presented in 1929 by Struwe. In 1970 Eastham and Jancar reported that macrocytosis increases with age in patients with Down's syndrome.

In 1986 Hewitt and Jancar studied psychological and clinical aspects of 23 Down's syndrome patients aged over 50, who were closely matched for age with 23 non-Down's syndrome patients, and revealed that significant intellectual deterioration had occurred in middle age at an average of 49 years. Intellectual deterioration was independent of sex, initial mental age or length of hospital stay, but was associated with hearing loss, decreasing visual acuity and macrocytosis. Clinically there was no evidence in any patient of active physical illness, focal neurological illness or dementia.

Dupont et al. reported in 1986 a survey based on the Register of all Down's syndrome patients in the Danish National Services for the Mentally Retarded in the period January 1976 to 31 December 1980, followed up until 31 March 1984 (a total of 2412 Down's syndrome patients – 1273 males and 1139 females).

The difference in mortality for the patients in institutions and living outside was significant, with a higher mortality for women with residence in institutions than women living outside. Among males the mortality rate was not significantly different between the two types of residents.

In the study by Baird and Sadovnick in 1988 life expectancy for adults with Down's syndrome was calculated from data of 1610 affected individuals and survival to 68 years of age was predicted.

In 1988 there were 48 Down's syndrome patients in the Stoke Park Group of Hospitals, of whom 24 were over 50 years of age: 18 patients aged 50–59 years and six patients aged 60–69 years. Two male patients died at 68 and 69 years of age respectively.

It has always been thought that Alzheimer's disease and Down's syndrome are linked because the deposits in an Alzheimer's patient look very much like those found in the brains of elderly Down's syndrome patients. The new work focuses on isolation of the gene for B-amyloid protein which is found as deposits in the brains of individuals with Alzheimer's disease and of older Down's syndrome patients. The latest results strongly suggest a defect in a gene on chromosome 21 or its regulation in Alzheimer's disease and points to the over-expressing of this gene as the course of the Alzheimer's disease like histopathological features in Down's syndrome (Fraser, 1988).

Takashima and Becker reported in 1985 basal ganglia calcification in Down's syndrome localized in constant area of globus pallidus and becoming more prominent with increased age.

In 1987 Kinnell et al. studied 111 adult Down's syndrome patients for thyroid dysfunction and found very high rates of thyroid hypofunction (9%), hyperthyroidism (1.8%) and the presence of thyroid microsomal antibodies (29%). They recommended that thyroid function testing should be routine in older Down's syndrome patients, especially in those with microsomal antibodies present.

Cancer

The total number of deaths of mentally handicapped patients at the Stoke Park Hospitals from 1936 to 1975 was 1125. Of these patients 81 (7.2%) died of cancer.

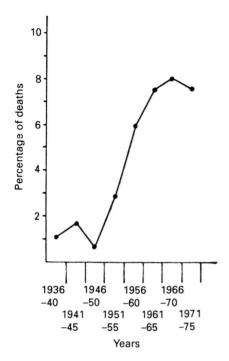

Figure 18.3 The percentage of deaths from cancer of gastro-intestinal tract (males and females) during four decades

From 1956 to 1975 the incidence of cancer, particularly gastrointestinal cancer, was higher than in the normal population (Figure 18.3). Further studies have confirmed this previously reported trend. It is interesting, however, that the average age at death due to carcinoma, which was 56.5 years in previous studies, rose to 65 years in 1982. Similarly the percentage of deaths due to cancer rose from 7.2% to 10.4% which is comparable with the figure of 10.7% reported in the study by McLoughlin in 1988. The increasing longevity of the mentally handicapped population may result in more patients surviving. Nevertheless the increase in particular of gastrointestinal carcinoma may reflect factors other than increasing longevity alone.

Although cholesterol levels in the mentally handicapped were lower than those in the general population, an association was found between relatively low serum cholesterol levels and mortality due to cancer of the colon (Jancar *et al.*, 1984).

In 1980, Jancar studied 288 epileptic patients. No case of cancer of the liver was observed, but one case of hepatoma and one case of carcinoma of the gall-bladder among non-epileptic patients was noted, neither having received any drugs. All the epileptics were taking anticonvulsant drugs for many years. Similarly a number of patients were for many years receiving various tranquillizing drugs for superimposed psychotic illnesses and for severe behaviour disorders. It therefore appears that prolonged use of various anticonvulsant and tranquillizing drugs, sometimes in high dosages, did not have a carcinogenic effect on the liver in the epileptic patients.

Only three patients (two males and one female) had died from lung cancer out of a total of 81 cases of cancer deaths. All the patients had had, as a preventative measure against pulmonary tuberculosis, an annual medical examination and regular chest X-rays, and more recently, frequent mass radiography, therefore very few pathological processes of the lungs would remain undetected. A number of patients in the survey were smokers, some very heavy, smoking both manufactured and home-made cigarettes.

Interestingly, none of the 115 patients in the survey suffering from Down's syndrome died from cancer. However, there was one male patient with some features of Down's syndrome who died of cancer of the stomach and one patient who suffered from cancer of testes (seminoma), and recently another similar case was reported in the literature.

Diabetes mellitus

In a survey of 1116 mentally handicapped patients in 1982, it was found that 23 were diabetic (13 females, 10 males). At the time of the diagnosis the age range was from 24 to 75, with a mean of 56.7 years. Diabetes was associated with the following conditions: Down's syndrome, achondroplasia, Potter's syndrome, tetraploidy, familial microcephaly, atrioseptal defect and Dupuytren's disease. Complications were identified in 34% of patients (repeated infections, hypertension, blepharitis, cataracts, retinopathy and neuropathy). There was a family history of psychiatric disorders in five cases and of diabetes mellitus in two. The prevalence of diabetes mellitus appears to be higher in the mentally handicapped than in the general population.

Diabetes mellitus is believed to represent an heterogeneous group of conditions characterized by a chronically elevated blood glucose. Clinically there are two forms, insulin dependent (IDDM) which is usually of juvenile onset, and non-insulin dependent (NIDDM) which tends to occur in later life. It is thought that these two forms represent different genetic, hormonal and immunological entities. The survey shows three IDDM and 20 NIDDM patients.

With the patients' increasing longevity it is important that diabetes mellitus is detected early and proper treatment instituted (Jancar and Lansdall-Welfare, 1986).

Fractures

A recently concluded survey revealed a high incidence of fractures in 731 mentally handicapped hospitalized patients over 40 years of age (366 males and 365 females). There were 54 males with one or more fractures (72 fractures) and 62 females (110 fractures).

The main known causes of fractures were: osteoporosis, osteogenesis imperfecta, bone dysplasias, epilepsy, neurological lesion and psychotropic drugs. Other mental and physical disorders, diseases and genetic elements contributed to or caused fractures.

The reason to include in the study patients aged 40 years and over is mainly because of the higher incidence of osteoporosis in females. Peak bone mass in both sexes is usually reached at about 35–40 years of age, with women reaching a lower level. They are therefore nearer the critical fracture threshold associated with decreased bone mass and with an accelerated phase peri- and post-menopausally. Elderly women lose on average about 35% of trabecular and 50% of cortical bone mass at their lowest point, compared with no more than a quarter of bone mass lost in elderly men.

In the normal population, the most common fractures in females after 40 years

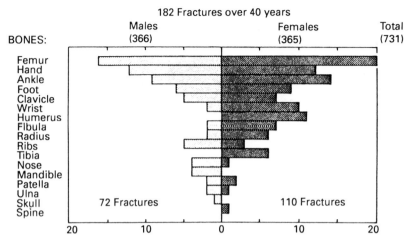

Figure 18.4 Number of fractures and bones involved in males and females over 40 years of age (Reproduced by permission of the editor of the *British Journal of Mental Deficiency Research*)

of age are wrist fractures followed by fractures of vertebral bodies. In our study the most common fractures in females over 40 years of age are hip fractures followed by fractures of metacarpals, ankle, metatarsals, clavicle, wrist and others (Figure 18.4).

To prevent or to minimize osteoporosis leading to fracture, it is essential for mentally handicapped people to be regularly examined physically and mentally to detect early signs of disorder and to provide specialist treatment as required.

Regular exercise throughout later life is essential to help to maintain skeletal mass. Nursing, physiotherapy, chiropody, occupational therapy and games must be provided to all according to their needs. All medication should be constantly monitored and adjusted according to age. Side-effects of drugs should be treated as soon as detected.

Genetic counselling should be available to the families with members suffering from congenital bone dysplasias and other disorders (Jancar, 1989).

Hepatitis B

Between 1976 and 1980 all the patients in the seven hospitals (four from the Stoke Park Group) and seven hostels for the mentally handicapped in the Bristol area were screened for markers of hepatitis B infection. Of 2239 patients, 123 (5.5%) were carriers of hepatitis B surface antigen (HBsAg) and a third of these were 'infectious' (negative for antibody to hepatitis Be antigen). Patients with Down's syndrome were 18 times more likely to be 'infectious' carriers than those without, and male patients were six times more likely to be 'infectious' carriers than female patients. The carrier rate *decreased* with age, but the proportion of carriers who were hepatitis Be antigen positive was *unaffected* by age.

It is therefore very important that monitoring of the hospital and community population of the mentally handicapped for hepatitis B is maintained and vaccination of the patients and staff carried out when appropriate (Clarke *et al.*, 1984).

Dupuytren's disease

In a survey carried out in the Stoke Park Group of hospitals in 1984 it was found that 36 of the 1092 mentally handicapped patients suffered from Dupuytren's disease (22 males, 14 females). Age ranged from 31 to 77 (mean 53.3 years) in males and 32 to 96 (mean 69.1 years) in females. Epilepsy was present in nine males and seven females, two males suffered from fragile X chromosome abnormalities and one female from diabetes. No Down's syndrome cases suffered from Dupuytren's disease, nor have any other abnormalities been detected so far (Jancar *et al.*, 1985).

Drugs

All drugs used for the elderly mentally handicapped population have to be very carefully monitored. Elderly people react to drugs differently because of age-related physiological changes. These include changes in drug absorption, distribution, metabolism, excretion as well as the presence of brain pathology. Therefore adverse drug reactions are more common and sometimes very severe in the aged.

James in 1983 reported a study of 270 patients in the four hospitals for the mentally handicapped who were receiving drugs affecting the central nervous system; 6% of the patients were aged 60 or more. He used modified Michel and Kolakowska guidelines for the reduction in the frequency and amount of drugs used as follows:

1. The need to avoid polypharmacy.
2. The reduction of the frequency of administration of those drugs with long duration of action.
3. A reduction or discontinuation of medication unless there was evidence that it was doing some good.

The study showed that regular and systematic application of simple guidelines for the prescribing and monitoring of drugs affecting the CNS can effect substantial reduction in the amount and frequency of medication and less side-effects of drugs. Considerable savings resulted both in nursing staff time devoted to drug administration and in drug cost.

Eye anomalies

In 1987 a survey of eye abnormalities of the mentally handicapped patients in Stoke Park Hospital was undertaken.

The total population was 367 patients (262 females and 105 males). Of the 367 patients reviewed, 216 were found to have one or more eye anomalies (including Down's group), which shows that more than half the patients suffered from eye disorders (59%).

The prevalence of the following anomalies was presented in detail: strabismus, refractive errors and cataracts. Corneal anomalies, nystagmus, retinopathy, glaucoma and other eye pathologies associated with various syndromes were noted.

Eye anomalies in 31 patients suffering from Down's syndrome in the sample were recorded.

The number of eye anomalies was found to be higher in the ageing group. There were 144 patients over 40 years of age of whom 62 suffered from more than one ocular defect (Figure 18.5).

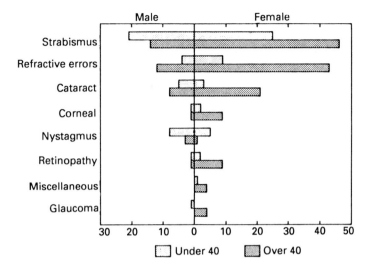

Figure 18.5 Eye anomalies in the hospital population

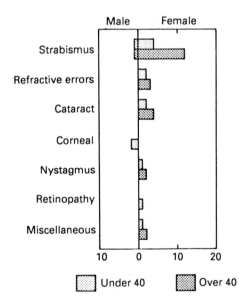

Figure 18.6 Eye anomalies in Down's syndrome patients

There were 26 female and five male patients, ages ranging from 21 to 65, recorded IQ extending from under 15 to 31 with a mean IQ of 19.

Over 40 years there were 19 female and three male Down's syndrome patients, again showing the high percentage of ageing in this group – 71%. The highest percentage was in the 50–60 age groups. Strabismus was the most common defect, followed by cataract and refractive errors (Figure 18.6).

Although this was a small selective study of the mental handicap population suffering from eye anomalies, it highlights the high incidence of pathologies and indicates the need for the regular assessment of the patients' sight and an early detection of diseases and disorders and provision of medical and surgical treatment (Aitchison *et al.*, 1989).

Retinitis pigmentosa (tapetoretinal degeneration) in the ageing mentally handicapped is often associated with blindness, deafness, neurological, psychotic and other clinical abnormalities (Jancar and Walters, 1974).

Defective hearing

In a survey by Cooke in 1988 of 222 patients over 45 years of age, 70 were found to suffer from defective hearing (31.5%), 36 had had an audiogram and 26 had been fitted with a hearing aid, but only seven were wearing one. This indicates one of the difficulties of treating hearing impairment in the elderly mentally handicapped, because of their reluctance to wear hearing aids. Out of 37 patients with Down's syndrome, 14 had various degrees of hearing loss.

Poor aural hygiene is thought to be one factor, as the severely handicapped may be unable to communicate their discomfort when suffering from middle ear infection or canal occlusion by wax, so it is important that their ears are examined regularly. Some conditions that cause mental handicap may also cause hearing deficit, in particular maternal infections such as rubella, but the most significant association is that with Down's syndrome.

The most striking finding in the study was an increasing prevalence of hearing loss with advancing age, and this has significant implications for service provision, with the increasing numbers of elderly mentally handicapped both within hospital and out in the community.

Previous studies have found a positive correlation between the existence of hearing deficit and the development of Alzheimer type dementia. Therefore treatment of a hearing deficit may have an important preventative role to play in this group (Cooke, 1988).

Dental care

The main problem in diagnosis and treatment of dental problems in the mentally handicapped is one of patient management. Very often patients are reluctant, unwilling or unable to communicate their symptoms.

The dental care in the ageing mentally handicapped patients can be discussed under two broad headings:

1. Routine dental care, e.g. construction of dentures, fillings and improving oral hygiene.
2. Specific oral problems, e.g. ulcers, white patches, difficult surgical extractions, fractures, pre-malignant and malignant conditions.

Regular dental examination and care is essential to prevent unnecessary pain and to improve mastication, speech and appearance.

Chiropody

The chiropodist has a great role to play in maintaining mobility and preventing and relieving pain and discomfort in the ageing mentally handicapped people. He or she is able to provide the following services:

1. Palliation of established deformities and dysfunction both as short-term treatment for immediate relief of painful symptoms and long-term management to secure optimum results.

   This requires the backing of effective appliances and footwear.
2. Curative foot care, including the use of various therapeutic techniques including minor surgical techniques such as partial or total nail avulsions, the prescription and provision of specialized and individual appliances/orthotics.
3. Preventative services to include inspection of feet and detection of foot conditions requiring treatment and advice, and foot health education.

In addition the chiropodist is able to recognize conditions that manifest themselves in the feet and to treat and alleviate the resultant foot condition, e.g. circulatory disorder, diabetic states and ulcerative conditions.

Community

Two community nurses, Colledge and Crook, surveyed a district health area population of 214 000 and identified 634 mentally handicapped patients living outside hospital, of whom 130 (20.5%) were 40 years of age or older (range 40–76 years). The majority of those older than 40 were less than 60 years of age, but 23 (3.6%) were more than 60 years old, and six of those were older than 70. Fourteen (10.8%) of those 40 years of age or older had Down's syndrome. Their ages ranged from 40 to 52 years.

Of the 130 mentally handicapped older patients, one-third were without some form of day care outside the home. A more detailed study of a random sample of 50 patients from the identified group revealed that more than half had some significant skill deficit or medical condition requiring treatment. Of those 50 patients, nearly half (48%) had lost both parents, 34% had only one living parent and in only 12% of cases were both parents alive (Colledge and Crook, 1986).

Carter in 1984 found that nearly 75% of all permanent hospital admissions of handicapped patients over a 10-year period were attributed to increasing parental age (consequently also increasing age of the mentally handicapped individual), parental illness or parental death (Carter, 1984).

The picture that emerges of ageing mentally handicapped people poses fundamental questions as to their future care, especially because many of these patients have been and continue to be released from hospital care to fend for themselves. With increasing age, these patients will need more care and treatment from a specialized multi-disciplinary team if their quality of life is to be maintained.

Diet

Diet plays a very important role in the care and treatment of the mentally handicapped in hospital and community alike. The caregiver must ensure that all nutrients, particularly protein, calories, minerals, vitamins, fibre, and trace elements, are in the right quantities. Balanced fluid intake is also essential to maintain the body's fluid levels.

Disorders and diseases associated with ageing require a special diet. Diet sheets should therefore be available to staff, relatives and caregivers to suit individual needs. It is in the interest of both patients and caregivers to supply the best possible diet so as to encourage an active, healthy and independent old age. This helps to reduce the cost and burden of nursing the sick handicapped elderly.

Environment

A suitable environment for the elderly mentally handicapped is a great contribution towards better and healthier care and living. When planning accommodation one has to take into consideration the increasing disabilities and disorders of ageing.

When the two units for the elderly were built at Stoke Park Hospital in 1983 they were placed in a peaceful environment at the edge of the hospital near the woodland with easy access to all the required hospital services. Units are homely, well lit and brightly coloured. The furniture and fittings, particularly the doors, were planned in such a way that the very disabled and wheelchair bound patients would be able to use the units with the minimum of discomfort. The heating of the units has been well planned to prevent hypothermia. Privacy for the patients and visitors has also been included in the plans. The garden and flower beds are within easy reach. The bird-table and feeding places for woodland animals provide great pleasure for the patients (Figure 18.7).

Therapeutic team

Besides the professionals already mentioned earlier other members of the therapeutic team are essential to provide proper care, treatment or amelioration of diseases or disorders of the elderly mentally handicapped either at home, in the community or in hospital.

Nurses

Nursing the elderly handicapped cannot be carried out in isolation. With the associated problems of old age comes the need for specialist skills and knowledge. Through the multi-disciplinary team problems will be identified and by using the nursing process as a tool, the nurse will assess, plan, implement and evaluate the care given to each person. The nurse will participate fully in some aspects of care while in other areas will find herself or himself acting as an agent for other specialities.

Physiotherapy

The physiotherapist's role with the ageing population is as follows:

1. *Acute conditions* – A varied and changing caseload, showing great similarity to normal ageing population. Work includes stroke rehabilitation, acute respiratory conditions, degenerative skeletal conditions like osteo-arthritis, fractures and terminal care.

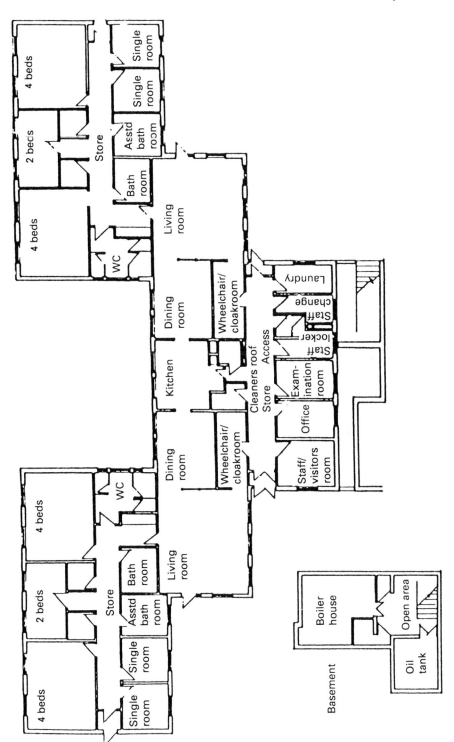

Figure 18.7 Plan of a unit for the elderly mentally handicapped

2. *Chronic conditions* – These are associated with handicap rather than illness, and are ongoing treatments continued through life to maintain mobility, to achieve good and changing positions, to slow down deterioration and to maintain function.
3. *Appliances* – Provision, maintenance and re-assessment of all appliances continues throughout life. Changes in requirements in later life now become apparent, especially in footwear. Wheelchair dependence and independence have to be considered and taught.
4. *Activities* – A wide range of therapeutic activities are used – including movement/music groups, keep fit classes, hydrotherapy – to help maintain mobility and function.

Occupational therapy

The Occupational Therapist provides a varied programme of activities and aids to satisfy the needs and requirements of the ageing mentally handicapped. Apart from their work in the hospital setting and community homes, their help is very much needed and appreciated in the patient's home.

Speech therapy

Communication problems in mentally handicapped people are often very acute and increase with ageing. Therefore the skills of the speech therapist are essential for this group of people. They are also very relevant in times of bereavement and terminal illness.

Visiting consultants

Visiting consultants from various branches of medicine are often called upon to give their expert advice and treatment when necessary to the patients, thus completing the therapeutic team. The hospital pharmacy and X-ray department also play an important part in the therapeutic team.

Research

Research in the field of ageing of mentally handicapped people in all aspects is of paramount importance. Without research we can neither improve the care, treatment and prevention of old age disorders and diseases nor can we plan proper provision of services and manpower which will be required for the future.

During the last few years great strides were made in the study of ageing in the fields of biochemistry, histopathology, neurophysiology, drugs, genetics and other specialties.

Conclusion

Many factors, as previously described in this chapter, are influencing the future care and treatment of the ageing mentally handicapped. Education as to the problems of longevity and all that old age brings with it is needed at all levels of professional training of those who work in the field of mental handicap. In addition it is important to present the problem of ageing to society at large and in particular to the planners of the future health services.

Whenever possible the elderly should be examined and treated in their own environment and by the people they know. Frequent medical and psychological examination with multidisciplinary assessment and proper placement will prevent unnecessary suffering and help with early diagnosis and proper treatment and care.

The number of terminally ill mentally handicapped is increasing. Special facilities and suitably trained staff are therefore needed to provide adequate care for those people, who should end their days in a peaceful environment among their friends and with familiar carers.

References

Aitchison, Christina, Easty, D.L. and Jancar, J. (1990) Eye abnormalities in the mentally handicapped. *Journal of Mental Deficiency Research*, **34**, 41–48

Baird, Patricia A. and Sadovnick, Adele D. (1988) Life expectancy in Down's syndrome adults. *Lancet*, **ii**, 1354–1356

Carter, G. (1984) Why are the mentally handicapped admitted to hospital? *British Journal of Psychiatry*, **145**, 283–288

Carter, G. and Jancar, J. (1983) Mortality in the mentally handicapped: a 50 year survey at the Stoke Park group of hospitals (1930–1980). *Journal of Mental Deficiency Research*, **27**, 143–156

Clarke, S.K.R., Caul, E.O., Jancar, J. and Gordon-Russell, J.B. (1984) Hepatitis B in seven hospitals for the mentally handicapped. *Journal of Infection*, **8**, 34–43

Colledge, A. and Crook, P. (1986) Community care for aging mentally handicapped people: a nursing survey. In *Science and Service in Mental Retardation* (ed. Berg, J.M.). Methuen, London, pp. 335–344

Cooke, Leila B. (1988) Hearing loss in the mentally handicapped. A study of its prevalence and association with ageing. *British Journal of Mental Subnormality*, **XXXIV**, 112–116

Day, K.A. (1985) Psychiatric disorder in the middle-aged and elderly mentally handicapped. *British Journal of Psychiatry*, **147**, 660–667

Day, K.A. (1987) The elderly mentally handicapped in hospital: a clinical study. *Journal of Mental Deficiency Research*, **31**, 131–146

Dupont, Annalise, Waeth, M. and Videbech, P. (1986) Mortality and life expectancy of Down's syndrome in Denmark. *Journal of Mental Deficiency Research*, **30**, 111–120

Eastham, R.D. and Jancar, J. (1970) Mean red-cell volume and patient's age. *Lancet*, **i**, 896

Fraser, J. and Mitchell, A. (1876) Kalmuc idiocy: Report of a case with autopsy, with notes on sixty-two cases. *Journal of Mental Science*, **22**, 169–179

Fraser, M. (1988) *Dementia: Its Nature and Management*, Wiley, Chichester, pp. 5–20

Heaton-Ward, W.A. (1977) Psychosis in mental handicap (Blake Marsh Lecture). *British Journal of Psychiatry*, **130**, 525–533

Hewitt, K.E., Fenner, M.E. and Torpy, D. (1986) Cognitive and behavioural profiles of the elderly mentally handicapped. *Journal of Mental Deficiency Research*, **30**, 217–225

Hewitt, K.E. and Jancar, J. (1986) Psychological and clinical aspects of aging in Down's syndrome. In *Science and Service in Mental Retardation* (ed. Berg, J.M.), Methuen, London, pp. 370–379

Hogg, J., Moss, S. and Cooke, D. (1988) *Ageing and Mental Handicap*, Croom Helm, London

James, D.H. (1983) Monitoring drugs for the mentally handicapped. *British Journal of Psychiatry*, **142**, 163–165

James, D.H. (1986) Psychiatric and behavioural disorders amongst older severely mentally handicapped in-patients. *Journal of Mental Deficiency Research*, **30**, 341–345

Jancar, J. (1979) Organic causes of mental illness in the mentally handicapped. In *Psychiatric Illness and Mental Handicap* (eds James, F.E. and Smith, R.P.), Gaskell Press, London

Jancar, J. (1980) Anticonvulsant drugs and cancer. *Lancet*, **i**, 484

Jancar, J. (1987) *Monograph on Medical Aspects of Aging in the Mentally Handicapped*. A Stoke Park Presentation. (Translated into Spanish, German and Japanese.)

Jancar, J. (1989) Fractures in older persons with mental handicap. *Australia and New Zealand Journal of Developmental Disabilities*, **12**, 329–335

Jancar, M.P. and Jancar, J. (1977) Cancer and mental retardation (a forty year review). *Bristol Medico-Chirurgical Journal*, **92**, 3–7

Jancar, J. and Lansdall-Welfare, R.V. (1986) Diabetes and mental handicap. A preliminary report. *Bristol Medico-Chirurgical Journal*, **101**, 82

Jancar, J. and Walters, Ruth M. (1974) Tapeto-retinal degeneration in three mentally retarded sisters with other disorders in the family tree. *Acta Geneticae Medicae et Gemellologiae (Roma)*, **23**, 175–180

Jancar, J., Eastham, R.D. and Carter, G. (1984) Hypocholesterolaemia in cancer and other causes of death in the mentally handicapped. *British Journal of Psychiatry*, **145**, 59–61

Jancar, J., Griffiths, H.E.D. and Sawdon, B. (1985) Dupuytren's disease and mental handicap. *British Journal of Psychiatry*, **147**, 211–212

Janicki, M.P. (1984) Comparisons of older mentally handicapped persons residing at home and institutions. A round table discussion '*At Home and Institutional Care*', at the *11th International Conference on Gerontology, Rome*.

Janicki, M.P. and Wisniewski, H.M. (eds) (1985) *Aging and Development Disabilities. Issues and Approaches*, Paul H. Brookes Publishing Company, Baltimore

Kinnell, H.G., Gibbs, N., Teale, J.D. and Smith, J. (1987) Thyroid dysfunction in institutionalised Down's syndrome adults. *Psychological Medicine*, **17**, 387–392

McCurley, R., MacKay, D.N. and Scally, B.G. (1972). The life expectation of the mentally subnormal under community and hospital care. *Journal of Mental Deficiency Research*, **16**, 57–66

McLoughlin, I.J. (1988) A study of mortality experiences in a mental handicap hospital. *British Journal of Psychiatry*, **153**, 645–649

Primrose, D.A.A. (1966) Natural history of mental deficiency in a hospital group and in the community it serves. *Journal of Mental Deficiency Research*, **10**, 159–189

Richards, B.W. and Sylvester, P.E. (1969) Mortality trends in mental deficiency institutions. *Journal of Mental Deficiency Research*, **13**, 276–292

Struwe, F. (1929) Histopathologische Untersuchungen uber Entstehung und Weses der Senile Plaques. *Zeitschrift fur des gesamtes Neurologie und Psychiatrie*, **122**, 291–307

Takashima, S. and Becker, L.E. (1985) Basal ganglia calcification in Down's syndrome. *Journal of Neurology, Neurosurgery and Psychiatry*, **48**, 61–64

World Health Organisation (1985) *Mental Retardation: Meeting the Challenge*, Offset Publication No. 86, WHO, Geneva

19

Statutory framework

19.1 Some ethical considerations

Mary Holland

Integration

When surveys are carried out on public attitudes towards care in the community, it is found that the vast majority support such policies. However, questions about people with mental handicap living next door receive a far more mixed response, usually couched in terms such as 'the roads might not be safe for them', 'yes, but the value of the property will decrease', 'I agree with integrated education, but it's not fair to them' or 'my child's education will suffer', 'they're happier with their own kind'.

Most people can choose where they live, and how they live, albeit dependent on financial circumstances, but do they extend this choice to people with mental handicap? Perhaps the first ethical issue of mental handicap is how people live with each other.

Profound handicap and life-threatening conditions

Modern advances in medicine have reduced the mortality rates of children with mental handicap, and for many their life expectancy will be near that of the general population. Nonetheless, there will be infants born with severe mental handicap and life-threatening conditions. Should life support systems and/or life giving operations be performed on these children? In 1981, the 'Hammersmith case' was widely publicized in the national press. In this case, the parents concerned felt unable to give permission for a life-saving operation for their mentally handicapped infant. The local authority then stepped in, taking responsibility for the infant. Mencap, the largest national parent organization for children and adults with mental handicap, agreed with this and made the following points:

'In recent times the advance of medical science has given parents of a mentally handicapped child a choice as to whether or not life-support systems are to be used or a life-giving operation is to be performed on that child. To help parents in reaching this agonizing decision every support and counselling must be offered by the medical, para-medical and social services. However, it is vital that other experienced parents of mentally handicapped children are involved in this counselling process for only they know, at first hand, the joys and sorrows as well as the practical problems ahead. If, after all this consultation, the parents concerned still feel unable to give permission for a life-saving operation to be performed on their mentally handicapped child, then a procedure similar to that carried out in the recent "Hammersmith case" should apply, with the full responsibility for the child's future being assumed by the Local Authority concerned. . .'

Antenatal screening and abortion

Over 2% of all live births are infants with congenital malformations. This statistic understates the number of infants with handicaps being born, as many disorders only become apparent later. Hereditary factors are the most common cause of congenital handicap, of which there are over 1500 different forms. The most effective way of diagnosing a handicap before birth is to study the chromosomes and genes of the fetus. The most widely used method is amniocentesis. A recent development is chorionic villus sampling (CVS). This can be carried out at around the 8th–10th week of pregnancy, and will detect some abnormalities. But, as with amniocentesis, if abnormalities are detected, the only option that can be offered is termination of pregnancy. Few issues provoke such extreme reactions as abortion. Surely the fundamental principle should be to enable those concerned to make their decision in accordance with their beliefs. Too often, this ethic is distorted by the judgement of others.

A new issue now confronts us: embryo research. Legislation will be brought forward in response to the Report of the Warnock Committee Inquiry into Human Fertilisation and Embryology. MPs will be asked to vote between two straight options:

1. That research on embryos should be permitted within the present time limit of 14 days, if it is licensed by a new statutory authority.
2. That all research on embryos, including research within the present limitation of 14 days, should become a criminal offence.

Most people have limited information about medical and scientific research. Exaggerated and emotive propaganda distorts the facts and causes confusion and anxiety. The purpose of pre-embryo research is to find out why problems occur during reproduction, such as miscarriage, infertility and genetic disorders, in order to prevent or treat them. Pre-implantation diagnosis of human pre-embryos holds great promise for carriers of genetic disease, and in the foreseeable future it may be possible to detect those pre-embryos that would develop specific disorders such as muscular dystrophy, Down's syndrome, cystic fibrosis, Hunter's syndrome, Hurler's syndrome and Huntington's chorea. If the presence of an abnormal gene or chromosomal defect could be detected in a pre-embryo, it would be possible to ensure that only non-affected pre-embryos were transferred back.

The forthcoming debate on embryo research will need to resolve difficult ethical dilemmas. When does life begin? What is the legal status of the pre-embryo? The debate could simply polarize prejudices or it could align religious and philosophical beliefs with current biological understanding and provide a framework to benefit both science and human life.

Growing up and growing on

In the past, people with mental handicap had little opportunity to explore and experience personal relationships. Their needs for physical and sexual contact were denied – because they were seen to be eternal children – or were forbidden through segregated living arrangements. Care in the community should mean wider opportunities for personal development and expression. It also will bring with it wider risks. Education, social skills training and instruction on the basic facts and consequences of sexual relationships can go a long way towards minimizing the risks. However, many people will continue to need supervision and support if they are to avoid exploitation or disaster. The questions confronting society are complex. During recent years, a number of cases involving women with mental handicap and the question of sterilization or abortion have been the focus of national attention. The debate at times has been muddled by emotion and lack of information. The fundamental issue is how to enable vulnerable individuals to have personal freedom and expression and, at the same time, the protection they need.

Many parents, carers and professionals agree that adults with mental handicap should be able to express and enjoy their sexual feelings. However, one great fear is that this will result in pregnancy – a pregnancy which would be unplanned and unwanted, and not understood by the woman involved. It could result in the newborn infant being immediately taken into care. Some propose that the best solution would be for the woman to be sterilized, therefore removing any risk of pregnancy. Others say that to perform a sterilization, for other than wholly medical reasons, is a denial of a woman's fundamental rights. What is the answer?

Every year, thousands of women in the UK choose sterilization as a permanent method of contraception. In the USA it is the second most frequently used form of contraception after the contraceptive pill. For these women, there is no hue and cry over their decision to opt for sterilization. The hue and cry arises when the decision is made *for* the woman, and not by her.

Decisions concerning medical procedures – especially abortion and sterilization – tend to raise the emotional temperature. Yet the contraceptive pill and the IUD do not provoke this reaction. It is, of course, true that sterilization and abortion are irreversible procedures, wheras the pill and IUD are not. Nonetheless, the question of being incapable of consenting to treatment is the fundamental issue.

If adults with mental handicap are unable to give consent to medical treatment, who should speak on their behalf? A number of organizations have debated the issues and produced reports making recommendations on how they should be tackled. An independent working party convened by Mencap produced a report, 'Competency and Consent to Medical Treatment' (March, 1989). This starts from the premise that the interests of the individual should be paramount. The report proposes principles for determining incapacity in an adult with mental handicap; criteria to be applied in deciding what is in an individual's interests; who should be party to the decision-making process; and the setting up of multi-disciplinary ethics committees. The debate continues, and it is hoped that action will be taken to establish clear procedures to be followed. Even when such procedures are established, the basic dilemma will remain: how can vulnerable people enjoy personal freedom and be protected from sexual abuse and exploitation?

Prosperity?

Many people have prospered in the 1980s in Britain. The average weekly wage is £216; the average weekly income (for a family of 3) is £303 (1989). This prosperity has meant more consumer purchasing power: videos, cars, washing machines etc. For many, two annual holidays are the norm. People dependent on benefits and income supports have not shared in this prosperity. The OPCS surveys of disability in Great Britain (1989) found that there are 6.2 million disabled people in Britain – 1 in 10 of the population. Three-quarters of disabled adults rely on state benefits as their main source of income, with an average weekly total income for adults living at home of £65.20 (1985). Less than one third of disabled people under pension age are in paid work, compared with 69% of the general population. Not only do disabled people have less money to spend, but their costs *because of disability* are higher than that of the general population.

One out of four disabled adults felt that because of their disability they needed to spend more than they were able to afford. High on the list of items that people needed but couldn't pay for were thermal underwear and bedding. This, combined with the fact that the most common item of additional expenditure on 'normal' items was fuel for extra heating or hot water, illustrates the link between poverty and disability. If people are unable to afford basic needs, how can they participate in the life of the community?

It must be remembered that the majority of people with mental handicap live with their families until their families are unable to continue to provide the care they need. Children and young people with mental handicap are entitled to education until the age of 19 years. When these young people leave school, what opportunities are available for them? The answer is 'very little'. There is no statutory obligation on local authorities to provide day services for people with mental handicap, and often there are no places available at adult training centres (ATCs).

In the general population, most young adults leave the family home and establish independent lives of their own. But for families with a mentally handicapped member this does not happen, and parents continue caring into their own old age, with the constant worry, 'What will happen when we die?'. Most parents would like to see their sons and daughters happily settled in a residential setting that is appropriate to their needs. Unfortunately, there is not enough residential care available. Likewise, parents need to have breaks from caring, but short-term/respite care is thin on the ground. Ironically, in the past years, as people have moved out of long-stay mental handicap hospitals, there has been an upsurge in the number of people going *into* long-stay mental handicap hospitals for short-term/respite care. If care in the community is to be a success for people with mental handicap, their families and carers, the financial, physical and social supports must be made available.

19.2 Legal aspects

Ros. Lyall

Introduction

Legislation affecting the care of people with a mental handicap rather than being solely concerned with management of their property appeared first in 1886 with 'The Idiots Act' which laid down conditions for admission to, discharge from, registration and inspection of institutions. Since then there have been many pieces of legislation which have impinged in one way or another on people with a mental handicap. Some of the enactments have had a very positive effect, for example to guarantee education for all children with a mental handicap until 16 years of age; others remain contentious in the light of contemporary thinking.

In 1983, an amended Mental Health Act came into force in England and Wales (a similar Act for Scotland came into force in 1984 and an Order for Northern Ireland in 1986). The new Act had several changes from the previous 1959 Act, not the least of which was the removal of the terms subnormality and severe subnormality, replacing them with mental impairment and severe mental impairment. The impetus for these changes was felt when the Bill was being considered by Parliament; a large amount of lobbying, especially by Mencap, to have mental handicap removed from the Act altogether, resulted in what at first sight is merely a semantic means of satisfying the pressure groups. The terms, however, are not meant to be just a less pejorative way of describing people with a mental handicap; they are further defined to include impairment of social functioning as well as intelligence, and this has to be associated with abnormally aggressive or seriously irresponsible conduct.

Under the terms of the 1983 Mental Health Act, therefore, we now have a new category of people with mental handicaps – those whose mental handicap is associated with abnormally aggressive or seriously irresponsible conduct. Those people who do not fulfil these criteria are not subject to the Act, unless they qualify under one of the other provisions – mental illness or psychopathic disorder, with the exception of Sections 2, 4, 5, 135 and 136 (see below).

Mental Health Act 1983

The Act covers 'the reception, care and treatment of mentally disordered patients, the management of their property and other related matters'. It principally refers to patients who have to be admitted to hospital on a compulsory basis, or placed under guardianship.

Mental disorder is defined as 'mental illness, arrested or incomplete development of mind, psychopathic disorder and other disorder or disability of mind'.

However, most purposes of the Act require a person to be suffering from one of four specific categories:

1. *Mental illness* – This is not further defined.
2. *Mental impairment* – A state of arrested or incomplete development of mind which includes *significant* impairment of intelligence and social functioning, and is associated with abnormally aggressive or seriously irresponsible conduct.
3. *Severe mental impairment* – A state of arrested or incomplete development of mind which includes *severe* impairment of intelligence and social functioning, etc.
4. *Psychopathic disorder* – A persistent disorder or disability of mind (whether or not including significant impairment of intelligence) which results in abnormally aggressive or seriously irresponsible conduct.

The distinctions between significant and severe in the definitions of mental impairment and severe mental impairment are important as they have a bearing on the grounds for detention and renewal of detention under certain circumstances (see below). It should also be noted that people may not be detained by reason only of promiscuity or other immoral conduct, sexual deviancy or dependance on alcohol or drugs.

Section 2 – Admission for assessment

This allows for admission for assessment for a period of up to 28 days. The application, by the nearest relative or approved social worker, must be supported by two medical recommendations, one from an approved doctor, which have to agree:

1. That the patient is suffering from mental disorder of a nature or degree which warrants the detention of the patient in hospital for assessment or assessment followed by medical treatment for at least a limited period.
2. That he ought to be detained in the interests of his own health or safety or with a view to the protection of other persons.

There is a right of appeal against detention by the patient to a Mental Health Review Tribunal within the first 14 days and the nearest relative, Responsible Medical Officer (usually the Consultant) or the managers of the hospital can discharge the patient with the 'safeguard' that the RMO can bar discharge by the nearest relative. The patient must be discharged after 28 days unless further detained for treatment under Section 3 or agreeing to remain on an informal basis.

It should be noted that Section 2 requires only that mental disorder is present and does not require that this is further defined. In theory, therefore, people with a mental handicap without the 'abnormally aggressive or seriously irresponsible conduct' element of mental impairment or severe mental impairment could be liable to detention under Section 2.

Section 3 – Admission for treatment

This section allows for the admission and detention of a patient, in hospital for treatment, for a period of up to 6 months, with the possibility of renewal after that time. The application, by the nearest relative or approved social worker, must be supported by two medical recommendations as for Section 2. However, the medical recommendations must now state the grounds for their opinion and why other methods of dealing with the patient are inappropriate. The grounds must state:

1. Which form of mental disorder the patient suffers from – mental illness, severe mental impairment, mental impairment or psychopathic disorder and that it is of a nature or degree that makes it appropriate to receive treatment in a hospital.
2. In the case of psychopathic disorder or mental impairment the treatment is likely to alleviate or prevent a deterioration of the disorder.
3. That it is necessary for the health or safety of the patient or for the protection of others that he receive such treatment and it cannot be provided unless he is detained under this Section.

Discharge may be effected by the nearest relative after giving 72 hours notice unless barred by the RMO, by the RMO, or by the managers of the hospital. The nearest relative may also, if barred from discharging the patient, apply to the Mental Health Review Tribunal within 28 days. The patient has the right to apply to the Tribunal on one occasion during any period of detention. The hospital managers must refer any patient whose detention is renewed to the Tribunal if he has not previously applied.

Section 4 – Emergency admission for assessment

An emergency application for admission for assessment for 72 hours may be made by the nearest relative or an approved social worker, and supported by one medical recommendation, given preferably by a doctor who knows the patient. The grounds are the same as for admission under Section 2, and contain a statement to the effect that it is urgently necessary to admit the patient and that admission under Section 2 would involve undesirable delay. The Order lasts for 72 hours, but detention can be continued under Section 2 if the second medical recommendation has been made before the expiry of the Order.

Section 5(2) – Application in respect of a patient already in hospital

The application is made by report from the doctor in charge of the case if it appears that an application for compulsory detention in a hospital should be made as the patient is presenting a danger to himself or others. As with Section 4, it lasts for up to 72 hours.

Section 5(4) – Nurses holding power

This section allows for nurses of a prescribed class (equivalent to RMN, RNMH) to detain a patient already in hospital for a period of up to 6 hours while a doctor is found. The patient must appear to the nurse to be suffering from mental disorder to such a degree that it is necessary for his health or safety or for the protection of others, for him to be immediately restrained from leaving the hospital and also that it is not practicable to obtain the immediate attendance of a doctor for the purposes of Section 5(2).

Section 7 – Application for guardianship

This section provides for a patient (over 16 years of age) to be placed under the supervision of a guardian. As with application for detention in hospital, the applicant may be the nearest relative or an approved social worker: the application is made to the local social services authority. It must be supported by two medical recommendations, one of which is that of an 'approved' doctor, and they must have each seen the patient within 5 days of each other. The patient must be suffering from one of the forms of mental disorder and it must be stated that it is necessary in the interests of the welfare of the patient or for the protection of other people that he should be received into the guardianship of an individual or local authority. The Order lasts 6 months and is renewable. Discharge is by RMO, local authority or nearest relative. The patient may apply to a Tribunal once during each 6-month period of the Order.

Section 8 – Powers of guardian

1. To require the patient to reside at a specified place.
2. To require the patient to attend at specified places and times for medical treatment, occupation, education or training.
3. To require access to the patient to be given, at the patient's residence, to any doctor, approved social worker or other specified person.

The guardian has no other statutory powers. Further mention of guardianship will be made later in the chapter.

The Mental Health Act also makes provision for mentally abnormal offenders, some of whom are likely to have a mental handicap.

Section 35 allows a Crown Court or Magistrates Court to remand an accused person to hospital for a report. The person must be thought to be suffering from one of the forms of mental disorder and to be accused of an imprisonable offence, or convicted and awaiting sentence. The Order lasts for 28 days and is renewable up to 12 weeks.

Section 36 allows the Crown Court (only) to remand an accused person to hospital for treatment, providing it is an imprisonable offence and not murder. In this case the person must be suffering from mental illness or severe mental impairment only. Again the Order is for 28 days renewable up to 12 weeks.

Section 37 – Empowers a Court to order hospital admission or reception into guardianship of an individual found guilty of an imprisonable offence (except murder). The grounds for admission are as for Section 3 excluding the necessity in terms of the patient's health or safety or safety of others. The Order is for 6 months, and may be renewed. Rights of appeal to a Tribunal operate from the second 6-month period.

This is by no means an exhaustive account of the relevant sections of the Mental Health Act; however, with regard to detention in hospital it covers those with the most relevance to people with a mental handicap.

Consent to treatment – Sections 57 and 58

The Act lays down regulations governing consent to treatment of mental disorder by detained and informal patients. The Mental Health Act Commission has responsibility for implementing these regulations and a discussion of this can be found in Section 19.3.

The Act also allows for review of such treatment when detention is renewed. Consent to non-psychiatric treatment will be discussed later.

Section 62 – Urgent treatment

It may, under certain circumstances, be necessary to give treatment otherwise restricted by Sections 57 and 58 urgently. In these cases, if the treatment is immediately necessary to save the patient's life or not being irreversible or hazardous is immediately necessary to prevent a serious deterioration in the patient's condition or to prevent serious suffering to the patient or it represents the minimum interference necessary to prevent the patient from behaving violently or being a danger to himself or others, it may be given to a detained patient without the need for formal consent or a second opinion under this section.

Other aspects of the Mental Health Act will be discussed later.

Mental Health (Scotland) Act 1984

The provisions of the Mental Health (Scotland) Act are broadly similar to the 1983 Act. There are some important differences which will be highlighted in the following summary of the main provisions. It should be noted also that mental handicap, as a term, is used in addition to mental impairment and severe mental impairment.

In the Scottish Act, mental disorder is defined as 'mental illness or mental handicap however caused or manifested'. Mental impairment and severe mental impairment have the same definitions as the Mental Health Act. There is no separate category for psychopathic disorder. Mental illness is not further defined; however, treatment provisions are included in certain circumstances.

Where the mental disorder from which he suffers is a persistent one manifested only by abnormally aggressive or seriously irresponsible conduct, such treatment is likely to alleviate or prevent a deterioration in his condition; or in the case where the mental disorder from which he suffers is mental handicap, the handicap comprises mental impairment (where such treatment is likely to alleviate or prevent a deterioration of his condition) or severe mental impairment.

As with the Mental Health Act, the health or safety of the person must be at risk or there must be a need for protection of other persons.

Section 18 – Admission to hospital

This Section provides for an application by the nearest relative or a mental health officer (equivalent to approved social worker) for the admission of a person to hospital. It must be accompanied by two medical recommendations, one of which must be from an approved doctor, and submitted to the Sheriff for approval. The Sheriff may choose to have a hearing, has to have a hearing if the nearest relative or mental health officer objects to the application, or may just scrutinize the forms. Once approved by the Sheriff, the Order lasts for up to 6 months, it can then be renewed for a further 6 months and thereafter annually.

There is a right of appeal to the Sheriff and/or to the Mental Welfare Commission of Scotland during each period of detention. (See Chapter 23 for further discussion about the Mental Welfare Commission.)

Discharge may be effected by the Responsible Medical Officer (usually the consultant in charge of the patient), by the Mental Welfare Commission, by the managers of the hospital, by the Sheriff or by the nearest relative. As with the Mental Health Act, discharge by the nearest relative can be barred by the RMO.

Section 24 – Emergency admission to hospital

Section 24 allows a person with mental disorder to be admitted to hospital urgently on the recommendation of any medical practitioner. Where practicable, the consent of the nearest relative or of a mental health officer must be obtained. The period of detention is 72 hours from the time of admission to hospital and in addition there is a period of 3 days during which admission to hospital may be effected. Further detention under Section 24 is not permissible immediately after expiry of the initial period of detention. The definition of 'immediately' with regard to time has not been stated. If further detention is required then a Section 26 is applied (see below). Section 25(1) is essentially the same as Section 24 but applies to patients already in hospital informally.

Section 26 – Short-term detention

This section, which can only be applied to a patient detained under Section 24 or 25(1), allows for further detention for a period of 28 days. It requires a recommendation from an approved doctor (psychiatrist) and again, where practicable, the consent of the nearest relative or a mental health officer. The patient has the right of appeal to a Sheriff and/or to the Mental Welfare Commission.

Section 25(2) – Nurses holding power

In contrast to the Mental Health Act, the time allowed for detaining a patient under this Section is only 2 hours – as previously noted, for Section 5(4) of the Mental Health Act in England and Wales the time allowed is 6 hours. Otherwise, provisions are much the same: the nurse must be of a prescribed class, the patient already in hospital and the Section ceases to have effect when a doctor sees the patient.

Guardianship in Scotland

The powers and requirements of Guardianship are broadly similar to those in the Mental Health Act. However, in Scotland the patient need only be said to suffer from mental disorder and although it is further defined on the Statutory forms, it is only either mental illness or mental handicap (cf. Mental Health Act), and not one of the specified forms of mental disorder. The welfare ground is similarly slightly different in that it only requires to be 'necessary in the interests of the welfare of the patient', there is no mention of a need to protect other people. The application, supported by two medical recommendations, has to be approved by a Sheriff. As with compulsory detention there are rights of appeal to the Mental Welfare Commission.

Mentally abnormal offenders

Under Part VI of the Act, provision is made for dealing with mentally abnormal offenders. The Sections that professionals in the field of mental handicap are liable to encounter are the relevant Sections from the Criminal Procedures (Scotland) Act 1975 which are included in the Mental Health (Scotland) Act. The Sections are divided into those referring to people charged under (1) Solemn procedure and those under (2) Summary procedure. The most commonly used sections are: 25 and 330, which allow for remand to hospital instead of custody pending trial; Sections 175 and 376 (Hospital or Guardianship Order), the Court makes an order for the admission and detention in hospital of a person convicted of an offence punishable with imprisonment, or the Court may make a Guardianship Order. Under Sections 178 and 379 the Court may add a further order that the patient is subject to special restrictions:

1. Solemn procedure refers to offences which are tried in the High Court.
2. Summary procedure refers to offences which are tried in a Sheriff Court.

Consent to treatment (see also Section 19.3)

See Sections 97 and 98 Mental Health (Scotland) Act 1984.

Part X of the Scottish Act governs consent to treatment. The provisions apply *only* to detained patients (Sections 26 and 18). The regulations are otherwise as in the English Act.

Section 102 covers emergency treatment (cf. Section 62 Mental Health Act) for mental disorder.

Mental Health (Northern Ireland) Order 1986

The Northern Ireland Order is in essence a hybrid of parts of the English and Scottish Acts, although it has its own unique provisions. It has four categories of mental disorder – mental illness, mental handicap, severe mental handicap and severe mental impairment. The mental handicap definitions rely totally on impairment of intelligence and social functioning and only 'severe mental impairment' includes a requirement for abnormally aggressive or seriously irresponsible behaviour.

For a person with a mental handicap who may be detained under the Order, the consequences are determined by the category in which his handicap falls. Thus, someone said to be suffering from 'mental handicap' may be admitted for assessment, detained for 48 hours under the doctor's holding power or for 6 hours under the nurse's holding power or removed to a place of safety for 48 hours. However, he may not be placed under guardianship or detained in hospital for treatment unless classified as severely mentally impaired or severely mentally handicapped. Consent to treatment provisions are similar to the English Act.

The reader wishing to learn in more detail about the three Mental Health Acts is advised to look at the Acts themselves in conjunction with the official Notes or Guides issued by the Departments of Health and the Codes of Practice when they are published. Where the Acts have a bearing on other legal matters discussed below, the relevant sections will be noted.

Other provisions of mental health acts with particular reference to people with a mental handicap

Section 127 makes it an offence for staff or managers of a hospital or mental nursing home to 'ill treat or wilfully neglect' both in-patients and out-patients and for any individual to 'ill treat or wilfully neglect' a mentally disordered person subject to guardianship or who is otherwise in that individual's custody or care.

The Sexual Offences Acts 1956 and 1967 are amended by the Mental Health Act. It is an offence for a man to have unlawful sexual intercourse with a woman who is severely mentally handicapped unless he did not know or had no reason to suspect that the woman was severely mentally handicapped. It also is an offence for a man to have homosexual intercourse or other forms of homosexual activity (gross indecency) with a man who is severely mentally impaired. Again, if the man did not know or had no reason to suspect then it is not an offence.

The Mental Health Acts make it an offence for any member of staff in a hospital or home to have unlawful sexual intercourse with a female in-patient or out-patient, or under guardianship or otherwise in his custody and care under the Mental Health Act (Section 128, Section 107(5)).

Guardianship

As already noted, guardianship is covered by the Mental Health Acts. In general, its powers are limited, there are no powers of compulsion in the Acts so that some element of compliance is seen to be necessary. Neither do the powers extend beyond residence, attendance at various places or allowing access, so that a person with a mental handicap on a guardianship order may fulfil all the requirements and yet still be at risk because of where he goes to spend his leisure time, for example. Whilst the guardian may be able to advise the client not to go to certain places, there are no powers under the legislation to prevent the client ignoring this advice. The other major area of an individual's life not governed by guardianship is that of property and finance. Management of individual's property when that person is under guardianship is specifically excluded from the powers.

Many people have suggested that guardianship does not go far enough in protecting people with a mental handicap. Recently, in Scotland, an old common law has been used in one case to appoint a 'tutor', in essence to appoint someone (in this case the parents) to continue to act as a parent or tutor to a person with a mental handicap beyond the age of 18 years, who is incapable of managing his affairs in the widest sense. Not all the powers available were requested or granted, but the appointment allowed the tutors generally to decide on place of residence, to act in legal proceedings on his behalf (excepting in the case of the individual's estate), to consent to health care, to decide on daytime occupation, and to provide the person with care, support and guidance.

Management of property and estate

Court of protection – England and Wales

This is an office of the Supreme Court authorized by the Mental Health Act which is empowered to administer the property and affairs of a patient deemed to be incapable of managing his own affairs by reason of mental disorder. In effect the Court appoints an Official Receiver who may control or manage a patient's property, sell or acquire property, enter into contracts and conduct legal proceedings on behalf of the patient. In doing this, the Receiver is expected to do all that is necessary or expedient for the patient for his benefit and also for members of his family if appropriate. There are disadvantages in that the patient is deemed incapable of managing *all* his affairs whereas in practice he may be perfectly capable of managing his weekly benefit, etc. There have been calls for some years to make the system more flexible (Section 93).

In Scotland, patients declared Incapax – incapable of managing their affairs by reason of mental disorder – have a Curator Bonis appointed, usually a solicitor or accountant, if their estate is over £10 000 (this figure is currently under review). If they are in hospital and their estate is below £10 000 then the hospital managers are allowed to manage their affairs. The powers of the hospital managers are set out in the Mental Health (Scotland) Act (Section 94). There is a major gap in arrangements for managing the estate of a person who is Incapax and living in the community as appointment of a Curator Bonis is not financially viable under £10 000.

As in England and Wales, the problem with the curatory system is that it is an 'all or nothing' procedure, although some curators are beginning to be more flexible. However, the powers of a curator are not as wide ranging as that of the Court of Protection, e.g. the curator cannot make a will on behalf of the client. Curators are supervised by the Accountant of Court to whom they have to submit regular accounts.

Wills

The making of a will and its legality depends on testamentary capacity. The person making the will must be able to understand and know the extent of his property, and to whom and how it should be dispersed. The majority of people with a mild or borderline degree of handicap will be perfectly capable of making a will. In England those whose affairs are managed by the Court of Protection can have a will drawn up for them by their Official Receiver. As stated above, people subject to curatory in Scotland cannot have a will made for them by the Curator and there is currently some debate as to whether a person subject to a curatory is automatically deemed incapable of making a will.

Consent to medical treatment

Recent legal proceedings have sought to clarify the position of doctors in relation to giving medical treatment to adults who are mentally incapable and therefore unable to give consent. It should be clearly understood that with the exception of a tutor appointed under Scots Law who takes that particular power no one can give consent for another adult. So the practice of asking relatives to consent, whilst important for many reasons, has no legal status and therefore cannot be legally valid.

The case of F, a woman with a mental handicap living in a hospital for whom a sterilization operation was planned has led to the Courts attempting to fill the gap in the law on consent to treatment. The Appeal Court has stated:

'the violability of a person's body was not an absolute right, it had to coexist with other rights, such as the right to skilled medical treatment. Where there were gaps in the statute law on consent to medical treatment for incapable adults, the common law would fill them, in the interests of society as a whole.'

However, it has held that controversial treatments such as sterilization, abortion and donation of organs through surgical intervention will still require the approval of the Court. As far as other treatments are concerned, the Court stated:

'Ability to consent must not be dismissed as desirable but inessential; it was crucial to all medical treatment. If it was unavoidably absent, whether temporarily in an emergency or permanently in the case of mental disability there had, other things being equal, to be greater caution in deciding whether to treat and how.'

It is recommended that the medical profession draw up ethical guidelines for the treatment of mentally incompetent adults. So, the decision about treatment of mentally incapable adults, in general, rests solely with the doctor proposing the treatment and no one else can give consent on the patient's behalf. Approval from the Court must, however, be sought for treatments such as sterilization.

Marriage

Marriage is a voluntary contract between two people, if the consent of either party is not voluntary then the marriage can be declared void by a court. It could be argued that consent is lacking if one of the parties is of unsound mind when the marriage takes place. There is no law that prevents people with a mental handicap from marrying, the only bar is if they are declared to be of unsound mind. There is nothing in law to prevent those subject to the Court of Protection or Curatory from marrying. The burden of proof rests with proving the existence of 'unsound mind' and not the other way round. In practice, people with a severe mental handicap will almost certainly be deemed of unsound mind and unable to give voluntary consent to marriage.

Voting rights

Prior to 1983, people resident in hospitals for people with mental disorder were unable to vote. This restriction extended to people in 'hospital hostels' as well. Since then, informal patients have been granted the right to vote if they can make a 'patient's declaration'. The bar to electoral registration was because of Section 4(3) of the Representation of the People Act 1949, which does not allow a hospital or hostel address to be used for registration purposes. This is still the case; however, residents in hospital can now be registered if they can give an address outside the hospital at which they would be resident if not in hospital or an address at which they resided prior to admission and complete a 'patient's declaration' without assistance. The declaration is meant to be a test of the competence of the individual's capacity with regard to voting. 'Without assistance' implies that a patient must be able to understand the information required to make the declaration and communicate that information to the person responsible for attesting the declaration. It applies only to the making of the declaration and does not mean that there can be no assistance in filling in the form, e.g. if the person is blind or unable to read or write, nor does it preclude the person from asking questions in order to clarify points. The declaration must be attested by a member of staff at the hospital, who will usually be a first-level nurse trained in mental illness or mental handicap nursing.

There is still a common-law duty placed on the electoral registration officer to exclude from the right to vote anyone who cannot discriminate between the candidates and who cannot answer simple questions about his residence or identity in an intelligible manner. The changes in the regulations do not apply to anyone subject to formal detention under the Mental Health Acts.

Community charge

In Great Britain the rating system ('the Rates') has been replaced by the Personal Community Charge. Previously, people with a mental handicap often avoided paying rates if they lived in the community because their income was low enough to entitle them to a rebate or to have their rates paid by the DSS. However, under the Community Charge regulations, everyone has to pay at least 20% of the charge unless they can claim exemption. Exemption, obtained by means of a doctor's certificate, and entitlement to one of a list of specific State benefits and allowances, and the agreement of the registration officer, has created quite a considerable amount of controversy; in particular over the grounds for the granting of a doctor's certificate – severe mental impairment. The definition of severe mental impairment in the context of the community charge is *not* the same as that of the Mental Health Acts. It includes arrested or incomplete development of the mind involving severe impairment of intelligence and social functioning, and also brain injury and those who have suffered severe strokes. The inclusion of dementia has now been agreed by the Government. It is meant to exclude people with mental illness. Not unnaturally, the whole process of obtaining exemption has caused anger amongst people with a mental handicap and those who work with and for them as it is seen as unnecessary, pejorative labelling. It also means that many people with a mental handicap who do not qualify for exemption will have even less disposable income and therefore be financially worse off. However, any person detained in hospital under the Mental Health Act, or liable to be detained, i.e. on leave of absence, is not liable to pay the Community Charge.

The 'Tom Clark' Act (Disabled Persons (Services and Consultations and Representation) Act 1986)

This Act, which has not yet been implemented in full, was the result of pressure from various organizations who felt that the 1970 Chronically Sick and Disabled Persons Act was not being fully implemented in spirit. The new Act is significantly different and stronger. Its main elements are:

1. The appointment of *representatives* for disabled people.
2. The requirement on local authorities to *assess needs* of disabled people.
3. The duty of local authorities to *consider* these needs.

4. The requirement for health boards and local authorities to arrange *assessments* of those with mental disorder who have been in hospital for 6 or more months.
5. The duty of the local authority to take into account the ability of the *carer* to provide care when assessing the needs of the disabled person.
6. The requirement that *information* be made available to disabled people on local authority services and other services.
7. The requirement that local authorities consult with and encourage *representation* of bodies who represent the interests of disabled people.
8. The *monitoring* of in-patient and community care services for the mentally ill and handicapped by annual reports to Parliament by the Secretary of State.
9. Arrangements for *assessment* of disabled people in Special Education and notification of their leaving.

To date, the only sections of the Act that have been implemented are Section (8(1) which refers to the ability of carers (see (5) above), Section 9 which refers to information of services (see (6) above), Sections 10 and 11 ((7) and (8) above) and in part Section 4 ((2) and (3)), excluding the sub-section referring to the request for assessment by a representative. There has been no date set as yet for the implementation of those parts of the Act which refer to representation (1) or to assessment after discharge from hospital (4). The earliest date is probably 1990.

Advocacy

The Act referred to above requires representation or advocacy for disabled people. In Britain, the Jay Report (1979) encouraged it and the Advocacy Alliance started in 1982 to promote a one-to-one scheme of friendship protection and representation for many isolated people living in long-stay Mental Handicap Hospitals. Not until the Tom Clark Act was advocacy provided for by government. In general, three forms of advocacy are recognized:

1. *Self-advocacy* – Such as in *People First*.
2. *Legal advocacy* – Lawyers and other skilled individuals help mentally ill and mentally handicapped defend their rights.
3. *Lay advocacy/citizen advocacy* – People appointed on a one-to-one basis to foster respect, give voice to individuals' concerns and aspirations, and see that everyday services (social, recreational, health, etc.) are provided. This is the type of advocacy envisaged in the 'Tom Clark' Act.

Miscellany

Driving licences – People who are detained under the Mental Health Acts, or receiving in-patient treatment for mental disorder, or who have severe mental impairment or whose estate is governed by the Court of Protection by reason of mental disorder or mental defect, may not be granted a driving licence (Road Traffic Act 1972.)

Travel abroad – Many countries have specific regulations which may exclude people with mental disorder from entering them. This also applies to people with criminal records; e.g. for travel to the USA, people with a mental handicap may have difficulty if not travelling with a parent or guardian, or if they have been detained under the Mental Health Act.

This chapter had covered most of the major legal issues which impinge directly on people with a mental handicap, by virtue of that handicap. It has not covered the entitlements to benefits such as Severe Disablement Allowances, Mobility Allowance, etc. Of necessity, the chapter is not exhaustive, and the reader is advised to consult the regulations themselves if further information is required.

References

Bluglass, R. (1983) *A Guide to the Mental Health Act 1983*, Churchill Livingstone, Edinburgh
DHSS (1979) *Report of the Committee of Enquiry into Mental Handicap, Nursing and Care*, Cmnd 7468, HMSO, London
DHSS (1986) *The Mental Health (Northern Ireland) Order 1986: A Guide*, HMSO, London
DHSS (1986) *Mental Health Act 1983. Memorandum on Parts I–VI, VIII and X*, HMSO, London
Gostin, L.O. (1975) *A Human Condition*, MIND, London
Gostin, L.O. (1983) *The Court of Protection*, MIND, London
Mental Health Act (1983) HMSO, London
Mental Health (Scotland) Act (1984) JMSO, London

Further reading

Royal Society for Mentally Handicapped Children and Adults (1989) *Consent to Medical Treatment*, Mencap, London

19.3 Role of the Commissions

Hector Fowlie

The Commissions which are appointed in the United Kingdom with, *inter alia*, particular responsibility for overseeing the care of people with mental handicaps are derived from provisions made in the different Mental Health Acts for England and Wales, Northern Ireland and Scotland. Although the Commissions may have a common purpose they are, because of their separate legal origins, quite different in some very important aspects concerning their composition and in the execution of their distinctive duties.

There are three Commissions. They are the Mental Health Act Commission for England and Wales, the Mental Health Commission for Northern Ireland and the Mental Welfare Commission for Scotland.

It is immediately important to notice that their titles are different for this underlines the fundamental differences between the Commission in Scotland and the other two Commissions in the rest of the United Kingdom.

In England and Wales the Commission is restricted in its work with people with mental handicap to a concern for the care of those who are detained compulsorily under some provision of the Mental Health Act 1983 and who are, or have recently been, in hospital care. In Scotland and Northern Ireland, on the other hand, the Commissions have a wider frame of reference for they can concern themselves with the welfare of persons with mental handicap, whatever their legal status, provided they are in hospital. In Scotland this duty extends even further to persons with mental handicaps whether they are in hospital or in the community.

This distinction greatly increases the importance of the Scottish Commission for of course the great majority of people with mental handicaps are neither detained nor are they in hospital. In Scotland the care of all people with mental handicaps can fall within the Commission's remit whereas in England and Wales and in Northern Ireland the care of the great majority is outwith the scrutiny of the respective Commissions.

All three Commissions can trace their origins to the middle of the nineteenth century when Boards of Commissioners in Lunacy were established to oversee the work of District Boards of Lunacy which were then responsible for providing accommodation and care for the mentally unsound, a category which included those who would nowadays be termed as people with mental handicaps. Although legislation in the next 100 years or so made minor modifications to the duties of these Boards and, during the time of the First World War, changed the name to Board of Control, it was not until the mid-1950s that substantial change was made. At that time public opinion and concern for the mentally disordered had been so heightened that new more liberal legislation was introduced. This was probably in part a consequence of dissatisfaction with the standards of care provided by local authorities prior to the establishment of the National Health Service in the late 1940s and, in part, a response to the public's growing sense of moral obligation towards its less fortunate members.

However, at that time in England and Wales and in Northern Ireland the Board of Control was disbanded so that there was for the next 25 years no body statutorily charged with the important task of monitoring the care, rights and welfare of people with mental handicaps in these parts of the United Kingdom.

In Scotland, however, the Board of Control, after a brief administrative hiatus, was replaced by the Mental Welfare Commission for Scotland which has persisted to this day so that in Scotland there has been an uninterrupted period of 130 years or so during which there has been some kind of independent scrutiny of the lives of people with mental handicap.

Some people have said that this difference between England and Wales, where there was no scrutiny for 25 years, and Scotland, where there was, accounts for the fact that there occurred in England and Wales in the 1960s and 1970s a number of episodes of grossly deficient care which were revealed by public enquiries whereas there were none of these in Scotland.

There may be some substance in this but it should not be thought that Scottish services for people with mental handicap were necessarily significantly better for during that same period the Mental Welfare Commission in Scotland held a number of private statutory enquiries which dealt with similar, though perhaps not such widespread, neglect and abuse.

Be that as it may, in 1962, the Mental Welfare Commission for Scotland was established by the terms of the Mental Health (Scotland) Act of 1960. Its duties and composition were revised and enlarged by the Mental Health (Scotland) Act of 1984 of which Part 2 deals exclusively with the Commission.

It is the Scottish Commission's duty:

'Generally to exercise protective functions in respect of persons who may, by reason of mental disorder, be incapable of adequately protecting their persons or interests.'

The Scottish Commission is, in effect, a standing Royal Commission for its members are appointed by the Queen on the recommendation of the Secretary of State for Scotland who, before he makes recommendations, is obliged to consult interested bodies.

There must be at least 10 Commissioners of whom three must be women, three must be medical practitioners and one must be a lawyer or advocate. But these are minimal numbers. In 1989 there were 19 Commissioners in Scotland of whom five were women and four were medical practitioners. One, who was the Chairman, was a lawyer and another was an advocate. Three were nurses, three were social workers, one was a clinical psychologist and one an occupational therapist. Some Commissioners had interests in education and in health service administration; others were connected with or worked for a variety of voluntary agencies concerned with mental health.

In Scotland three Commissioners (two psychiatrists and one social worker) have full-time salaried appointments. The rest, who have part-time appointments, are paid an annual honorarium (about £300 in 1989) and give an average of between 30 and 40 days per year to the work of the Commission.

The Scottish Commission also employs professional staff – one full-time and two part-time medical officers and one full-time social work officer. The secretary of the Commission in Scotland is a seconded civil servant as are the other administrative and clerical staff who process the work of the Commission.

By contrast the Commissions in England and Wales and in Northern Ireland are special health authorities whose members (Commissioners) are appointed by the respective Secretaries of State for Health who may direct the Commission in the performance of its duties. The Scottish Commission is not subject to direction in this way.

The principles governing appointment to the three Commissions and the range of interests and professional expertise of those appointed are essentially similar. There is, however, no minimal number, no requirement as to medical membership or female representation and no statutory requirement to consult interested bodies before making appointments in either England and Wales or in Northern Ireland. Unlike Scotland there are no full-time Commissioners nor professional officers in either England and Wales or Northern Ireland where all Commissioners are part time and are paid, not an honorarium but a fee for each attendance to carry out the duties of a Commissioner.

With the exception of the independence and wider remit enjoyed by the Scottish Commission (which are seen to be extremely important, however) the above are differences of detail which are of little importance. One other difference, however, is most important.

The Scottish Commission has a significant role to play as an appellate body to which detained patients may appeal against liability to detention and guardianship.

The general duty of the Mental Welfare Commission quoted above is extended in these terms:

> 'And where those persons are liable to be detained in hospital or subject to guardianship under the following provisions of this Act their functions as aforesaid shall include in appropriate cases the discharge of such patients in accordance with the said provisions.'

The provision which allows the Commission to discharge a patient is contained in Section 33(3) of the Mental Health (Scotland) Act 1984 where it states:

> 'The Mental Welfare Commission shall make an order for discharge in respect of a patient where ... they are satisfied that:
> (a) he is not suffering from mental disorder of a nature or degree which makes it appropriate for him to be liable to be detained in hospital for medical treatment or
> (b) it is not necessary for the health or safety of the patient or for the protection of other persons that he should receive such treatment.'

In this regard the Commission in Scotland carries out work similar to that of the Mental Health Review Tribunals in England and Wales and Northern Ireland. These tribunals have no counterpart in Scotland where however patients, in addition to their right of appeal to the Mental Welfare Commission, have periodic rights of appeal against liability to detention to a sheriff.

It will be recalled from the preceding section that there are three types of detention in Scotland. Emergency detention (which lasts for up to 72 hours) under Section 24 of the Mental Health (Scotland) Act 1984; detention under Section 26 of the Act for a period which may last up to 28 days and what is sometimes called 'full detention' under Section 18 of the Act which may last for up to 6 months and may be further extended under the powers of Section 30 of the Act.

It is a serious anomaly of the Scottish legislation that there is no effective appeal against detention for up to 72 hours under Section 24 of the Act. Although empowered to do so the Commission cannot in practice respond within that period of time and although it may be theoretically possible to have some emergency hearing before a sheriff within the 72 hour period the writer is not aware of this ever having been done.

In effect therefore the Commission must hear any appeal against liability to detention which has been lodged with it within certain time limits from any patient who has been detained for more than 72 hours.

Where the Commission thinks it proper to do so it may discharge these patients from liability to detention so that, if they remain in hospital, they do so by their own wish as informal patients. However, in the case of a patient who is detained (under Part V of the Act) following criminal proceedings in court, and upon whose discharge a Restriction Order has been placed, only the Secretary of State has the power to discharge. The Commission may, however, on request from such a patient or someone acting for him, undertake a review of the case and may recommend to the Secretary of State that the patient be discharged.

The Secretary of State need not act on this recommendation, however, and in this regard it has to be realized, particularly in the case of a person who is suffering from mental handicap, that the grounds for detention rest upon the assertion that the patient is suffering from a mental disorder and not that the patient suffers from one of the sub-categories of mental disorder.

In the cases of some detained patients whose detention had been the subject of a Restriction Order, and who at the time of appearance in court were said to be suffering from a mental disorder which was mental handicap, it was subsequently shown that improvement in their condition had been such that they could no longer be regarded legally as mentally handicapped. The Commission's subsequent recommendation that they should be discharged has not been acted upon, however, because the Secretary of State has held that the patient has been and is also suffering from a mental illness (usually personality disorder) which, though not explicitly specified in court, nonetheless existed then and was, by implication, part of the mental disorder which was the justification for detention.

This is an unsatisfactory state of affairs and the Commission's periodic confidential representations about the injustice inherent in such situations is a good example of one of the ways in which the Commission in Scotland exercises its general duty to care.

In Scotland a patient may appeal against liability to detention to the Commission by telephone message or by letter, and anyone acting for the patient may intimate the appeal verbally or in writing. The patient need not put forward any stated case. It is sufficient that a detained patient says merely 'I don't want to be here' for the Commission to initiate the appeal process. The Commission reacts very promptly, in a matter of days rather than weeks. A medical officer will visit to examine the patient, to scrutinize the legal and medical documents and to interview the Responsible Medical Officer and others who were principally concerned with the care of the patient. Relatives and friends may also be interviewed. A formal written report and recommendation is then made to the Commission. If the medical officer is of the opinion that the Commission should discharge the patient a Medical

Commissioner also personally examines the patient, makes such further investigations as seem appropriate and makes a separate report. The Commission does not as a body interview the patient and neither the patient nor his advisers have a right of audience with the Commission.

If, in the view of the Commission as a whole, the patient should be discharged from liability to detention the Commission will do this and advises the patient and the Responsible Medical Officer within about 2 days.

The Commission rarely finds it advisable to discharge a patient. The explanation for this is two-fold. First, because no stated case need be made before the Commission starts the appeal process it is a fact that in the great majority of cases there has been no significant change in the patient's condition and very often only a very brief period has intervened since the detention order was made or renewed. Second, very frequently a medical officer or Commissioner investigating an appeal against liability to detention will, in discussion with the Responsible Medical Officer, reach a situation where the Responsible Medical Officer is prepared to discharge the patient from liability to detention rather than having the Commission discharge the patient against the apparent wish of the Responsible Medical Officer. The Commission prefers that this should happen for it believes that it is more likely that the patient and doctor will remain in a helpful therapeutic relationship which might be damaged if the Commission is seen to be overruling the Responsible Medical Officer. Nevertheless, the Commission does not shirk from so overruling the Responsible Medical Officer where it thinks it appropriate and necessary to do so.

Discharge from liability to detention does not of course imply that the detention has been improper: only that in the opinion of the Commission as a whole it is no longer necessary.

Certain duties are laid upon all three Commissions. They are, in general, required to respond to allegations of ill-treatment, deficiency of care, deficiency of treatment, and loss or damage to property belonging to the mentally handicapped person but the Scottish Commission is also empowered to initiate enquiry into any such alleged circumstance.

Allegations of ill-treatment may be made by a person or group of people with mental handicaps or by someone on their behalf. Depending on the circumstances alluded to in the allegation, the Commission may call for reports from those who are clinically or managerially responsible or may send one or more Commissioners or officers to make its own informal enquiry into the circumstances. Most allegations of ill-treatment are investigated by one or other or by a combination of these two methods but all three Commissions are careful to allow Management to make its own investigation and response to the allegation before the Commission intervenes:

> During a routine visit by the Scottish Commission to a large hospital for mentally handicapped persons a number of patients requested private interview with Commissioners. Amongst other things three or four patients complained of sexual harassment by other patients in a particular ward. These complaints, combined with other matters which came to light during the Commission's visit, caused the Commission such concern that within 24 hours it had paid an unannounced night visit to the hospital and in the ensuing week had interviewed privately every patient in the ward concerned. The allegations made by patients were, in the view of the Commission, substantiated. Such was the Commission's

concern about this and other matters that it sought an urgent meeting with the Hospital Board concerned. Following this the Board concerned took prompt action to remedy the immediate unsatisfactory situation in the ward concerned and the Commission's intervention probably played a significant part in the Board's subsequent determination to improve conditions in the hospital as a whole.

Where the Scottish Commission thinks it appropriate it may conduct a formal enquiry at which evidence may be taken on oath or it may appoint some other person or persons to do this on its behalf. This has very rarely been done. Between 1972 when this power was given and 1984 there were three such enquiries, all of which were brief and held in private. There has been no such enquiry since 1984 when, in Scotland, regularly recurring visiting of institutions by Commissioners was instituted. This power is not enjoyed by the other Commissions.

Allegations of deficiency of care or of treatment can be made by any person in respect of an individual or group of people with mental handicaps. Such allegations about patients are difficult to investigate, for, especially in the field of treatment, which is a medical responsibility, as opposed to care, which is usually a nursing responsibility, the Commissions tread on the thin ice of professional independence, responsibility and culpability. Nevertheless the Commissions do not where it is appropriate shy from making a judgement about these matters for the Commissions have within themselves a considerable range of professional expertise and can take evidence on these matters from expert witnesses where this is thought appropriate:

> On a number of successive visits to a large hospital for the mentally handicapped (not that referred to above) the Scottish Commission was increasingly concerned by the evidence of a general lack of any planned or structured therapeutic programme for the vast majority of patients and by the persistingly poor standards of accommodation which combined to afford patients what was considered to be an unacceptably low quality of life. Repeated representations were made both to the local management and to the health board concerned. Unhappily the Commission remained dissatisfied with the responses to these representations to an extent that it felt it necessary to describe the conditions about which it was concerned and to name the hospital in one of its Annual Reports to Parliament.
>
> Although the hospital board and local management formulated and put into effect ambitious and far-reaching plans for improvement in the hospital and for the development of services for people with mentally handicapped in the community, the Commission insisted ultimately on meeting the health board to point out that although understandably these plans would only come to fruition over the period of a number of years the conditions under which some patients were living remained quite unacceptable. After that meeting there was evidence that the board had been persuaded of the urgency of immediate as well as long-term improvements in its services.

All three Commissions will investigate any complaint of loss or damage to property. The Scottish Commission may do this even though the property is in the community:

> During a hospital visit a patient with mental handicaps complained to a Commissioner that she had been transferred from a part of the hospital where she had enjoyed the privacy of her own room to another ward which did not

have that facility. The Commission could not intervene in the clinical and managerial decision to transfer the patient, for it was management policy to close the original ward. However, in the original ward the patient had been able to gather personal possessions which she cared for, regularly used and valued. In the transfer from one ward to another certain of these personal possessions had been lost. Various administrative explanations had been given to the patient but no compensation was offered until the Commission insisted that this be done.

The Commissions are required to visit regularly patients who have been detained, and in Scotland the Commission regularly visits patients who are living in the community on leave of absence or on guardianship.

There are few patients with mental handicap who are on leave of absence but a not inconsiderable number of patients are on guardianship. Visiting by the Commission affords an opportunity for independent review of the extent to which care is or is not being given to the mentally handicapped person concerned:

A man with mental handicaps living with unrelated guardians in Scotland was found during a visit by the Commission living in what was little more than a garden hut and obliged to use dry sanitation. Some aspects of his accommodation were thought to be dangerous but in addition it was in such stark contrast to the comfortable conditions of the guardians that the Commission made immediate complaint to the Social Work Department whose responsibility it was to supervise the Guardianship Order. As a result steps were taken initially to improve the man's accommodation and ultimately to move the man to more appropriate, modern sheltered accommodation.

The English and Scottish Commissions are informed when mail addressed to a patient in a special hospital in England or the State Hospital in Scotland is withheld and if the patient objects to this the Commission is required to investigate the circumstances and is empowered if it thinks it appropriate to instruct that the withheld mail be delivered to the patient.

The three Commissions are now required to make reports to Parliament which are published and available to the public. This is done at varying intervals: periodically in Northern Ireland, every 2 years in England and Wales and annually in Scotland.

The Commissions are not required to do so but where they think it appropriate they may bring any matter about which complaint has been made to the Commission to the notice of the appropriate Secretary of State, health board, local authority or any other person or authority which has an interest in the matter. The Scottish Commission may proffer advice and bring matters to notice even though these have not been the subject of complaint to it.

The Scottish Commission, in what was to prove a controversial decision, made an exceptional public statement in 1987 on the topic of the staffing levels in hospitals for mentally disordered patients. The Commission had, over the previous 3 years, noted with mounting concern that in many instances level of staff available to patients including those with mental handicap was such that although safe care was being provided no pretence could be made that therapeutic care was being carried out. Repeated comment had been made privately to health boards but the evidence of what amounted to neglect was so compelling that the Commission felt it necessary to bring this to the notice of the public at large. Shortly thereafter, and coincidentally, it was announced that increased funding would be made available for staff in hospitals for the mentally disordered and the Commission's public statement probably helped subsequently to further improve the situation in many hospitals.

A complaint was made to the Scottish Commission by the parents of a handicapped child about their dissatisfaction with the way in which evidence of an assault upon the child had been investigated by the local authority which was responsible for the child's care. In what proved to be an extremely complex case it transpired that the child was living in a hostel run by the local authority social work department and was attending a school run by the local authority education department. School staff noted that the child was bruised and there was prima facie evidence that this had been the result of an assault sustained while the child was in the social work department hostel. The authority's investigation was extremely protracted (it was compounded by the fact that two departments were concerned and that there was a possibility of litigation) and it was not until the Commission intervened in response to the parents' complaint that the authority was prepared to make even a qualified explanation of the circumstances which had resulted in bruising.

The Manager of a privately run home for persons with mental handicaps sought the support of the Scottish Commission in his resistance to complying with certain requests made by a local authority. When these people with mental handicaps were visited the Commission, far from supporting the manager, found, reported and was instrumental in having rectified certain specific deficiencies of care and made known its concern about some aspects of the accommodation and general care being afforded to these handicapped people. Periodic visiting over a period of about 3 years probably influenced an improvement in the living conditions but demonstrated how important it is to recognize the tension between the handicapped person's contentment and the enhanced self-image which derives from relative self-sufficiency on the one hand and the denial to that person of an enhanced quality of life because the potential for that fuller life is not perceived by either the immediate carers or the handicapped person himself.

The three Commissions have developed different styles of work which allow them to carry out these duties. The English Commission, because of its widespread geographic responsibilities and the number of Commissioners (approximately 100), organizes itself into a Central Policy Committee with three Regional Committees which carry out the actual work of the Commission. The Commissions in Northern Ireland and in Scotland do not require such a Committee structure. In England and Wales responsibility for investigation and follow-up of any matter arising out of a complaint or a visit remains with the particular Commissioners to whom the work has been delegated whereas the Commissions in Northern Ireland and in Scotland receive reports of these activities and, as a whole, instruct such further action as seems necessary either by the Secretariat or, in Scotland, by its full-time professional staff.

It will be apparent from examples of work given above that the Commissions make regular visits to hospitals in which there are detained patients and in Northern Ireland and Scotland to every hospital dealing with mentally ill patients or people with mental handicap. Usually several Commissioners go on each visit primarily for the purpose of interviewing every patient who has been detained more than 2 years and any other detained patient who requests this.

During these visits the Commissioners in England and Wales and in Northern

Ireland will scrutinize the medico-legal documentation of detained patients but in Scotland that is not necessary since such documents are in any case copied routinely to the Commission whose officers scrutinized their detailed accuracy.

In Scotland, in addition to these annual visits to hospitals, a second visit each year is paid to allow patients the opportunity of interview and, of course, Commissioners visit any patient as a matter of urgency when the circumstances seem to merit this. Officers of the Scottish Commission also visit at least once a year all patients who are on guardianship; and patients who are on leave of absence but still liable to detention are visited at least annually after they have been on leave of absence for 6 months. A patient who is subject to guardianship is required to live at an address approved of by the guardian:

> When such a patient was visited by the Scottish Commission it was discovered that the patient was required to reside in a hospital for the mentally handicapped. This seemed to be an inappropriate use of the powers conferred on a guardian (which in this case was the Local Authority Social Work Department), the more so since the intended temporary admission to hospital had been prolonged over a period of several months while the Social Work Department sought unsuccessfully to find a more appropriate placement for the patient in the community. The Commission's intervention in the case almost certainly lent such urgency to a reconsideration of the case that an appropriate place was shortly thereafter found in the community for this mentally handicapped person who had no need of hospital care.

The Scottish Commission has reported to it accidents, incidents and the unexpected death of patients, particularly detained patients, but it must be noted that there is no requirement on hospital authorities to make reports on these matters. As a consequence the Commission cannot speak with any authority about prevalence or trends in these matters. Nevertheless, the custom, which is of long standing, has enabled the Commission to remind hospital authorities of such matters as the importance of safeguarding poisonous domestic fluids and of regulating access to fire escapes:

> It was reported to the Commission that a man with mental handicaps had been injured while he was a patient in a mental handicap hospital. He had been working with agricultural machinery and, either because the machinery was insufficiently safeguarded or because the supervision given to him was insufficient, he sustained an injury which resulted in the loss of a fingertip. The Commission advised that legal advice should be furnished to the patient as to whether a possible action for negligence on the part of the Hospital Board should be raised. Possibly as a result of this an *ex gratia* payment, the amount of which seemed satisfactory to the patient's legal advisers and to the Commission, was made to the patient.

> An alleged sexual assault on a female patient was reported to the Commission. In the context of that report it became apparent that the alleged perpetrator was a fellow patient, a man with mental handicaps, who had been charged with the offence and who had appeared in court without benefit of legal representation. The Commission immediately instructed that a lawyer be made available to the patient and manifested its continuing interest in both parties by attending court to observe the subsequent proceedings.

All three Commissions have selected some topics of psychiatric practice in which they have had a special interest and about which they have made special enquiry during their visits to hospitals. These topics have, most importantly, centred on the theme of the deprivation of liberty and, especially in England and Wales, on the rights of Ethnic and minority groups. The Scottish Commission has surveyed and reviewed practices concerning the seclusion of patients, the use of locked wards and the use of time-out from positive reinforcement which is a technique of behavioural therapy which, in some instances, involves the deprivation of liberty.

The legal and ethical implications of managing some informal patients and residents in accommodation which is locked has exercised professional staff, management, voluntary organizations and the Commissions to a considerable degree. The issues are complex and the Mental Welfare Commission in particular has thought it important to point out that any resolution of the problem should not, to an even greater extent, disadvantage any individual or group of people with mental handicap.

In its report for 1985 under the heading 'De Facto Detention' the Scottish Commission said:

'The Commission thinks it will be helpful to say that it has formed a view about the vexed question of *de facto* detention by which is meant the physical protection of informal patients who do not object to it, or who are incapable of objecting to it, by caring for them in closed wards.

'The Commission thinks it entirely appropriate and believes that relatives and the public would expect that the exits from wards in which such patients are nursed should be under close staff surveillance and where that cannot be guaranteed the Commission accepts that it will be necessary to keep these patients under lock and·key.

'Such patients do not seem to the Commission to be advantaged in any way by being legally detained in order only to legitimize the locking of a door in front of them. To detain these patients would be to stigmatize them. In any case these informal patients or someone acting on their behalf can complain to the Commission which also regularly visits these wards in which they are living if it is felt that they are being improperly cared for.

'These patients do not therefore seem to the Commission to be significantly or materially deprived of any human right in being so safeguarded by an informal process of *de facto* detention. Indeed it could be argued that failure so to safeguard them would be reprehensible.'

The review which the Commission in Scotland undertook of the practice of time-out from positive reinforcement is most relevant to the care of persons with mental handicaps. The Commission concluded in its Annual Report for 1985 with the following comment:

'Time-out procedures would appear from the returns given by hospitals to be used in just under one-third of Scottish psychiatric and mental handicap hospitals. In these hospitals the vast majority of situations in which the procedures were used, related to patients with a mental handicap rather than a mental illness. Time out is reported to be used in fewer hospitals than is seclusion (12 as opposed to 16 hospitals); seclusion is more commonly used in psychiatric settings as well as in those relating to mental handicap. However, the Commission has formed the strong view that a number of hospitals reporting the use of time out were in practice carrying out seclusion. The Commission arrived at this view from either a study of the policy or practice statements included in the questionnaire returns; or as a result of discussions with staff during hospital visits; or both. The Commission are at a loss to provide an adequate explanation for this finding; it is likely that confusion over the precise nature of the two procedures exists in some hospitals; it is possible that one procedural label (time out) is considered (albeit erroneously) to be more "therapeutically respectable" than the other (seclusion); or it is possible that an intention to conduct time out procedures was imperfectly realized in practice.'

The Scottish Commission had, in 1985, reviewed the practice of seclusion in hospitals caring for people with mental handicaps. Eight such hospitals permitted seclusion while 7 did not. Three years later when the practice was again reviewed no hospital caring for people with mental handicaps reported that seclusion was still permitted.

All three Commissions have responsibility for operating those parts of the relevant Mental Health Acts which deal with Consent to Treatment. It is vitally important to realize that it is only treatments for mental disorder which have been specified by the relevant Secretaries of State in regulations which are governed by these Acts.

Surgical and medical treatments for other conditions of a surgical or medical nature which may coincidentally affect a person with mental handicaps in the same way as they affect any other person are not included in these legal provisions. There are other considerations regarding the ability of a person with mental handicap to give consent to such operations and treatments but these have been dealt with in the preceding section.

The provisions of the three Mental Health Acts which deal with Consent to Treatments for mental disorder are detailed and must be followed meticulously. Here it is possible only to give a general outline of them. In practice the relevant Acts, the associated Notes of Guidance and Codes of Practice; and any advice given by the relevant Commission should be consulted at a very early stage in the consideration of these treatments.

There are two classes of these treatments. The first comprises two different kinds of treatment. These are the treatment of mental disorder by the surgical removal of brain tissue and the surgical implantation of a hormone or hormones for the purpose of altering male sex drive.

In England and Wales and in Northern Ireland the regulations concerning these treatments apply to any patient whereas in Scotland they apply only to detained patients. In Scotland, however, the treatment could not be given lawfully to a non-consenting informal patient. The only difference is therefore that in Scotland it is not necessary (though it will always be prudent) to have independent confirmation of the patient's consent and need for the operation.

The three Acts are otherwise the same. Before such operations can be carried out the patient must freely request it in the sense that he must understand the nature, purpose and likely effect of it and consent to it; and his ability to understand and consent must be verified by a group of three people appointed by the Commission. Two of the people must not be medically qualified. The medically qualified Commissioner must, in addition, be of the opinion that, having regard to the likely effect of the treatment in alleviating or preventing deterioration in the patient's condition, the treatment should be given.

In practice these operations are not presently indicated for the treatment of mental handicap. Although it is possible that a patient with mental handicaps might have an associated mental disorder for which one of these treatments was indicated, the writer knows of no such occurrence. Indeed in Scotland no such treatment has been carried out on any detained patient since 1984.

The second class of treatments with which this part of the Acts are concerned is the giving to detained patients either ECT at any time or the continuous use of medicines for the treatment of mental disorder for longer than 3 months.

If a patient can understand the nature, purpose and likely effects of the treatment and consents to it, the treatment can be given once the responsible medical officer has signed a certificate of consent to that effect.

Where such a treatment is proposed for a patient who either cannot understand the nature, purpose and likely effect of the treatment or who objects to it, the treatment cannot be given unless and until a doctor appointed by the Commission (and colloquially known as a Second Opinion Doctor) certifies that the treatment should be given.

These are not treatments for mental handicap *per se* but it is not uncommon for people with mental handicaps to suffer from an associated mental illness for which these treatments are indeed indicated. Staff who are dealing with detained patients with mental handicaps should therefore be familiar with the Acts, the more so since there is an indication in each Act that in addition to medical staff who have been concerned in the treatment of the patient other, non-medical staff should be consulted by the Second Opinion Doctor before a Certificate of Treatment is issued.

The Certificate of Treatment or of Consent will specify the nature of the treatment or the plan of treatment. Staff should be aware also that, other than in situations of urgency which call for separate Certification, a treatment for mental disorder which is not included in the specification of the treatment or the plan of treatment cannot be given to a patient who objects or who does not understand.

In the early days of the operation of these Acts this led to much confusion which is not, even yet, entirely resolved. If a Responsible Medical Officer or Second Opinion Doctor precisely specifies the dose and frequency of administration of a drug rather than specifying treatment with that drug within certain limits then the drug should not be administered in a dose or at a frequency other than those appearing on the Certificate of Consent or of Treatment. Medical staff who prescribe these treatments should be aware of the limitations imposed by the Responsible Medical Officer or the Second Opinion Doctor and should not place nursing staff and others in the invidious position of being invited to carry out what is in fact an unlawful instruction.

Each of the three Commissions operates this part of the Act in essentially the same way though the nature of the Commissions permit slight variations. In Scotland the Commission receives a copy of each Certificate of Consent or of Second Opinion and has therefore been able to monitor very closely the way in which these treatments are being given to detained patients. It is likely that the operation of this part of the Act and the way in which the three Commissions have exercised their responsibilities have resulted in some changes in medical practice. There is some evidence that the frequency of use of ECT in any one patient has lessened; that the use of medicines for the treatment of mental disorder in doses in excess of those recommended by manufacturers has been virtually eliminated other than in extremely difficult or intractable cases; and that the simultaneous use of two or more drugs for the treatment of mental disorder has become less prevalent.

The three Commissions review treatments given under this part of the Act in different ways. In Scotland, for instance, the Commission instructs a further second opinion on any detained patient who has understood the nature, purpose and likely effect of a treatment which has persisted for more than 3 years. The initial results of this review indicate that the treatment is seldom stopped or radically altered and this, together with the high rate of agreement between Responsible Medical Officers and Second Opinion Doctors, has led to scepticism about the effectiveness of the system amongst those who oppose such treatments and about the necessity for the system by those who oppose such treatments and about the necessity for the system by those who see merit in these treatments.

In this chapter it is possible only to give an outline of the work of the three Commissions. For a fuller account of this it is necessary to go to the periodic formal reports of the Commission. Each Commission also publicizes its work in various ways – by contact by the media, by contributing to professional teaching programmes and scientific meetings and in Scotland by the publication and wide distribution of a series of leaflets for patients or residents and for staff in hospitals and institutions as well as for the relatives and friends of people with mental handicaps.

Appendix I

Milestones of speech and language acquisition

Average age		
Birth	Vocalizations	Profoundly mentally handicapped
6 months	Babble	
10 months	Reduplications appear: 'Ma-ma' – 'Ba-ba'	
1 year	One-word sentences	
18 months	Two-word utterances	Severely mentally handicapped
20 months	Telegrammatic speech	
2 years	Pre-sleep monologues	
2½ years	50-word lexicon, 5-word sentences, I, personal pronoun	
3 years	Plurals established, 250 words	
3½ years	'p', 'b', 'm', 'w', 'h' pronounced. How? Why? questions	
4 years	Tells story; still many morphological erros	
4½ years	't', 'k', 'd', 'ng', 'y' pronounced. Asks what words mean	
5½ years	'f', 'z', 's', 'v' pronounced	Language established
6½ years	'sh', 'zh', 'l', 'th' pronounced. Adult morphology complete. Listens to another's standpoint in conversation	
8 years	'ch', 'r', 'wh' pronounced	Normal intelligence

Appendix 2

Diagnostic categories and clinical conditions

Ronald MacGillivray

Categorization

The clinical varieties of mental handicap may be considered as follows:

1. Mental handicap following infections:
   (a) Gastro-enteritis in the newborn.
   (b) Meningitis.
   (c) Congenital syphilis.
   (d) Encephalitis.
   (e) Congenital rubella syndrome.
   (f) Cytomegalic inclusion disease.
   (g) Toxoplasmosis.
2. Mental handicap following injury or physical agents:
   (a) Pre-eclampsia and eclampsia.
   (b) Excessive intra-uterine irradiation.
   (c) Birth injury.
   (d) Rhesus incompatibility.
   (e) Drugs and the newborn.
   (f) Lead poisoning.
3. Mental handicap associated with disorders of metabolism:
   (a) Disorders of lipid metabolism:
       (i) Amaurotic family idiocy (cerebromacular degeneration).
       (ii) Niemann–Pick disease.
       (iii) Gaucher's disease.
       (iv) Metachromatic leucodystrophy (sulphatide lipidosis).
   (b) Disorders of amino-acid metabolism:
       (i) Phenylketonuria.
       (ii) Tyrosinaemia.
       (iii) Homocystinuria.
       (iv) Histidinaemia.
       (v) Maple syrup urine disease.
       (vi) Hartnup disease.
       (vii) Hyperuricaemia.
   (c) Disorders of carbohydrate metabolism:
       (i) Gargoylism (Hunter/Hurler).
       (ii) Galactosaemia.
       (iii) Hypoglycaemia.
   (d) Disorders of endocrine metabolism: cretinism.

    (e) Disorders of mineral and electrolyte metabolism:
        (i)   Wilson's disease (hepatolenticular degeneration).
        (ii)   Diabetes insipidus (nephrogenic).
        (iii) Hypomagnesaemia.
    (f) Disorders of nutrition in the infant: malnutrition.
4. Mental handicap associated with brain disease:
    (a) Neurofibromatosis.
    (b) Sturge–Weber syndrome.
    (c) Tuberous sclerosis.
    (d) Schilder's disease.
5. Mental handicap associated with disease and conditions due to prenatal factors:
    (a) Acrocephalosyndactyly.
    (b) Craniostenosis.
    (c) Hydrocephalus.
    (d) Hypertelorism.
    (e) Microcephaly.
    (f) Laurence–Moon–Biedl syndrome.
    (g) Ichthyosis.
    (h) De Lange syndrome.
    (i) Rubinstein–Taybi syndrome.
    (j) Smith–Lemli–Opitz syndrome.
6. Mental handicap with chromosomal abnormalities:
    (a) Down's syndrome.
        (i)   Regular (trisomy).
        (ii)   Translocation.
        (iii) Mosaic.
    (b) Cat-cry syndrome.
    (c) Trisomy 13 (Patau's syndrome).
    (d) Trisomy 18 (Edwards' syndrome).
    (e) Sex chromosome abnormalities:
        (i)   Klinefelter's syndrome.
        (ii)   Turner's syndrome.
        (iii) Triple-X syndrome.
        (iv) XYY syndrome.
        (v)   Fragile X.
    (f) Prader–Willi syndrome.
7. Mental handicap associated with prematurity:
    (a) Prematurity.
    (b) Kernicterus.
    (c) Cerebral palsy.
8. Unclassified mental handicap.

1. Mental handicap following infections

(a) Gastro-enteritis in the newborn

In the newborn fluid loss and dehydration in gastro-enteritis may be so severe that brain damage with permanent mental handicap results. Intracranial venous thromboses are usually found in such cases.

(b) Meningitis

Meningitis is an infection of the coverings of the brain. The common types are bacterial and tuberculous meningitis.

The onset in bacterial meningitis is acute, with headache, increasing irritability and pyrexia. Projectile vomiting occurs. Muscle rigidity is found with stiffness of the neck. Mental handicap may develop as a direct result of meningitis causing severe brain damage or following the development of hydrocephalus, when inflammatory lesions block the flow of cerebrospinal fluid. Can be lethal in hours, hence accurate diagnosis and antibiotic treatment are urgent.

Tuberculous meningitis
This usually develops insidiously. Irritability alternates with drowsiness. There is loss of appetite with vomiting and constipation. During the terminal stage hyperpyrexia occurs with coma and paralysis. With antituberculous drugs the majority of infants recover from the infection, but damage to the central nervous system and mental handicap are still too often found.

(c) Congenital syphilis

Congenital syphilis is preventable and occurs only in untreated pregnant women. It occurs before birth and is due to the passage of the organism, *Treponema pallidum*, across the placenta from the mother to the infant. Shortly after birth the infected infant becomes pale and wasted and fails to thrive. A rash is visible on the skin and the nailbeds are infected. There are usually moist lesions on the skin around the mouth, anus and genitals. A characteristic feature is 'snuffles' due to infection of the bones of the nose, with nasal obstruction and purulent and blood-stained discharge; collapse of the nasal bridge occurs with the formation of the saddle-nose deformity. When the nervous system is involved, signs of meningeal irritation develop and convulsions and hydrocephalus may occur. Late manifestations of syphilis may appear from 1 to 10 years after birth, with maldevelopment of the teeth, damage to the eyes, spastic paralysis, convulsions and mental handicap. Thorough antisyphilitic treatment is essential when the diagnosis has been made.

(d) Encephalitis

Encephalitis is an infection of the brain substance. It may occur following infections with measles, rubella, chicken-pox, mumps, epidemic encephalitis lethargica, herpes simplex and herpes zoster. The onset of encephalitis is usually sudden with severe headache and drowsiness, progressing to deep coma. However, the onset can be insidious with a gradually increasing headache, convulsions or behaviour disorders. In young infants mental handicap, nerve palsies and behaviour disorders are likely to be severe and permanent.

(e) Congenital rubella syndrome

Rubella (German measles), if contracted within the first 3 months of pregnancy, may cause in the infant mental handicap, deafness, cataract and congenital heart disease. Immunization which is now available should reduce the incidence. There is no treatment, so prevention is of paramount importance.

(f) Cytomegalic inclusion disease (CMV)

This virus disease in the mother is usually mild. Infection of the fetus, however, gives rise to mental handicap, often with microcephaly and enlargement of the liver and spleen with jaundice. Inclusion bodies can be recognized in tissue cells and in urine and cerebrospinal fluid. Cytomegalic virus (CMV) occurs in 0.4–2.2% of all live births in most populations, this infection being the commonest cause of microbial central nervous system defects. Infection can occur in the uterus, during birth, or from breast milk. No treatment, but virus vaccine under investigation.

(g) Toxoplasmosis

Infection with a boat-shaped protozoon is transmitted to the offspring either late in pregnancy or at birth. It causes mild hydrocephalus or microcephaly, spastic deformities, convulsions and enlargement of liver and spleen. Diagnosis is made by blood tests. It has been estimated that in the UK about 1200 women contract Toxoplasma every year and about 40% of their babies are affected. The usual source is soil contaminated with cat faeces. Commoner in France and Austria, perhaps reflecting the popularity of undercooked meat containing tissue cysts. Routine blood testing is available in certain countries. Treat mother or child with sulphonamides or pyrimethamine.

2. Mental handicap following injury or physical agents

(a) Pre-eclampsia and eclampsia

Pre-eclampsia and eclampsia are conditions which may affect a mother in the last 3 months of pregnancy. There is a rise in maternal blood pressure accompanied by severe headache and oedema of the limbs with kidney and liver disorders. Continuous epileptic seizures occur in eclampsia. Stillbirths are common in this condition and live births may show severe brain damage with mental handicap and epileptic attacks later in life.

(b) Excessive intra-uterine irradiation

During the first 3 months of pregnancy irradiation of the uterus may result in microcephaly and mental handicap of ranging degrees of severity. This is becoming much less common now that pregnancy tests are carried out as a routine before irradiating a woman of childbearing age. While irradiation readily produces congenital malformations experimentally, its teratogenicity in man is less clear.

(c) Birth injury

Prematurity, anoxia (an inadequate supply of oxygen to the tissues) and difficult labour are important factors in birth injury. Prematurity itself may be a cause of intracranial haemorrhage and anoxia is common in premature infants. Anoxia due to delay in breathing after birth can cause direct damage to the brain cells and gives rise to spastic paralysis and mental handicap. Anoxia can result from the administration of large doses of anaesthetic to the mother, from the inhalation of mucus or from the constriction of the windpipe (trachea) by the cord being twined tightly around the neck of the infant. Other obstetric difficulties, such as instrumental delivery, multiple births, hydramnios, precipitate labour or breech delivery, may produce damage to the brain of the baby.

(d) Rhesus incompatibility

About 85% of people carry the Rhesus factor in their red cells ('Rh positive'). The other 15% do not have this factor and are called 'Rh negative'. The condition of rhesus incompatibility occurs when the mother (usually Rh negative) and the fetus (usually Rh positive) are of different groups. Fetal blood enters the mother's circulation and stimulates the production of substances called 'antibodies'. Later in pregnancy these antibodies return across the placenta to destroy the fetal red blood cells; a condition known as 'haemolytic disease in the newborn'. The fetus may die *in utero* or be born with kernicterus, survivors having mental retardation, choreo-athetosis and deafness. Hence antenatal screening for blood and Rh type first in the pregnant mother, and if Rh negative then in the husband.

(c) Drugs and the newborn

Some drugs taken by the mother during pregnancy and by the infant after birth can affect the development of the infant and give rise to mental handicap.

Excessive intake of vitamin D can cause infantile hypercalcaemia. Children so affected become ill shortly after birth with vomiting and constipation. Muscle weakness occurs with thirst and increased output of urine. The blood calcium is raised. Many of these children have elfin faces with low-set ears and prominent epicanthic folds. Heart murmurs are found and the child is usually mentally handicapped.

Enzyme systems in the liver of the infant can be affected by excess of vitamin K and by some antibodies giving rise to jaundice and kernicterus with possible brain damage. Drugs given to the mother to control endocrine, physical or emotional disorders may cause fetal damage. Hypoglycaemia (low blood sugar) usually occurs in these infants and brain damage may follow. Cretinism may develop in the child of a mother who has had treatment for hyperthyroidism (oversecretion of the thyroid hormone) during her pregnancy. Fetal phenytoin syndrome develops in about 11% of children whose mothers receive phenytoin during pregnancy. Features include mental retardation, microcephaly, growth failure, facial abnormalities and cardiac defects. Sodium valproate is also sometimes teratogenic, but it is not always possible to change to carbamazepine currently thought to be the drug of choice.

(f) Fetal alcoholism

There are around 75 000 women alcoholics of child-bearing age in Britain today, whose pregnancies are likely to result in babies with some mental retardation and physical abnormalities. The first 12 weeks of pregnancy, as usual, are the most critical period. At birth a degree of microcephaly is common, physical and mental growth is slow and they never catch up with their contemporaries. They sleep badly, shake and cry a lot, a situation that can go on for years and one that many alcoholic mothers find difficult to cope with, resulting in baby battering, child neglect and accidents in the home.

Drugs in pregnancy should be avoided except where absolutely necessary. An Edinburgh survey showed 80% of women were taking drugs of various kinds other than iron in pregnancy. The mean birth weight of infants born to mothers who smoke cigarettes during pregnancy is 170 g (6 oz) less than that of infants born to non-smoking mothers. The incidence of spontaneous abortion, stillbirth and neonatal death may also be increased in pregnant women who smoke.

(g) Lead poisoning

Ingestion of lead by children may lead to mental handicap. Lead may be absorbed from paint, toys, ointments and cosmetics. A major source in Scotland is the soft water reacting with lead-lined water tanks and pipes. Lead from petrol fumes may contribute. The symptoms include loss of appetite, constipation, headache, irritability, delirium and convulsions. Diagnosis is by estimation of lead in blood and urine and treatment by chelating drugs after withdrawal from exposure. It has recently been suggested that the association between lead and mental retardation extends over a wider range than hitherto considered and that small amounts of lead can be an aetiological factor in mild and borderline cases of mental handicap, particularly with aggressive behaviour. It is therefore suggested that raised lead levels should be considered in the examination of all children suspected of mental retardation. The US government estimates that 4% of children under the age of 6 years have a dangerously high blood concentration of lead. Annual screening of children is therefore recommended, but only 3% are being tested at present.

3. Mental handicap associated with disorders of metabolism

An ever-increasing number of discrete metabolic diseases are now known where abnormalities of lipid, protein or carbohydrate metabolism are associated with mental defect. Some can be detected by simple urine tests, others require elaborate biochemical procedures.

(a) Disorders of lipid metabolism

These conditions form a group of diffuse and progressive disorders of childhood which have a common feature of progressive mental deterioration. They are storage diseases in which various lipids are deposited in the cells of the central nervous system and the tissues of the body.

(i) Amaurotic family idiocy
One example is Tay–Sachs disease. This is a rare condition due to an autosomal recessive gene. There is a deposition of a lipid material within the nerve cells, leading to their degeneration. Tay–Sachs disease is the commonest form and is a disease that mostly affects the Jewish race. The child is normal at birth and develops normally until about the end of the third month when spasticity, generalized weakness, and muscle wasting occur. A characteristic feature is that the infant is easily startled by loud noises. There is progressive loss of vision leading to complete blindness. A 'cherry-red' spot is found in the macula of the retina.

Death usually takes place within 4 years of the onset of the disease. Other types of amaurotic family idiocy have similar presentations but develop later in life. There is no treatment, but the disease can be diagnosed both antenatally and postnatally and the carrier or heterozygote accurately detected.

(ii) Neimann–Pick disease
The onset of this disease caused by a recessive gene is during infancy and death often occurs before the second year. The disease is characterized by mental deterioration and handicap with the physical features of wasting, profuse sweating and yellowish pigmentation of the skin. The liver, spleen and lymph-glands are enlarged. There is loss of vision and hearing. A lipid (sphingomyelin) accumulates in the reticuloendothelial cells and can be demonstrated in biopsy specimens or tissue culture. Treatment is only palliative.

(iii) Gaucher's disease
This is an uncommon familial disorder of lipid metabolism. The cells of the reticulo-endothelial system contain deposits of abnormal glucocerebrosides which lead to an enlargement of the liver, spleen and lymph nodes. In cases with an acute onset the brain may be involved, resulting in mental handicap.

   Treatment – Sometimes splenectomy; blood transfusions for anaemia. Enzyme replacement is under study.

(iv) Metachromatic leucodystrophy (sulphatide lipidosis)
Metachromatic leucodystrophy is a familial disease found in late infancy which causes severe brain damage. The child appears normal for the first year or two but then progressive muscular weakness and inco-ordination develop. Death usually occurs between the third and sixth years in this disease. Metachromatic lipids accumulate in the brain and kidneys, and the accumulation of these substances interferes with normal brain function. Diagnosis is by sophisticated techniques of enzyme analysis and tissue culture.

(b) Disorders of amino-acid metabolism

(i) Phenylketonuria (PKU)
Phenylketonuria is an inborn error of metabolism due to an autosomal recessive gene and commonly accompanied by severe mental handicap. The basic fault is deficiency of the enzyme normally responsible for converting the amino-acid phenylalanine to the amino-acid tyrosine so that phenylalanine, phenylpyruvic acid and their toxic products accumulate in the blood and are subsequently excreted in the urine. Incidence: 1 in 16 000 live births.

   The patient affected with phenylketonuria is nearly always fair-haired with light blue eyes, from pigment deficiency. The skin is fair, soft, smooth and fine in texture. There is frequent occurrence of eczema and there is often cyanosis of the hands and feet due to poor circulation. The patient is dwarfed and a slightly reduced head circumference is not uncommon. The gait is stiff, short-stepped and on a broad base. The incisor teeth are widely spaced. Some phenylketonurics show stiffness in their limbs. Epilepsy occurs in most patients. Repetitive finger movements are seen in the lower-grade patient. Dermatitis is not unusual.

After the newborn has consumed a moderate amount of milk (the source of phenylalanine) for at least 48 hours he should be screened. The Guthrie test which is a bacteriological method detects raised levels of phenylalanine. Use of a dried capillary blood spot on special filter paper permits a punched-out paper disc to be used for simultaneous testing of other conditions (galactosaemia, maple-syrup urine disease, congenital hypothyroidism, etc.). Equipment is semi-automated so a single laboratory may receive specimens from an entire country or state. Another simple screening test involved addition of 10% ferric chloride to a urine sample. A deep blue–green colour is positive. Best after the neonatal period and should be repeated regularly if there is a family history of PKU. When the blood phenylalanine concentration rises above $4\,mg/100\,ml^{-1}$ a diagnosis of phenylketonuria is considered.

Phenylketonuria, when detected at birth, is treated with a low-phenylalanine diet which prevents mental, physical and neurological complications so that affected individuals may live a normal life span. Maternal PKU if untreated has a profound effect on the fetus.

(ii) Tyrosinaemia
There are two types of disorder of tyrosine metabolism in the newborn. Transient tyrosinaemia is the condition in which there are increased plasma tyrosine values which decrease as the child gets older. Usually the only reason why these infants come to notice is that a positive test for tyrosinaemia is found when testing for phenylketonuria in the newborn. Infants with transient tyrosinaemia are physically normal in all respects. The more permanent disorder of tyrosine metabolism is tyrosinosis. Within a few days of birth children affected with this disorder develop severe vomiting and diarrhoea. They fail to thrive and progressive liver failure and severe kidney damage occur. Children who survive may suffer from mental handicap. Treatment is by diet low in phenylalanine and tyrosine.

(iii) Homocystinuria
Homocystinuria is an inborn error of sulphur amino-acid metabolism. The amino-acid methionine is increased in the blood and the amino-acid homocystine appears in the urine. In homocystinuria the patient has certain signs and symptoms, some mild, some severe. These symptoms are dislocated lenses; fine, sparse hair; convulsions; arterial thrombi; malar flush; knock-knees and mental handicap.

Treatment – Massive doses of pyridoxine (B6), control methionine intake.

(iv) Histidinaemia
Histidinaemia is caused by an enzyme defect in the metabolism of the amino-acid histidine. Urine from these patients shows a positive test with ferric chloride, but phenylpyruvic acid is not present in the urine. Affected patients have a speech defect and some are mentally handicapped.

Treatment – Low-protein diet, controlled histidine intake.

(v) Maple syrup urine disease
This condition is so called because the sweet smell of the urine is said to resemble the smell of maple syrup. The blood and urine contain abnormal amounts of the amino-acids valine, leucine and isoleucine.

Affected patients show clinical symptoms shortly after birth. There is difficulty in feeding, and respiration is irregular. Stiffness of the limbs is found. Rapid physical deterioration occurs and the infants die within a few weeks or months.

The condition can be treated with a diet which is deficient in the amino-acids valie, leucine and isoleucine.

(vi) Hartnup disease

This condition resembles pellagra, is inherited as an autosomal recessive and is an abnormality in the metabolism of the amino-acid tryptophan leading to a pellagra-like skin rash, temporary cerebellar ataxia, constant aminoaciduria and the excretion of large amounts of indole substances. Some patients affected have been mentally handicapped while others are emotionally unstable or even psychotic. Treatment is by nicotinamide.

(vii) Hyperuricaemia (Lesch–Nyhan disease)

Only male infants have been described with this condition. The child is normal at birth, but after a few weeks develops hypertonic attacks. Increasing spasticity develops and with eruption of teeth these children mutilate their fingers and bite their lips away. As in gout, the serum acid levels are high and the urine shows a heavy deposit of orange urates. Urinary calculi are frequent. The basic enzymatic defect is known and cases and carriers are detected by biochemical studies on cultured cells.

(c) Disorders of carbohydrate metabolism

(i) Gargoylism (Hunter–Hurler syndrome)

Gargoylism is a rare type of mental handicap characterized by the deposition of mucopolysaccharide in the tissue cells of the brain, liver, heart, lungs and spleen. There are two main types of gargoylism. In the first type (Hurler syndrome), autosomal recessive, both males and females are equally affected and cousin marriages are frequent precipitating factors. Clouding of the cornea and dwarfism occur. The second type (Hunter syndrome) is a sex-linked recessive. Only males are affected. Corneal clouding does not occur and only one-third of patients are small of stature. Half of the patients affected are deaf.

The name 'gargoylism' is evocative and describes the grotesque appearance of the affected patients. The head is enlarged and the forehead protrudes. The eyebrows are bushy and the nose is saddle shaped. The abdomen is protuberant and there is usually an umbilical hernia. Considerable enlargement of the liver and spleen is found. The degree of mental handicap varies. The affected hemizygous male and heterozygous female can be detected biochemically and the affected male fetus antenatally through enzyme assay of cultured amniotic fluid cells.

(ii) Galactosaemia

This is a rare congenital and familial disorder in which the sugar galactose is not converted into glucose in the normal manner due to enzyme defect. It is caused by an autosomal recessive gene. Incidence in United Kingom is 1 in 80 000 live births. Gene situated on short arm of chromosome 9. The infant with this condition appears normal at birth but after a few days' milk feeding loses his appetite and has persistent vomiting. In severe cases death occurs from malnutrition. Those who survive are, at 3 months of age, undernourished and small in stature. Mental handicap and cataracts occur. Examination of the urine shows a constant presence of the sugar galactose and an increased excretion of amino-acids and protein. If diagnosed shortly after birth a galactose-free diet should be instituted and maintained until puberty.

(iii) Hypoglycaemia in the newborn

Hypoglycaemia or low blood-sugar in the newborn has many causes. It is found in premature infants and in twins and in small-for-age infants. It can be familial and mothers with diabetes mellitus and toxaemia of pregnancy may give birth to infants with hypoglycaemia.

Infants with hypoglycaemia are pale and reluctant to feed. They are irritable and the infant is said to be 'jittery'. Convulsions may occur. Treatment is by correction of the cause, by diet, cortisone, intravenous infusion of glucose, as if untreated neurological damage will occur.

(d) Disorders of endocrine metabolism

Cretinism (hypothyroidism)

The condition of cretinism is due to a defect of the thyroid gland resulting from various enzyme disturbances. The early signs of the disease are feeding difficulties, noisy respiration, constipation and jaundice. The child's growth is retarded. He is apathetic and he does not readily smile or laugh and is slow to suck. The tongue becomes large and protrudes as the condition progresses. The skin becomes yellowish, loose and wrinkled, with marked puffiness of the eyes and thickening of the eyelids, nostrils, lips, hands, feet and back of neck. Prominence of the abdomen with an umbilical hernia is common. The hair on the scalp and eyebrows is often very scant. The child has a peculiar hoarse cry. With the lapse of time the child makes little attempt to sit up, stand or walk. Speech may not appear until 7 or 8 years of age. The characteristic features of untreated cases are severe mental handicap, dwarfed stature, bowed small legs and stumpy hands and feet. The eyes are set widely apart and the lips are pouting. The nose is broad and flattened. Puberty is usually late and the external genitals remain infantile. Diagnosis requires a high index of suspicion and is greatly aided by routine determination of serum T4 and TSH in umbilical cord blood, or filter paper blood spots taken at 2–5 days of age.

Prompt treatment with thyroid (no later than the first 7–10 days of the post-natal period) prevents or reduces abnormalities in mental development. Treatment is monitored by measuring serum T4 and TSH and changes in the symptoms and signs such as macroglossia and slow growth rate which may take many months to normalize. Caution must be taken not to over-treat and produce hyperthyroidism. Juvenile hypothyroidism is characterized by growth retardation, delayed dentition and mental defect. Symptoms and signs of adolescent hypothyroidism are similar to those of adults; additionally there may be short stature and precocious puberty with an enlarged sella turcica.

(e) Disorders of mineral and electrolyte metabolism

(i) Wilson's disease (hepatolenticular degeneration)

This rare often familial condition is accompanied by a decrease of blood copper and a low level of the copper-containing protein, caeruloplasmin, in the serum.

Urine copper excretion is increased. The age of onset can be from 5 to 40 years, with ascites, jaundice and enlarged liver. Involuntary choreiform movements and tremor develop with progressive difficulty in articulation and swallowing. Rigidity of the muscles of limbs, trunk and face occur resulting in contractures and muscle wasting. A smoky brownish ring (Kayser–Fleischer ring) forms at the outer margin of the cornea. There is progressive mental and physical deterioration. Detection as early as possible is vital. Siblings should have periodic blood tests. Suspect the disease in children or young adults with the above signs. Treat. Avoid foods high in copper. Use chelating agents to mobilize copper, D-penicillamine or trietine.

(ii) Nephrogenic diabetes insipidus (NDI)
This condition is due to an X-linked recessive gene. It affects males who are unable to control the passage of water from the blood to the kidneys, and are completely unresponsive to antidiuretic hormone (vasopressin). In early infancy the child develops an excessive thirst and passes large amounts of urine. He becomes dehydrated and may run erratic fevers. Brain damage with permanent mental retardation occurs if the condition is unrecognized. This is prevented by continuous large intakes of water and administration of thiazide diuretics and indomethacin.

(iii) Hypomagnesaemia
Infants born to mothers who are suffering from magnesium deficiency may develop convulsions in the neonatal period. Hypomagnesaemia also develops when severe malnutrition is complicated by chronic diarrhoea. These convulsions, especially if complicated by dehydration and malnutrition, are liable to cause permanent brain damage. Adequate replacement of the deficient magnesium rapidly relieves the condition, by i.v. or i.m. magnesium sulphate with careful blood and ECG monitoring.

(f) Disorders of nutrition in the infant

(i) Malnutrition
There is considerable experimental evidence that vitamin deficiencies in pregnant rats and rabbits may result in brain damage in the offspring, similar to that seen in human infants. The possibility that protein malnutrition may be a factor in limiting mental development has also been put forward and this might act antenatally or postnatally. The occurrence of severe impairment of brain growth has been documented in infants subjected to severe protein malnutrition for socio-economic reasons and this limitation of mental capacity means in the end an impossibility of improving socio-economic development.

This is a major concern in developing countries where famine and hunger are commonplace. Malnutrition coupled with environmental deprivation (lack of the physical, emotional and cognitive support required for developmental growth and social adaptation) may be the most common cause of mental handicap world-wide.

4. Mental handicap associated with brain disease

(a) Neurofibromatosis (von Recklinghausen's disease)

This is the commonest disorder inherited as an autosomal dominant trait, the disease is characterized by pigmentation of the skin and tumours of the nerve-trunks and skin. Malignancy may develop in both skin and nerve tumours. About 20% of cases are mentally handicapped. Central neurofibromatosis with bilateral acoustic neuromas is also dominantly inherited. The genes for peripheral and central neurofibromatosis have been located on chromosomes 17 and 22 respectively.

(b) Sturge–Weber syndrome (naevoid amentia)

The causative factor is unknown. The condition is characterized by naevus of the face on one side only, meningeal angioma, possible calcification in this and the cerebral cortex, epilepsy, contralateral hemiplegia and often severe mental handicap. Treat the epilepsy; neurosurgery for removal of the naevus.

(c) Tuberous sclerosis (epiloia)

This condition is due to an autosomal dominant gene or to mutation. The three classic signs of this condition are mental handicap, epilepsy and adenoma sebaceum, although on occasion all may be absent.

Most patients are severely mentally handicapped and, as they grow, they undergo progressive mental deterioration and many die before reaching maturity. Epileptic fits, which may be major, minor or Jacksonian, occur from the first year of life and continue with increased severity. Nodular growths occur in the brain and may undergo malignant change or calcify. Status epilepticus is a common cause of death. Adenoma sebaceum (butterfly rash) is a rash arranged symmetrically on both cheeks and involving the nose. It is due to an overgrowth of sebaceous glands of the skin. Post-mortem examination often reveals multiple tumours of various internal organs and of the brain. Treat the epilepsy; sometimes neurosurgery. Linkage has been shown with chromosome 9 markers in some families and fibromata may be present in otherwise healthy family members indicating a carrier state.

(d) Schilder's disease (adrenoleukodystrophy)

The condition is due to a recessive gene. Defective synthesis of myelin is associated with axon degeneration, neuronal overgrowth and adrenal atrophy.

This disease usually makes its appearance in childhood or adolescence and occurs only in boys. Clinical features consist of progressive failure of vision and hearing, spastic paralysis, convulsive attacks, mental deterioration, muscular inco-ordination of limbs, and tonic and clonic spasms. There is laboratory evidence of adrenal cortical dysfunction. Death invariably occurs in 1–5 years.

5. Mental handicap associated with diseases and conditions due to prenatal factors

(a) Acrocephalosyndactyly

A rare condition due sometimes to an autosomal dominant gene and showing marked association with paternal age. The two commonest features are an abnormally high or pointed head and varying degree of fusion of fingers and toes.

Not all cases are mentally handicapped. Reconstructive hand and foot surgery is frequently indicated.

(b) Craniostenosis

This is an uncommon condition occurring predominantly in males. There is premature closure of the cranial sutures resulting in malformations of the skull with secondary effects on brain and eyes. Mental handicap and cranial nerve defects follow. Cleft palate, syndactyly and congenital heart disease are sometimes associated. Treatment, by surgical creation of artificial sutures in the early months, is not generally accepted.

(c) Hydrocephalus

Hydrocephalus ('water on the brain') refers to an increased volume of cerebrospinal fluid within the skull. The excess cerebrospinal fluid may be within the ventricles or in the subarachnoid space. In the infant the head expands to accommodate the excess fluid; as a result the circumference of the head may increase to as much as 90 cm, the normal average adult circumference being 55 cm. A genetic factor is sometimes involved, while intracranial haemorrhage at or around birth may lead to hydrocephalus. Rare causes are tumours or cysts in childhood.

The hydrocephalus may be primary or secondary. Primary hydrocephalus results from developmental abnormalities causing excessive secretion of the cerebrospinal fluid and a low or absent absorption of the secreted fluids. Secondary hydrocephalus is caused by lesions within the system of ducts which drain away the cerebrospinal fluid. Blockage of these ducts causes an obstruction to the flow of fluids. Those commonly affected are the aqueduct of Sylvius and the foramina of Luschka and Magendie. Hydrocephalus at birth is usually associated with meningomyelocele. The hydrocephalus may be active, producing progressive deterioration. The patient will suffer from blindness, deafness and convulsions, be severely wasted, bedridden and paralysed. Evaluate with skull X-rays or CT scan. The latter will show the ventricular size and the site of obstruction. Ultrasonography can document progression of the hydrocephalus when congenital infection is suspected, do serological studies for toxoplasmosis, syphilis, cytomegalovirus and rubella. Treat. Medical treatment with acetazolamide, glycerol or lumbar punctures sometimes help temporarily. Progressive hydrocephalus requires a shunt procedure to reduce pressure. Type depends on surgeon's preference; ventriculoperitoneal often preferred as fewer complications. Monitor progress after operation. Some non-progressive arrest spontaneously.

(d) Hypertelorism (Greig's syndrome)

Hypertelorism is a rare form of mental handicap. There is abnormal development of part of the sphenoid bone of the skull and this thrusts the brow forward, separating the nasal bones more widely than normal. The distance between the eyes is increased and in extreme cases the eyes tend to disappear on the side of the face. Harelip, congenital heart disease, and cleft palate may occur.

Ocular hypertelorism occurs more frequently as part of other syndromes involving the upper mid-face than as an isolated defect. These include Down's syndrome, gargoylism and acrocephalosyndactyly.

(e) Microcephaly

Microcephaly is the name applied to mentally handicapped persons whose cranium on completion of development is less than 42.5 cm in circumference. This condition may be due to a single recessive gene which determines the inability of the brain to develop to its normal size or be secondary to untreated pregnancy in a phenylketonuric mother, alcoholic mothers, cytomegalovirus, toxoplasmosis or rubella.

The head is reduced in size so that a relatively normal nose and chin and large ears contrast with the receding forehead and flattened back of head. There is overlapping of the sutures of the skull and thick ridges of bone can be felt. The scalp is sometimes loose and wrinkled longitudinally as though too big for the skull. Spastic diplegia is common. About 50% of such persons are epileptic. Mentally they vary from severely to moderately handicapped and may be restless and vivacious with considerable powers of mimicry.

(f) Laurence–Moon–Biedl syndrome

This is a very rare condition due to an autosomal recessive gene and characterized by obesity, hypogenitalism, extra fingers and toes, eye defects – which include pigmentary degeneration of the retina, nystagmus, optic atrophy, poor night vision and progressive visual defect – and severe mental handicap. Close relatives of the patients may show some of the signs.

(g) Ichthyosis

Ichthyosis is a congenital skin disease characterized by scaling and hyperkeratosis and is a common complaint in the general population. Several genes may cause it. The most frequent is an autosomal dominant. There are two syndromes associated with mental handicap, of which ichthyosis is an essential part. The Sjögren–Larsson syndrome is characterized by spastic diplegia, ichthyosis and mental handicap and an autosomal recessive gene. Rud's syndrome is characterized by ichthyosis, sexual infantilism, epilepsy and varying degrees of mental handicap.

(h) De Lange syndrome

This syndrome consists of severe mental handicap, short stature, bushy confluent eyebrows and general hirsutism, wide prominent upper lip and abnormalities of digits. No consistent cytogenetic abnormality or known pattern of inheritance has been found.

(i) Rubinstein–Taybi syndrome

This is a complex of congenital defects which is indicated by the findings of pathologically broad out-turned thumbs and toes, narrow beaked nose, epicanthal folds and downward-slanting eyes, in association with moderate to severe mental handicap. There is no known chromosome abnormality, although affected siblings are reported.

(j) Smith–Lemli–Opitz syndrome

This autosomal recessive syndrome shows itself in infancy with vomiting and failure to thrive. Ears are low set; there are epicanthic folds associated with a wide nasolabial distance and abnormalities of the digits, often syndactyly of second and third toes. There is ptosis, anteverted nostrils, hypospadias and mental retardation.

6. Mental handicap with chromosomal abnormalities

A human being originates in the union of two sex cells (gametes), the ovum and the spermatozoon, and is built up of single units called 'cells'. Each cell is composed of a cell membrane surrounding the complex cell structures which include the cytoplasm (a substance surrounding the nucleus) and the nucleus itself – a compact object containing the hereditary material, chromosomes which are rod-like structures.

The genes – the basic units of heredity – are molecules of deoxyribonucleic acid (DNA). The capacity of DNA to replicate itself constitutes the basis of hereditary transmission. DNA also provides the genetic code which determines the development of cells by controlling the synthesis of ribonucleic acid (RNA). The many thousands of genes are carried on the chromosomes. Genes are 'blueprints' for the development of the individual. The position of the gene on the chromosome is called its 'locus'. Genes occasionally change their character giving rise to new genes. This process is called 'mutation'.

The hereditary material in the cells of man is divided into 46 sections of varying lengths making 23 pairs of different chromosomes. When the genes of a pair of like chromosomes ('homologous') contain comparable sets of loci then they are said to be 'homozygous'. If they do not agree they are 'heterozygous'.

These arrangements apply to 22 pairs of chromosomes (the 'autosomes'); the sex chromosomes in the male differ, one being an X and the other Y, whilst in the female they are a homologous pair, XX.

Transmission of the hereditary material from one generation to another takes place through the germ cells, the spermatozoa in the male and the ova in the female. These cells, unlike the other cells of the body, have each only one-half the normal complement of chromosomes, 23 in number. When fertilization takes place the sperm and the ovum unite together to form a new individual and called the 'zygote'. Thus each individual has received one-half of his chromosomes from each of his parents.

Disorders caused by a defect in a single gene follow the patterns of inheritance described by Mendal. Individual disorders of this type are rare, but important because they are numerous and risks within an affected family are high and may be calculated by knowing the mode of inheritance and the family pedigree. Autosomal dominant disorders affect both males and females and can be traced for generations. Affected people transmit the gene for the disease to half their offspring whether male or female. The disorder is not transmitted by family members who are unaffected themselves.

Autosomal recessive disorders occur in a patient whose healthy parents both carry the same recessive gene. The risk of recurrence for future offspring of such parents is 25%. Although the defective gene may be passed from generation to generation the disorder usually appears only within a single sibship – within one group of brothers and sisters. In X-linked recessive conditions only males are affected, and the disorder is transmitted through healthy female carriers. A female carrier will transmit the disorder to half her sons, and half her daughters will be carriers. All the daughters of an affected male are carriers whereas none of the sons are affected. However, many X-linked recessive disorders are so severe and lethal that the affected males cannot reproduce.

There are two other types of genetically determined disorders, first polygenic or multifactorial conditions, in which genetic conditions involving more than one gene and non-genetic factors interact in ways that are not always clearly recognizable and second chromosomal abnormalities which include both structural defects and deviations from the normal number.

Chromosomal abnormalities are particularly common in spontaneous abortions. About 15–20% of all conceptions are estimated to be lost spontaneously, and about half of these are associated with chromosomal abnormality. Most chromosomal abnormalities lead to spontaneous abortion, some inevitably so – for example trisomy 16 is commonly found in aborted fetuses but never in liveborn infants. In liveborn infants chromosomal abnormalities occur in about six per 1000 births. The incidence of abnormalities of autosomes and sex chromosomes is about the same. Detailed examination of malformed stillbirths and fetuses is essential if parents are to be accurately counselled about the cause of the problem, the risk of recurrence and the availability of antenatal tests in future pregnancies.

By amniotic puncture (amniocentesis) it is possible to obtain a specimen of the fluid surrounding the fetus and to examine the cells and biochemistry. This makes it possible to tell in early pregnancy whether a baby is suffering from certain conditions, such as translocation mongolism, where the risk of a second affected child is high. A decision about termination may then depend on the mother's feelings, and the law.

Complications of amniocentesis at 16 weeks are uncommon. Fetal loss due to the procedure occurs in about 1 in 200 amniocenteses. Infection is rare. Although amniotic fluid leak, haemorrhage (fetal or maternal) or both occur in 1–2% of cases, they usually cease after bed rest. In Down's syndrome a detection rate of 35% could be achieved if all women over 35 had amniocentesis. The rate of detection can be improved by incorporating the results of measuring serum alpha fetoprotein, unconjugated oestriol, and human chorionic gonadotrophin concentrations with maternal age to give a composite risk value, but this refinement is not universally available as a screening programme.

Screening for neural tube defects is offered by many centres. In more than 80% of cases of anencephaly and open neural tube defects alpha-feto-protein is significantly elevated in the maternal serum at 16–18 weeks gestation. Surveys in the USA and UK have shown that such screening for all women who wish to participate is feasible, accurate and cost-effective.

Chorionic villus sampling (CVS) is an antenatal diagnostic procedure where a sample is obtained by passing a catheter through the vagina and cervix and advancing it to the site of fetal implantation under ultrasound guidance. An advantage is that this is done at 8–10 weeks gestation (2 months earlier than amniocentesis) and results are available in hours or days rather than weeks. If termination is elected, it is easier and safer. The main problem is that the degree of risk is not known. Data indicate a miscarriage rate of 2–6% and there is possibility of harm to the fetus that goes on to term.

Fetoscopy is a highly specialized technique using a fibre-optic endoscope. The procedure is carried out in the second trimester in cases in which the fetus must be seen directly. It is possible to take fetal blood and skin samples under direct ultrasonographic guidance without using an endoscope and as the number of disorders amenable to DNA analysis increases and more tests can be performed by CVS, indications for fetoscopy are diminishing.

(a) Down's syndrome (mongolism)

Although Langdon Down first described mongolism more than a hundred years ago it is only in 1959 that it was recognized that the condition is the result of chromosome abnormality. Down's syndrome is the commonest autosomal trisomy, although more than half conceptions with trisomy 21 do not survive to term.

1. Regular (trisomy)
The chromosome count is 47 instead of the normal 46, the extra chromosome being one of the smaller chromosomes. Accounts for about 95% of cases. The risk of recurrency of an abnormal live infant is 1%.

2. Translocation
The chromosome count remains at 46; the extra small chromosome has become attached to another chromosome making the chromosomal count appear normal. There is actually genetic material for 47 chromosomes – the additional chromosome 21 is transferred and attached to 14 or occasionally 21. Blood from both parents should be analysed to see if either is a translocation carrier, then genetic counselling.

3. Mosaic
The chromosome count is 46 in one cell line and 47 in the other cell line. The relative proportion of each cell line is variable both between individuals and within different organs within the same individual. The proportion of trisomic cells influences the severity of the physical signs and intelligence.

Down's syndrome accounted for 10% of all patients admitted to hospitals for the mentally handicapped. The incidence in the general population is 1 per 600 births. Cases tend to be born at the end of large families and the frequency is related closely to the age of the mother, the risk of giving birth to a child with Down's syndrome rising with the age of the mother. A low serum alpha-fetoprotein in the pregnant woman indicates an increased risk. More than one case can occur in a family. Other chromosomal abnormalities such as Klinefelter's syndrome, Triple-X syndrome and Turner's syndrome have been found in association with Down's syndrome. Leukaemia and cancer are more prevalent in Down's syndrome than in the general population. High incidence of hepatitis B and many remain carriers. It has been suggested that hepatitis B vaccination be offered before starting school with periodic checks on surface antibody.

Principal features of Down's syndrome
These are stunted growth, a small round head with flat face and occiput, florid complexion and obliquely set eyelids, with upper lids having an extra fold at the inner margin (epicanthic fold). There may be eye defects such as squint, nystagmus, cataract and speckled iris ('Brushfield's spots'). The ears are small and do not possess the natural folds. The nose is stubby and depressed at the bridge;

the tongue in most cases is large and flabby with well-defined fissures. The hair is dry and scanty. The hands are broad and clumsy looking and have a curious 'boggy' feeling. The little finger is curved and ends midway between the last and middle interphalangeal joints of the third finger. The palm creases are abnormal; a single transverse crease often runs across the palm of the hand. The feet are marked by a large cleft between the first and second toes and often a crease runs from this cleft down the sole of the foot. Supernumerary toes and webbing of the toes are seen occasionally. The abdomen is protuberant and umbilical hernia is common. The joints have abnormal range of movement due to laxity of the ligaments and hypotonus of the muscles. The more 'floppy', the worse the prognosis. The circulation is usually poor, the extremities being blue and cold and susceptible to chilblains. Congenital heart disease is common. Mongols are usually mouth breathers and are prone to respiratory infections.

The traditional stereotype of Down's syndrome, of equable temperament and loving disposition, is only statistically true for females aged 3–12 years. Patients often develop dementia early in life. Typical neuro-pathological changes of Alzheimer's disease appear in virtually all patients aged over 40. This has led to the search for an 'alzheimer gene' on chromosome 21. Some of the plasma amino-acids are raised.

(b) Cat-cry syndrome (cri-du-chat)

In this condition affected infants are mentally handicapped and have a characteristic mewing cry from which the syndrome gets its name. In appearance they are obviously abnormal, with small heads, wide-spaced eyes, epicanthic folds, abnormalities of the ears and mouth, and eyes slanting downwards. The condition is due to a deletion of the short arm of chromosome 5. A significant number survive to adulthood when facial asymmetry and malocclusion lead to a grotesque appearance.

(c) Trisomy 13 (Patau syndrome)

This chromosome defect is not only always associated with profound mental handicap, but also with early death. The characteristic features are seen in the face and consist of broad nose, cleft-palate and micrognathia. Microcephaly is the rule. The infants are small for age and associated abnormalities of the ear, heart, kidneys are common, as are polydactyly and microphthalmia. Some have patches of atrophic hairless skin on the scalp. It occurs in about 1 per 5000 births. Diagnosis is by cytogenetic examination. Mainly due to non-dysjunction with low risk of recurrence.

(d) Trisomy 18 (Edwards' syndrome)

Diagnosis is contingent upon cytogenetic study. Again there is profound mental handicap and early mortality. Mid-line facial defects are common, as well as micrognathia. The head is microcephalic sometimes with a prominent occiput. The nose takes off from the forehead and is straight or upturned. The index finger overlays the third finger in a characteristic fashion. Associated anomalies of heart and kidneys are known. Occurrence rate is about 1 in 3000 births. Risk of recurrence is low unless due to a parental translocation. Incidence increases with maternal age.

(e) Sex chromosome abnormalities

Numerical abnormalities of the sex chromosomes are more common than with autosomes and cause less severe defects. They are brought about by non-disjunction and are often detected at amniocentesis or during investigation for infertility. Risk of recurrence is low. When more than one additional sex chromosome is present mental and physical abnormalities are more likely.

The sex chromosome abnormalities are as follows:

(i) Klinefelter's syndrome

The patient is a male whose sex chromatin is positive. The sex chromosome constitution is XXY and the total chromosome count is 47. After puberty, patients with this constitution present with sterility and have small testicles. The breasts may be feminine in appearance and eunuchoidism may occur. The degree of mental handicap varies but is usually mild; often intelligence is within the normal range. Testosterone replacement treatment sometimes required. Incidence 2.0 per 1000 live-born males.

(ii) Turner's syndrome

The patient is female with complete or partial absence of one of the two X chromosomes. The cells have only a single X chromosome and the total chromosome count is 45. The patients are dwarfed and congenital abnormalities are found, particularly webbing of the neck. At puberty secondary sexual development is absent due to lack of ovarian tissue and hormones. The degree of mental handicap is usually mild. Often intelligence is within the normal range. Treatment is by oestrogen-replacement therapy. Incidence: 1.0 per 1000 live female births; 95% are said to miscarry; those who survive to the second trimester can be detected by ultrasound.

(iii) Triple-X syndrome

The patient is female and often there are no abnormal physical characteristics. The sex chromosome constitution is XXX and the total chromosome count is 47. The tissue cells are chromatin positive and some cells contain two sex chromatin bodies. Incidence: 0.65 per 1000 live born female infants and is often a coincidental finding. Taller than average, they are physically normal. Mean IQ lower than controls. Many require remedial teaching. Premature ovarian failure may occur.

(iv) XYY syndrome

These male patients are of interest, as the majority have been diagnosed in the high security hospitals. They are usually tall, with a tendency towards aggression and violence, but this association is less strongly marked than previously thought and many remain undetected clinically. Mild mental retardation and behavioural problems can occur. Incidence 1.5 per 1000 newborn males.

(v) Fragile X chromosome

The reason for the excess of males over females affected by mental handicap may be an X-linked genetic defect called the fragile X chromosome, characterized in most cases by a tiny, almost detached piece towards the end of the long arm of the X-chromosome. It had been suggested for many years, that X-linked genes should be considered in the causation of non-specific mental handicap, but only recently have laboratory methods become fastidious enough to demonstrate the fragile site on the X-chromosome.

There appear to be at least three distinct forms of X-linked mental handicap which breed true in families. Firstly, boys with the market X chromosome tend to have large heads, large ears and lower jaws. The most specific finding is macro-orchidism generally present at puberty, but sometimes at birth. Specific speech delay is common and the boys often have a characteristic speech rhythm called litany speech. Epilepsy is only found in the most severely retarded. Secondly, there are members of families who do not show the marker chromosome, but have the above clinical features without the macro-orchidism. Thirdly, Renpenning seems to have described a separate syndrome with microcephaly, small testes, severe mental handicap and no marker chromosome.

Mild to severe mental retardation occurs in around 30% of heterozygous female carriers. Not all female carriers show the chromosomal abnormality on testing, which makes counselling difficult. Pregnancies at risk can currently be monitored by CVS and fetal blood sampling for chromosomes, but in future DNA analysis will probably become the preferred method. Incidence in males is 1.8 per 1000, and next to Down's syndrome it is the most common cause of mental retardation that can be specifically diagnosed.

(f) Prader-Willi syndrome (PWS)

Recent work has shown cytogenic abnormality on the long arm of chromosome 15 in more than 55% of cases, while the others have apparently normal chromosomes. Associated mental handicap ranges from mild to severe, the main clinical features in the child being obesity, hypogonadism, short stature and high incidence of diabetes mellitus. Hypotonia is a prominent early sign, and this disorder and Down's syndrome provide good examples of the association of cerebral intellectual defect and profound infantile hypotonia. The obesity is due to polyphagia – the patient is only satisfied with large amounts of food – the diametric opposite of anorexia nervosa, and premature preventable death is thus common in the late twenties.

7. Mental handicap associated with prematurity

(a) Prematurity

Previously by definition any infant weighing 2500 g or less at birth was termed premature; now any infant born before 37 weeks gestation, since many infants weighing less than 2.5 kg are actually mature or post-mature; 5–10% of all births are in this category. Premature infants are particularly liable to develop severe respiratory distress at birth and this is associated with a higher mortality rate. Infants with a birth weight less than 1500 g show an association between respiratory distress and the development of mental handicap and neurological abnormalities. Prematurity may be found in association with maternal toxaemia, congenital anomalies and multiple pregnancy. Premature children also have a liability to kernicterus and also hypoglycaemia which may lead to mental handicap. Small-for-dates infants have an increased incidence of mental handicap. Prematures of less than 32 weeks gestation who weigh less than 1500 g, have a 10–50% chance of being retarded, depending on weight, perinatal events and quality of care available. Infants at risk require close developmental observation during the first few years.

Hypoxic premature babies suffer much greater structural brain damage than hypoxic full-term deliveries. The latter often only have damage to the 'watershed' areas of blood supply which include the language areas and memory areas such as the hippocampus and mamillary bodies, while hypoxic prematures often suffer destruction of major structures such as the cortex, or parts of the thalamus. They may therefore fail to thrive or be wholly decorticate.

(b) Kernicterus

Kernicterus occurs in prematurity, infantile malnutrition and when some drugs are given to the infant or to the mother. With the breakdown of haemoglobin bilirubin is produced and deposited in the basal ganglia and brain-stem nuclei. Kernicterus thus occurs in haemolytic disease of the newborn especially when there is Rhesus antibody incompatibility. Sepsis, intrauterine infections, blood diseases and metabolic abnormalities can all produce hyperbilirubinaemia. The affected infant may be jaundiced at birth or becomes jaundiced a few days later. The infant is ill and fails to thrive. There is respiratory distress and death may occur at this stage in respiratory failure. The liver and spleen are enlarged. Cyanotic attacks occur and in some cases severe anaemia results from haemolysis. With recovery, athetoid movements may be noted as early as 6 months of age. Motor development is poor, high-tone deafness is frequent, disorders of balance and epilepsy may occur during early childhood. Clinical signs may be absent in preterm infants and develop later in childhood.

(c) Cerebral palsy (CP)

Cerebral palsy is a permanent disorder of movement and posture, due to a non-progressive defect of the brain occurring in early life. The incidence of cerebral palsy is about 1 per 500 live births. Mental handicap and cerebral palsy are commonly found together, the same cerebral insult accounting for both effects. Neurologically pyramidal signs are most commonly observed and may show as hemiplegia, diplegia, quadriplegia and as a variety of clinical pictures. In some cases extrapyramidal signs are seen including ataxia and athetoid movements. Many patients are epileptic.

Cerebral palsy may be found in association with prematurity, difficult birth, multiple birth and kernicterus. Severe systemic disease during early infancy (meningitis or other infections, water or salt depletion) may also cause a CP syndrome.

Children with spastic hemiplegia or paraplegia frequently have normal intelligence and a good prognosis for social independence; spastic quadriplegia and mixed forms are often associated with disabling mental retardation. Laboratory tests are useful in excluding progressive biochemical disorders involving the motor system such as Tay–Sachs. Athetosis, self-mutilation and hyperuricaemia in boys identify the Lesch–Nyhan syndrome while skin or eye abnormalities may indicate tuberous sclerosis, neurofibromatosis, Sturge–Weber which are usually progressive.

8. Unclassified mental handicap (non-specific)

Unclassified mental handicap applies to those cases in which there is no gross evidence of structural or biochemical abnormality. Approximately 65% of all cases of mental handicap still have to be placed in this group. However, more sophisticated microscopic examination of the neocortex showed that there are in many cases insufficient branching and spines on the nerve axons and what is described as 'ectopic' dendrogenesis (connections in the wrong places).

Unclassified mental handicap can be divided into two groups. The genetic contribution to disease varies, some disorders are wholly genetic and some entirely environmental. Many disorders have an appreciable genetic contribution without following a simple family pattern of inheritance. The term polygenic or multifactorial inheritance is used. Traits so inherited include height and intelligence. Thus mild mental retardation (IQ 50–90) is a polygenic trait representing the lower end of the normal distribution of intelligence. The intelligence quotient of offspring is likely to be around the mid-parental mean.

One or both parents of a mildly retarded child are often retarded themselves and have other retarded children. Intelligent parents with one mildly retarded child are unlikely to have another similarly affected child. In contrast parents of a child with severe retardation (IQ < 50) are usually of normal intelligence. A specific cause is likely when mental retardation is severe and can include chromosomal and genetic disorders. Risk of recurrence depends on diagnosis, but in severe non-specific retardation is about 3% for siblings, rising to 25% after the birth of two affected children.

The above classification does not pretend to be comprehensive as some of the extremely rare syndromes either associated with chromosome abnormalities such as deletion of short arm of chromosome 4 or those with eponymous names Marinesco, Wilderwanck, Noonan and Aicardi have been deliberately omitted. An exception, because of topicality, can be made for Rett syndrome, an overlooked disorder occurring as frequently as one in 12 500 girls. The disease probably results from mutation of a gene on the X chromosome. Pregnancy and birth are normal. Hand use never progresses beyond a late infancy level and language beyond one or two word utterances. Birth head circumference is within or close to normal range, followed by suboptimal growth. Imaginative and imitative play are lacking. There is regression with loss of skills in speech, manipulation and locomotion followed by a long stable plateau period with increasing muscle tone and scoliosis. Repetitive simple hand movements are present with little voluntary hand use. Mental handicap is profound. Music therapy and movement therapy improve management. The subcultural group is more complex, comprising genetic and environmental factors. Below-average parents and adverse home circumstances and upbringing give rise to this subcultural group of mentally handicapped people with intelligence quotients in the range 50–70. Social changes should eventually bring about a reduction in this type of mental handicap. Of normal appearance, they are easily led, being exploited either sexually or by unscrupulous employers. There is no social class bias among children with brain damage, whereas the subcultural group is almost confined to social groups four and five. Incidence is increased in the poorer areas of large cities with overcrowding, poverty, problem families, parents in debt and careless of property. Many receiving special education will have a sibling or parent who also needed special education. Parents generally will not have sought help prior to school and do not regard the child as abnormal.

Appendix 3

The use of drugs in mental handicap

Ronald MacGillivray

It is important for professionals to have a knowledge of the more common drugs in use today. The list given here is by no means complete since the wide variety of compounds available includes many examples of groups of drugs where usefulness, advantages and disadvantages overlap to a very considerable degree and the ultimate choice by the clinician of a particular preparation is determined largely by fashion and personal preference. The major tranquillizers are a striking example of a group where such duplication occurs.

It is also important to be aware that advances are being made and that certain newer drugs are found to be better than their predecessors in some way or another. Here an example can be found among the tranquillizers where buspirone which is distinct from the benzodiazepines has been found to have fewer unwanted effects, less abuse potential and does not interact with CNS depressants. For this reason prescribing policy must never be static, but instead it must be kept under constant review as new compounds become available.

Drugs in common use are divided for convenience into certain classes according to the prominent action produced by them. The drugs included here are listed according to this system of classification and set out in tabular form as follows:

1. *Sedatives* (See Table A3.1) – These drugs are mainly to help sleep.
2. *Anticonvulsants* (see Table A3.2) – These are drugs used to treat the various forms of epilepsy. Current opinion favours the use of one anticonvulsant only rather than the use of combinations of two, three or more drugs as has been employed in the past.
3. *Antispasmodics* (see Table A3.3) – These are drugs that are used in psychiatric practice to control the disorders of movement and muscle tone which can occur as an unwanted effect of the major tranquillizers.
4. *Tranquillizers* (see Table A3.4) – These are drugs that calm the patient and reduce tension, agitation and anxiety. Major tranquillizers are used mainly when there is a psychotic background and they have a specific antipsychotic effect, but they can also be given to non-psychotic patients to control anxiety symptoms. Minor tranquillizers are for use in non-psychotic patients. Caution is needed as they are usually addictive.
5. *Antidepressant drugs* (see Table A3.5) – These can be used to elevate mood in all kinds of psychiatric illness, but are less effective when the mood change is an understandable response to definite environmental factors.
6. *Miscellaneous* (see Table A3.6) – In the miscellaneous group lithium is used to reduce mood fluctuation in affective illnesses while ECT continues to have a unique and invaluable role in the treatment of severe depression.

Table A3.1 Sedatives

Drug	Trade name	Average daily dose	Indications	Side-effects	Nursing care
Amylobarbitone	Amytal	100–200 mg	Sleeplessness	Physical addiction with delirium tremens or epilepsy on sudden withdrawal	Treatment for overdosage. Aim to maintain respiration and eliminate the drug by stomach lavage and i.v. fluids
Chloral hydrate		0.3–2 g	Sleeplessness	Dyspepsia and gastric irritation	Must be given as a mixture well diluted: withdrawn from patient gradually
Chloral betaine	Welldorm	650 mg–1.3 g	Sleeplessness	Skin rashes, nausea	
Paraldehyde		10–20 ml	To quieten and induce sleep in the mentally disordered. Status epilepticus	Erythematous rash, gastric irritation, toxic hepatitis. May cause abscesses by i.m. use. Plastic syringes contraindicated	
Nitrazepam	Mogadon	5–10 mg	Sleeplessness	Morning drowsiness	Avoid administration over long periods because of dependency. For over-dosage: gastric lavage or emetic strychnine 8 mg hypodermically. Artificial respiration. Intravenous fluids
Triazolam	Halcion	0.125–0.25 mg	Sleeplessness	Short-acting dizziness	Do not use in nursing mothers
Temazepam	Normison	10–30 mg at bed-time	Sleeplessness	Morning drowsiness	
Flurazepam	Dalmane	15–30 mg at bed-time	Sleeplessness	Morning drowsiness	

Table A3.2 Anticonvulsants

Drug	Trade name name	Average daily dose	Indications	Side-effects	Nursing care
Ethosuximide	Zarontin	500–1500 mg	Epilepsy – petit mal	Gastro-intestinal disturbance, agranulocytosis	Frequent blood count
Phenytoin sodium	Epanutin	200–600 mg	Epilepsy – grand mal and focal	Gum hyperplasia, ataxia, nystagmus, tremors, rashes, headache, blood disorders including megaloblastic anaemia	15 mg folic acid daily for megaloblastic anaemia. Avoid in pregnancy if possible
Primidone	Mysoline	Adults: 0.5–2 g Children:0.25–1.0 g in divided doses	Epilepsy – grand mal and focal	Mild and transitory giddiness, nausea and vomiting. Occasionally megaloblastic anaemia	15 mg folic acid daily for megaloblastic anaemia
Carbamazepine	Tegretol	Initially 100 mg once or twice a day. 800–1200 mg daily for adults	Grand mal and focal epilepsy. Trigeminal neuralgia	Drowsiness, dizziness, rashes, dermatitis, aplastic anaemia, jaundice. Do not give in early pregnancy. Do not give with MAOI therapy	Regular blood counts

Clonazepam	Rivotril	4–9 mg daily in adults. Infants (0–1 year) 0.5–1 mg daily. Ampoules for status	All clinical forms of epilepsy in infants, children or adults, especially typical or atypical petit mal	Fatigue, somnolence, coordination disturbances, salivary hypersecretion, bronchial hypersecretion	Avoid alcohol and driving. Do not give in pregnancy
Diazepam	Valium	15–30 mg daily for adults. Ampoules for rectal i.v. or i.m. use in status. 0.15–0.25 mg (kg body weight)$^{-1}$. Can be repeated 1 hour later; may be put in a drip	Status epilepticus	Ataxia with big doses: i.v. injection rarely causes collapse, hypotension and apnoea	With i.v. injection have facilities for resuscitation available (Lorazepam can be given rapidly i.v.)
Sodium valproate	Epilim	600–1600 mg daily in adults	All types of epilepsy including petit mal. In women of child-bearing age use only in severe cases or resistance to other drugs	Minor gastric irritation with nausea. Partiallay excreted in the urine in the form of ketone bodies, hence false positives when testing the urine of possible diabetics	Well tolerated with other anticonvulsant drugs. May potentiate MAOI. Teratogenic in animals, therefore avoid in pregnancy unless essential
Phenobarbitone	Luminal	30–120 mg	Grand mal and focal epilepsy	As for amylobarbitone sodium. Paradoxically may cause hyperkinetic behaviour in children and confusion in the elderly	As for amylobarbitone sodium. Sudden withdrawal from epileptic patient may lead to further seizures

Table A3.3 Antispasmodics

Drug	Trade name	Average daily dose	Indications	Side-effects	Nursing care
Benzhexol	Artane	5–20 mg in divided doses	Drug-induced, parkinsonism	Drowsiness, dryness of mouth, nausea and vomiting. Delusions and confusion	May precipitate acute glaucoma
Orphenadrine	Disipal	50–150 mg	As for benzhexol	As for benzhexol	As for benzhexol
Benztropine	Cogentin	0.5–6 mg	As for benzhexol	As for benzhexol	As for benzhexol
Procyclidine hydrochloride	Kemadrin	Oral 7.5–30 mg in divided dose, i.m. 10–20 mg	As for benzhexol	As for benzhexol	As for benzhexol
Tetrabenazine	Nitoman	75–200 mg in divided doses	Tardive dyskinesia. Abnormal movement in Huntington's chorea	Drowsiness, dyspepsia, hypertension, parkinsonism in high dosage	Should not be given with MAOI drugs

Table A3.4 Tranquillizers

Drug	Trade name	Average daily dose	Indications	Side-effects	Nursing care	Remarks
			(a) Major tranquillizers (oral)			
Chlorpromazine	Largactil	75–800 mg orally daily. 25–100 mg by injection, repeated as required three or four times in 24 hours	Excitement or extreme agitation in psychoses, mental tension, excitable states in the mentally handicapped person	Drowsiness, hypotension, parkinsonism, dry mouth, jaundice, light sensitivity, blurred vision. May precipitate or potentiate epilepsy dystonia	Observe for the appearance of any side-effects and for the appearance of skin disorders. The nurse must take precautions and not handle the drug unless she is wearing rubber gloves	Patients have to be kept in a supine position for at least 1 h after injection
Thioridazine	Melleril	30–600 mg daily	Neurosis and psychosis	Drowsiness, dizziness, hypotension, dryness of mouth, transient oedema		Does not cause skin reaction in sunlight
Haloperidol	Serenace Haldol	1.5–40 mg daily	Psychotic disorders especially mania	Parkinsonism may be prominent		
Droperidol	Droleptan	5–15 mg i.v. Up to 10 mg i.m. 5–20 mg oral	Psychotic disorders especially mania – for rapid calming. In anaesthetics			(Not for severely depressed patients.) Useful for extreme and rapid action
Pimozide	Orap	2–20 mg once daily	Schizophrenia, chronic anxiety, monosymptomatic hypochondriacal psychosis	Extrapyramidal effects less common		Once daily dosage an advantage
Perphenazine	Fentazin	8–24 mg	Anxiety and agitated and excited patients	Dystonic reactions may be severe		More potent and less toxic than Largactil

Table A3.4 Tranquillizers (cont.)

Drug	Trade name	Average daily dose	Indications	Side-effects	Nursing care	Remarks
Trifluoperazine	Stelazine	Mild cases 2–4 mg daily chronic or acute cases 15–30 mg daily	Less sedative than chlorpromazine	Restlessness and akathisia		
			(b) Major tranquillizers (Depot)			
Fluphenazine enanthate injection	Moditen enanthate	25 mg every 2 or 3 weeks i.m.	As for chlorpromazine. Chronic schizophrenia	As for chlorpromazine	Watch for extrapyramidal symptoms which respond well to antispasmodics	Give small test dose before starting treatment
Fluphenazine decanoate injection	Modecate	25–50 mg every 1–3 weeks i.m.	As for chlorpromazine. Chronic schizophrenia	As for chlorpromazine	As above	As above
Flupenthixol decanoate injection	Depixol	20–40 mg every 2–4 weeks i.m. depot injections	Schizophrenia. Its alerting reaction is particularly useful in the withdrawn, apathetic or depressed patient	Extrapyramidal reactions less common	May cause overactivity	As above
Flupenthixol	Fluanxol	See below				
Zuclopenthixol decanoate	Clopixol	100–400 mg every 2–4 weeks i.m.	Psychosis associated with aggression			

Fluspirilene	Redeptin	2 mg/solution for injection. Given weekly up to 20 mg	Schizophrenia	Extrapyramidal reaction less common. Fatigue and upper gastro-intestinal symptoms such as nausea and vomiting can occur. May potentiate epilepsy		Drowsiness can occur and thus care should be taken with patients who drive or operate machinery

(c) Minor tranquillizers

Diazepam	Valium	8–40 mg in divided doses	Anxiety and tension in the absence of psychosis	Drowsiness, disinhibition, constipation		Dependency can occur with prolonged use. Abrupt withdrawal can precipitate epilepsy. Avoid alcohol
Chlordiaze-poxide	Librium	15–100 mg	As for diazepam	As for diazepam		As for diazepam
Lorazepam	Ativan	3–7.5 mg daily in divided doses	As for diazepam	As for diazepam	Intermediate acting	As for diazepam
Chlormethiozole edisylate	Heminevrin	1–4 g	Agitation and restlessness, delirium tremens and drug withdrawal states	Sneezing, conjunctivitis, nausea, hypotension		As useful sedative with anticonvulsant properties. Can lead to dependency with prolonged administration
Clorazepate potassium	Tranxene	15 mg	As for diazepam	As for diazepam	Long acting	As for diazepam
Buspirone hydrochloride	Buspar	10–30 mg	Anxiety	Dizziness, headache		A new anxiolytic not related to benzodiazepines so less abuse potential. May take 2 weeks to work

Table A3.5 Antidepressants

Drug	Trade	Average	Indications	Side-effects	Remarks
Monoamine oxidase inhibitors (MAOI)					
Phenelzine	Nardil	45 mg	Atypical depressions. Patients resistant to TCAD and agoraphobia	Oedema, hypotension, nausea	All MAOI drugs produce profound hypertension when taken with certain drugs (amphetamines, opiates, tricyclic antidepressants, barbiturates, tranquillizers) and foods containing tyramine (cheese, yeast, Marmite, broad beans)
Isocarboxazid	Marplan	40 mg		Coryza-like symptoms, oedema, hypotension, vertigo	
Tranylcypromine	Parnate	20 mg		Restlessness, dizziness, dry mouth, headache, agitation	
Tricyclic and related compounds (TCAD)					
Trimipramine	Surmontil	Up to 150 mg	Depression	Dry mouth, oedema, pruritus, hypotension, blurred vision, retention of urine, drowsiness, should not be given at the same time as or within 14 days of patient taking an MAOI	Sedating. Tricyclic and related drugs should be given only with extreme caution when antihypertensive medication is already being prescribed
Amitriptyline	Tryptizol	Up to 150 mg	Depression, enuresis	Dry mouth, oedema, pruritus, hypotension, blurred vision, retention of urine, drowsiness, should not be given at the same time as or within 14 days of patient taking an MAOI	Sedating. As above. Regular blood tests

Drug	Trade name	Dose	Indication	Side-effects/notes	Comments
Doxepin	Sinequan	30–150 mg	Depression		An effective anxiolytic
Imipramine	Tofranil	Up to 150 mg	Depression	Dry mouth, oedema, pruritus, hypotension, blurred vision, retention of urine, drowsiness, should not be given at the same time as or within 14 days of patient having an MAOI	Less sedating
Dothiepin	Prothiaden	Up to 150 mg	Depression		Elderly patients may tolerate this tricyclic better. Sedating
Mianserin	Bolvidon, Norval	Up to 120 mg	Depression		Causes fewer anticholinergic side-effects such as dry mouth, blurred vision and retention. Sedates
Maprotiline	Ludiomil	Up to 150 mg	Depression	Dry mouth, oedema, pruritus, hypotension, blurred vision, retention of urine, drowsiness, should not be given at the same time as or within 14 days of patient having an MAOI	Useful if there is coexisting cardiac disease. Anti-aggressive
Nomifensine	Merital	Up to 150 mg	Depression		
Clomipramine	Anafranil	Up to 150 mg	Depression		Sedating. Useful when phyobic or obsessive/compulsive features are present. May be more rapid if given i.v.
Tryptophan	Pacitron	Up to 6 g	Depression	When given along with MAOI it may provide a reaction resembling alcohol intoxication	Has a different mode of action from all other antidepressants in that it is a precursor of one of the neurotransmitters
Flupenthixol	Fluanxol	Up to 3 mg	Depression	Not recommended for over-active, agitated patients. May cause restlessness or parkinsonism	May be more rapid in action
Trazodone	Molipaxin	Single dose up to 100 mg	Depression	Sedating	Useful when there is coexisting heart disease

Table A3.6 Miscellaneous group

Drug	Trade name	Average daily dose	Indications	Side-effects	Nursing care
			(Ensure consent of patient)		
Benperidol	Anquil	0.25–1.5 mg in divided doses	Control of deviant and antisocial sexual behaviour. Adults only	May potentiate the action of opiates, barbiturates and other neuroleptics	Regular blood counts and liver function tests during prolonged therapy
Cyproterone	Androcur	Up to 200 mg	Excessive sexual drive in males when associated with deviance or violence	Tiredness, irreversible gynaecomastia, reversible infertility	Regular checks for liver function are required. Regular blood counts
			Lithium compounds		
Lithium carbonate	Camcolit	250–1500 mg in divided doses	Manic states and to prevent mood swings. Aggressive or self-mutilating behaviour	Vomiting, ataxia, drowsiness, coarse tremor, dysarthria, confusion and coma	Patient's dose controlled by regular blood tests to assess serum level
Baclofen	Lioresal	Up to 60 mg for adults	For spasticity. May reduce self-mutilation	Confusion, drowsiness, hypotonia	
Naltrexone	–	25 mg	Self-mutilation. Post-ictal confusion	Higher doses abolish effects	'Named' patients only

Index